FREE Study Skills DVD Offer

Dear Customer,

Thank you for your purchase from Mometrix! We consider it an honor and privilege that you have purchased our product and want to ensure your satisfaction.

As a way of showing our appreciation and to help us better serve you, we have developed a Study Skills DVD that we would like to give you for <u>FREE</u>. **This DVD covers our "best practices" for studying for your exam, from using our study materials to preparing for the day of the test.**

All that we ask is that you email us your feedback that would describe your experience so far with our product. Good, bad or indifferent, we want to know what you think!

To get your **FREE Study Skills DVD**, email <u>freedvd@mometrix.com</u> with "FREE STUDY SKILLS DVD" in the subject line and the following information in the body of the email:

    a.   The name of the product you purchased.

    b.   Your product rating on a scale of 1-5, with 5 being the highest rating.

    c.   Your feedback. It can be long, short, or anything in-between, just your impressions and experience so far with our product. Good feedback might include how our study material met your needs and will highlight features of the product that you found helpful.

    d.   Your full name and shipping address where you would like us to send your free DVD.

If you have any questions or concerns, please don't hesitate to contact me directly.

Thanks again!

Sincerely,

Jay Willis
Vice President
jay.willis@mometrix.com
1-800-673-8175

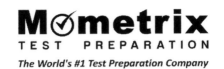

Cardiac/Vascular Nurse Exam

SECRETS

Study Guide
Your Key to Exam Success

Cardiac/Vascular Nurse Test Review for the Cardiac/Vascular Nurse Exam

Published by
Mometrix Test Preparation
Cardiac/Vascular Nurse Exam Secrets Test Prep Team

Written and edited by the Cardiac/Vascular Nurse Exam Secrets Test Prep Staff

Printed in the United States of America

This paper meets the requirements of ANSI/NISO Z39.48-1992 (Permanence of Paper).

Mometrix offers volume discount pricing to institutions. For more information or a price quote, please contact our sales department at sales@mometrix.com or 888-248-1219.

Mometrix Test Preparation is not affiliated with or endorsed by any official testing organization. All organizational and test names are trademarks of their respective owners.

ISBN 13: 978-1-60971-239-6
ISBN 10: 1-60971-239-0

Dear Future Exam Success Story:

Congratulations on your purchase of our study guide. Our goal in writing our study guide was to cover the content on the test, as well as provide insight into typical test taking mistakes and how to overcome them.

Standardized tests are a key component of being successful, which only increases the importance of doing well in the high-pressure high-stakes environment of test day. How well you do on this test will have a significant impact on your future, and we have the research and practical advice to help you execute on test day.

The product you're reading now is designed to exploit weaknesses in the test itself, and help you avoid the most common errors test takers frequently make.

How to use this study guide

We don't want to waste your time. Our study guide is fast-paced and fluff-free. We suggest going through it a number of times, as repetition is an important part of learning new information and concepts.

First, read through the study guide completely to get a feel for the content and organization. Read the general success strategies first, and then proceed to the content sections. Each tip has been carefully selected for its effectiveness.

Second, read through the study guide again, and take notes in the margins and highlight those sections where you may have a particular weakness.

Finally, bring the manual with you on test day and study it before the exam begins.

Your success is our success

We would be delighted to hear about your success. Send us an email and tell us your story. Thanks for your business and we wish you continued success.

Sincerely,

Mometrix Test Preparation Team

Need more help? Check out our flashcards at:
http://MometrixFlashcards.com/CardiacVascular

TABLE OF CONTENTS

Top 20 Test Taking Tips

1. Carefully follow all the test registration procedures
2. Know the test directions, duration, topics, question types, how many questions
3. Setup a flexible study schedule at least 3-4 weeks before test day
4. Study during the time of day you are most alert, relaxed, and stress free
5. Maximize your learning style; visual learner use visual study aids, auditory learner use auditory study aids
6. Focus on your weakest knowledge base
7. Find a study partner to review with and help clarify questions
8. Practice, practice, practice
9. Get a good night's sleep; don't try to cram the night before the test
10. Eat a well balanced meal
11. Know the exact physical location of the testing site; drive the route to the site prior to test day
12. Bring a set of ear plugs; the testing center could be noisy
13. Wear comfortable, loose fitting, layered clothing to the testing center; prepare for it to be either cold or hot during the test
14. Bring at least 2 current forms of ID to the testing center
15. Arrive to the test early; be prepared to wait and be patient
16. Eliminate the obviously wrong answer choices, then guess the first remaining choice
17. Pace yourself; don't rush, but keep working and move on if you get stuck
18. Maintain a positive attitude even if the test is going poorly
19. Keep your first answer unless you are positive it is wrong
20. Check your work, don't make a careless mistake

Assessment and Diagnosis

Methods of questioning that encourage the patient to give an accurate, in-depth personal history

Open discussion: Promotes patient comfort by encouraging questions and feedback during the interview.

Ask leading questions: Ask questions that require more than a "yes" or "no" answer and give clear permission for the patient to speak freely about his/her health.

Restate and summarize provided information in another way: Allows you to verify that your understanding of given information is correct.

Focus: Assist the patient to concentrate on identifying his/her highest healthcare needs or make connections between healthcare behavior and larger priorities.

Order and sequence: Verify cause and effect and timing of the events given in a patient history.

Encourage self-evaluation: Allow the patient to draw his/her own conclusions regarding information. Do not judge or try to educate at this point.

Make observations: Provide commentary on the patient's physical, mental and emotional demeanor to help him/her focus and give permission to discuss further aspects of his/her health or immediate needs.

Comprehensive cardiovascular patient assessment

1. Patient history: The best source of information about the history of his/her condition is the patient. Other resources might include past medical records and involved family members.
2. Physical exam: Execute a full, head-to-toe symmetrical exam including inspection, palpation, percussion and auscultation methods as appropriate.
3. Laboratory results: Typical laboratory tests include cardiac enzymes, clotting function, cholesterol levels and therapeutic medication levels.
4. Diagnostic tests: Diagnostic tests can include X-ray, computed tomography (CT) scan, magnetic resonance imaging (MRI), electrocardiogram (ECG), echocardiography (ECHO), myocardial perfusion imaging and cardiac catheterization.

General order of procedure for a physical examination

- Inspection: visual inspection with the naked eye and specialized equipment such as an ophthalmoscope to view physical features such as height, body mass, skin condition and color, breath frequency and quality, hair distribution, balance, gait and presence of tremors or physical injuries.
- Palpation: examination by touch for pulses, organ size and location, pain response, temperature, distinguishable masses.
- Percussion: further touch intervention utilizing the fingers to create sound.

- Auscultation: auditory assessment with and without the assistance of a stethoscope generally focusing on the cardiac, respiratory and digestive systems. Other useful tools might include the use of Doppler to locate pulses that were difficult to palpate.

This general procedure varies slightly during assessment of the abdomen, placing auscultation before palpation and percussion. Other systems may not require the use of all four examination elements.

Physical examination in patients with known or suspected peripheral artery disease (PAD)

- Blood pressure results taken from both arms as well as notations regarding hypertension and medications used to treat it.
- Carotid, femoral and extremity pulses assessed for presence, intensity and bruit.
- Abdominal auscultation and palpation for bruits or pulsation.
- Thorough skin examination, including bare feet, assessing color, temperature, perfusion, integrity, nail changes, hair distribution.
- Subjective history should include smoking, diabetes, extremity pain, numbness, exertion fatigue, reports of past slow-healing wounds, abdominal pain after eating, and family history of PAD or abdominal aortic aneurysm.
- Gather laboratory values for cholesterol levels and clotting times. Anticipate ultrasound evaluation of any abnormalities.

Risk factors associated with cardiovascular disease

Risk factors that the patient and his/her healthcare provider can exercise some control over are identified as modifiable. These can include smoking, excess weight, alcohol use, cholesterol levels, blood pressure, active management of diabetes, stress and the amount of exercise the patient engages in.

Risk factors beyond the patient's control include: age, male gender and genetic tendencies including race (Caucasian, black or Native American) and family history.

The greatest risk is to those who have already experienced a cardiovascular event or have been previously diagnosed with a cardiovascular disease such as peripheral vascular disease, aortic aneurysm or carotid artery disease. Others with high risk include those who have at least two of the modifiable or non-modifiable risk factors or type II diabetes.

Chronic obstructive pulmonary disease (COPD)

COPD and chronic heart disease (CHD) share a common causative factor: smoking. Priority preventive care and education would focus on smoking cessation for the patient presenting with COPD; this will in turn lower his/her risk of CHD.

The patient presenting with COPD is at a greater risk for cardiac and vascular problems such as pulmonary hypertension and right ventricular heart failure (cor pulmonale). Likewise, the patient with both cardiovascular problems and COPD is faced with a higher mortality rate than the patient with only one condition. COPD also complicates and slows recovery from chronic heart disease and surgical procedures that might be used in the treatment of CHD.

Diabetes

Diabetes mellitus is a significant risk factor for cardiovascular disease. The patient with diabetes should be treated as if he or she already has cardiovascular disease when addressing treatment and risk factor reduction. Approximately ⅔ of all individuals diagnosed with diabetes will die as a result of cardiovascular disease. This is particularly alarming when considering the rapid growth trends for newly diagnosed diabetics. Highest priority is given to maintaining an HbA1c level at or below 7. Complications such as retinopathy, microalbuminuria, neuropathy and elevated cholesterol levels can be reduced with tight blood sugar control. Careful blood sugar maintenance is also required after surgical procedures to reduce the risks of infection and delayed healing.

Cerebrovascular disease

Cardiovascular disease and cerebrovascular disease, most commonly chronic heart disease and carotid artery occlusive disease, are often coexisting because of their overlapping risk factors. Cardiovascular accident (CVA) is the third leading cause of death in the United States and can be directly linked to atherosclerosis. The patient experiencing dysrhythmia, MI or cardiopulmonary arrest is at increased risk for subsequent acute cerebrovascular injury. Cardiac and vascular surgeries can also result in CVAs. On the other end of the spectrum, the patient experiencing a CVA is less likely to survive if he/she also has chronic heart disease.

Pain that should be assessed in a thorough patient history

- Quality: Have the patient describe the quality of the pain using words such as dull, stabbing, sharp, aching, throbbing and burning.
- Severity: Pain can be rated on a scale of 1–10 or other assessment tool.
- Location: Where on the body is the pain located? Does it radiate or shift?
- Timing: When did the pain begin? Is it constant or does it come and go with a predictable or random frequency?
- Causative factors: Ask whether or not the patient is able to pinpoint a precipitating event prior to the onset of pain.
- Aggravating factors: Does the quality or severity of pain change with activity, position, stress level or other varying conditions?
- Alleviating factors: What effect do medication, position or other noninvasive treatment interventions have on the amount of pain?
- Related symptoms: Is the pain accompanied by nausea, dizziness, shortness of breath or other closely related symptoms?

Borg scale

Frequently used in outpatient and community exercise programs, the Borg scale is a method to evaluate patient exertion based on breath quality and perceived exhaustion. The subjective data—perceived increases in heart rate, respirations, sweating and muscle endurance—are rated on an ascending scale of 6–20. A mild physical effort would produce a lower number; extreme exertion would correlate with a higher number. This scale number also provides a fairly accurate estimate of the patient's actual pulse rate when multiplied by 10 (i.e., a rating of 9 [mild exertion] would correlate to a generalize pulse rate of 90). This method can be taught to the patient in order to assess his/her exertion level outside of a monitored, therapeutic environment.

Qualitative and quantitative methods of data collection

Qualitative: Seeks to identify generalities and answer initial questions regarding a situation or incident. Its focus is on exploring and observing to gain information. Answers and information are expressed in word and theory. Data gathered and conclusions made can be more subjective than quantitative data. It is generally used as a first step or in conjunction with more strictly defined quantitative studies.

Quantitative: Answers specific questions, tests theories, establishes cause and effect relationships, gauges impact and outcome of various conditions and can be translated into mathematical answers. Quantitative studies are generally easier to duplicate for credibility.

Age-related cardiovascular changes an older patient may experience

The risk for blockage by constriction of the vessels or blood clots increases with age, as does a tendency toward pooling blood in the legs and feet.

Cardiac output is reduced. Cardiac tissue and vessels can become hardened or brittle or become narrowed from plaque and inflammation buildup, all of which reduce cardiac efficiency and restrict blood flow.

Exercise endurance and oxygen perfusion is reduced. Many of these factors can be mitigated by maintaining an active lifestyle, with a focus on endurance training, as the patient ages.

Criteria, according to the AHA, for placing a patient on continuous cardiac (telemetry) monitoring

- Class I: These patients are under the highest risk for immediate, life-threatening cardiac events. They require continuous monitoring under the supervision of a practitioner highly skilled in both ECG interpretation and defibrillation. This level of care suggests intensive care treatment.
- Class II: This is a lower risk classification, suggested for patients on cardiac medications, minor surgical interventions such as angioplasty or pacemaker lead placement. These patients are normally found on a cardiac step-down or intermediate cardiac care unit.
- Class III: Patients carrying the lowest risk for cardiac events but requiring a short interval of increased monitoring, such as surgical and labor patients.

Uses of chest x-ray, computed tomography (CT) scan and magnetic resonance imaging (MRI)

Chest x-ray: Used for initial evaluation, x-ray provides a cursory view of the chest organs including size and position of the heart and health of the lungs.

CT scan: Without the use of contrast dye, this is still considered a noninvasive procedure utilizing concentrated x-rays. CT scans are useful for expanding the available view of an organ to a more 3-dimensional picture.

MRI: Uses a magnetic field to create a computerized 3-dimensional image without the use of harmful radiation; however, it is consequently the most expensive of the three procedures. MRI provides the most accurate and detailed information regarding the status of the soft tissue organs.

Expected pattern of creatine kinase (CK) results in the hours and days following a myocardial infarction (MI)

CK and CK-MB levels are evaluated every 6–8 hours in a suspected myocardial injury. Total CK and CK-MB (specific to cardiac cells) initially rise within the first 4–6 hours of an MI. A normal range would be 30 IU/L to 180 IU/L for CK and CK-MB totaling 0–5% of the CK level.

Assuming no further damage is sustained, peak levels (in excess of 6 times the normal range) are reached 12–24 hours after the injury.

CK levels will return to normal within 3–4 days of the event.

Small spikes in CK level might also occur following invasive cardiac procedures.

Typical changes that might be seen on an electrocardiogram (ECG) indicating the presence of heart disease

In a normal ECG, P waves are no taller than 0.25 mV and no wider than 0.11 seconds. A normal PR interval is 0.12–0.20 seconds. A normal QRS is 0.04–0.10 seconds. T waves gently curve upright and are no taller than 5 mm (10 mm in chest leads). U waves, when visible are also upright in the presence of myocardial injury, T waves turn upside down or become markedly tall. Higher T waves may be thinner than normal, or longer and followed by an inverted U wave.

ST segment drops below the baseline or measures wider than 0.12 seconds. The ST segment might not have a return to the baseline between S and T.

Q waves may measure greater than 0.03 seconds.

Aneurysms

An aneurysm is defined as a localized, blood-filled dilation of a blood vessel (artery or vein) caused by cardiac disease or weakening of the blood vessel wall. Aneurysms most commonly occur within the intracranial vessels, but are also found along the thoracic aorta, abdominal aorta, and in vessels of the extremities.

Aneurysms typically occur in elderly patients, but can present in patients of any age group. However, aneurysms are uncommon in individuals under 20 years of age. The risk of aneurysm increases with age and is most likely to occur in individuals between the ages of 50 and 80.

Aneurysms are more common in Caucasian patients than individuals of other ethnicities. Typically, men develop aneurysms more often than women do. However, women with aneurysms have a risk of rupture significantly higher than that of men.

Approximately 15,000 individuals in the United States die each year from ruptured aneurysms. Ruptured aneurysms are the 10th leading cause of death in men over age 50 in the United States.

Types of aneurysms
A peripheral aneurysm is more likely to affect individuals ages 60 to 80. Cerebral aneurysms are more likely to occur in people ages 35 to 60.

Approximately 0.2% to 3% of individuals in the United States with a brain aneurysm suffer from hemorrhage per year, with 10% to 15% of these individuals dying prior to obtaining care and over 50% dying within 1 month post rupture. Approximately half of patients surviving a rupture suffer from permanent neurological damage.

Abdominal aortic aneurysms are 4 times more common in men than in women and are most prevalent in Caucasians ages 40 to 70. Less than 50% of individuals with a ruptured abdominal aortic aneurysm survive.

Symptoms associated with aneurysms

Typically, aneurysms are asymptomatic until they grow large enough to cause symptoms. Associated symptoms vary by location of the aneurysm. Aneurysms located closer to the surface of body may present with swelling and pain; however, most aneurysms within the body are asymptomatic.

Aneurysms in the brain can present with symptoms of localized severe headache, intense pressure, nausea and vomiting, neck pain, blurred or double vision, pain in or around the eye, dilated pupils, sensitivity to light, and loss of sensation.

Aneurysms in the abdomen may present with a deep dull penetrating pain in the lower back or abdomen that lasts for days to hours.

Signs and symptoms of a peripheral aneurysm may include leg or arm cramping, coldness, and numbness or tingling in the feet due to blocked blood flow to the peripheral arteries.

Risk factors

Risk factors that can potentially lead to aneurysm formation: atherosclerosis, smoking, obesity, hypertension, head or body trauma, alcohol consumption, use of oral contraceptives, Marfan syndrome, tuberculosis, untreated syphilis, vasculitis, Caucasian ethnicity, male gender, and family history of aneurysms or heart diseases.

Smoking is a strong risk factor for the development of an aneurysm, with risk increasing according to the number of pack years. Increased blood pressure and atherosclerosis are also risk factors for aneurysms due to increased pressure within the blood vessels and damage to blood vessel walls.

Genetic disorders, including Marfan syndrome, can lead to aneurysm formation, as the disease affects connective tissue throughout the body, including the tissues of the blood vessels.

Another risk factor is a family history of aneurysms. Individuals with a family history of aneurysms typically develop aneurysms at an earlier age and should be monitored by a specialist.

Aneurysm diagnosis

Physical examination sometimes suggests aneurysms. For example, a pulsating abdominal mass suggests an aneurysm of the abdominal aorta. Medical imaging is used for definitive diagnosis including chest x-ray, ultrasound, magnetic resonance imaging (MRI), angiography, and computer tomography (CT) scan. Aneurysms are often incidentally found while imaging a patient for other reasons.

Patients at high risk for aneurysms should be followed regularly by a cardiothoracic, vascular, or neurological surgeon. Current guideline recommendations suggest that men who are 65 to 75 years old and are ex-smokers should be checked for aneurysms routinely. Men aged 60 and older with a family history of aneurysms should also consider routine screening.

<u>Aneurysm complications</u>
Aneurysm rupture can lead to complications such as sudden death, stroke, and brain damage. Signs and symptoms of aneurysm rupture include hypotension, rapid heartbeat, lightheadedness, fainting, nausea, vomiting, sweating, shortness of breath, chest pain, lower back/abdominal pain, and dizziness. The risk of death is high with aneurysm rupture, except for rupture in the extremities. Also, the risk of rupture increases as the blood vessel dilation increases.

Another complication of aneurysms is the risk of blood clots. The occlusion of blood flow can lead to complications such as brain damage, lack of peripheral blood flow to end organ systems or extremities, and sudden death. Blood clots can also dislodge from the site of origin and cause the above complications.

Atherosclerosis

Atherosclerosis is a disease caused by formation of plaque in the walls of arteries. Plaque formation is caused by a chronic inflammatory response and endothelial dysfunction where lipids, cholesterol, calcium, and other substances build up in the arteries. There is an imbalance between deposition of plaque and removal by low-density lipoproteins in smooth muscle cells. Two types of plaques can form in the arteries including stable plaques and unstable plaques. Stable plaques consist of a thick fibrous cap of smooth muscle cells that upon stimulation can lead to reduced blood flow to heart, lung, and other organ systems. Unstable plaques consist of a thin fibrous cap of smooth muscle cells that can rupture leading to a heart attack and/or stroke.

The disease can affect arteries in the heart, brain, lungs, and extremities. Therefore, based on the origin of the condition, atherosclerosis can be referred to as coronary heart disease, when present in coronary arteries, carotid artery disease when present in the carotid artery, and peripheral arterial disease when present in the arteries supplying the extremities.

In the United States, more than 11 million Americans have atherosclerosis. Atherosclerosis is the leading cause of coronary heart disease and stroke, with the disease responsible for more than half of the annual deaths. Over 1 million individuals in the United States annually are diagnosed with coronary artery disease and nearly 700,000 individuals suffer a stroke.

Atherosclerosis is a condition that develops over time, presenting symptoms in patients between the ages of 40 and 70 due to hardening of plaques, vascular remodeling, blood flow abnormalities, and diminished oxygen flow to end organ systems. Patients between the ages of 50 and 60 typically present with advanced complications of the condition as well as organ system dysfunction.

Individuals with an increased risk of atherosclerosis include men and patients with a family history of cardiovascular disease. The lower prevalence of atherosclerosis in women may be due to the protective effects of estrogen and progesterone. However, this hormonal protective effect has been shown to decrease after menopause, unless the individual is undergoing hormone replacement therapy.

<u>Risk factors and complications</u>
Factors that can increase an individual's risk for atherosclerosis include elevated low-density lipoprotein (LDL) cholesterol, decreased high-density lipoprotein (HDL) cholesterol, elevated

triglyceride levels, menopause, lack of physical activity, obesity, infection of the vascular smooth muscle cells, high blood pressure, history of smoking, and diabetes.

Smoking not only predisposes individuals to atherosclerosis, but it increases the progression of the disease. The progression of atherosclerosis itself also further increases the extent and degree of the condition, as further accumulation of lipids, cholesterol, and other substances stimulates the endothelium to produce other substances that cause increased plaque build-up.

Atherosclerosis leads to altered vascular function including coronary heart disease, myocardial ischemia and myocardial infarction, cerebrovascular insufficiency, stroke, peripheral vascular disease, limb ischemia, renal disease, aortic aneurysm, and vasculitis. The final mechanism of the above complications usually occurs via plaque rupture or severe vessel narrowing and blood clotting.

<u>Symptoms</u>
Typically, atherosclerosis is asymptomatic until plaques grow large enough to cause symptoms or rupture. The disease typically progresses slowly over time and the symptoms vary by location of the condition. The most common site of atherosclerotic formation is the lower abdominal aorta. Other sites include coronary arteries, popliteal arteries, descending thoracic aorta, internal carotid arteries, and other vessels.

Common symptoms include chest pain, peripheral pain, weakness, numbness, shortness of breath, dizziness, intermittent claudication, and erectile dysfunction in men. Specifically, individuals presenting with obstruction to coronary arteries experience chest pain, weakness, and fatigue. Individuals who present with obstruction of carotid arteries may experience weakness, numbness, and dizziness. Obstruction of peripheral arteries to extremities may result in intermittent claudication.

<u>Screening and diagnosis</u>
Physical examination often hints at atherosclerosis, but further blood testing and medical imaging is needed for diagnosis. For example, a bruit heard over the carotid artery or abdomen is suggestive of atherosclerosis in the carotids or abdominal aorta. Hairless legs are suggestive of peripheral atherosclerosis. Initial blood tests showing elevated low-density lipoprotein (LDL) cholesterol, low high-density lipoprotein (HDL) cholesterol, and elevated triglycerides also suggest it. Diagnostic tools used to determine the presence of plaque formation include electrocardiogram, exercise stress test, echocardiogram, nuclear scan, coronary angiography, electron beam computed tomography, coronary computed tomography (CT) angiography, and magnetic resonance angiography.

Screening for atherosclerosis includes annual blood tests in patients over 20 years of age with a history of cardiovascular disease. Patients 20 years or older should have cholesterol levels checked every 5 years including LDL cholesterol, HDL cholesterol, and triglycerides.

Assessment of other atherosclerosis risk factors should be done as well including modifiable risk factors such as smoking, uncontrolled diabetes, and obesity as well as unmodifiable risk factors such as family history and aging. Individuals with multiple risk factors should be followed on a more regular basis than every 5 years.

Buerger's disease

Buerger's disease, also known as *Thromboangiitis obliterans*, is a rare condition resulting impaired blood flow to extremities due to clot formation and inflammation in peripheral arteries and veins. The disease typically progresses from the hands and feet and extends to arms and legs.

The disease is more common in men than in women and typically occurs between 20 and 45 years of age. However, women over the age of 50 have more recently been diagnosed with the condition. The disease is most common in East Asia and the Middle East and rare in the Americas.

Complications of the disease include ulcerations, infections, and gangrene, which result from tissue damage.

Risk factors and complications

The main risk factor for Buerger's disease is smoking. The onset of Buerger's disease is dependent on the degree and extent of cigarette smoking. Nearly all cases of Buerger's disease occur in patients who are current smokers or tobacco users, previous smokers or tobacco users, or were exposed to smoke for an extended period.

Symptoms of Buerger's disease include pain and weakness in extremities, swelling of hands and feet, Raynaud's phenomenon, open sores on digits.

Complications of Buerger's disease include gangrene in digits, infection of the hands and feet, as well as amputation of digits/extremities. Symptoms associated with gangrene include black or blue digits, numbness or tingling in digits, and foul smell from infected area.

Diagnosis and screening

Physical examination, specifically distal ischemia and ulcerations, suggests Buerger's disease, especially in a male smoker under 45 years old. A positive Allen test also suggests the disorder. Blood tests are useful to rule out other etiologies. However, there are currently no definitive tests available to diagnose the disease and diagnosis is based on a process of elimination.

Diagnostic screening tools used to aid in diagnosis of Buerger's disease include blood tests to rule out scleroderma, lupus, diabetes and other blood clotting conditions. Allen test is used to assess blood flow to the hands and feet. Angiography, ultrasound, and echocardiography can be used to assess vascular flow.

The most commonly used criteria used for the diagnosis of Buerger's disease: individuals younger than 45 years of age, past or present tobacco use, presence of distal extremity ischemia (ischemic ulcers and gangrene), exclusion of autoimmune disorders, and consistent angiographic findings in extremities.

Raynaud's phenomenon

Raynaud's phenomenon is a condition where an individual's fingers and toes become discolored, pale, numb, and/or cold due to exposure to changes in temperature or emotional stress. Typical color changes are white, blue, and then red. The symptoms of Raynaud's syndrome occur due to the mechanism of action, where the small arteries carrying blood to the digits constrict and spasm. Thus, oxygen-rich blood is denied to the distal extremities and this causes the corresponding symptoms.

Raynaud's phenomenon is used to describe 2 conditions: 1) Raynaud's disease, also known as primary Raynaud's phenomenon, and 2) Raynaud's syndrome, also known as secondary Raynaud's phenomenon, where the condition is secondary to another comorbid disease.

Recent data has shown that Raynaud's syndrome is more common in women than men. Symptoms of Raynaud's syndrome typically present within the 4th decade of life, whereas symptoms of Raynaud's disease occur earlier in life.

Primary Raynaud's or Raynaud's disease is typically an inherited condition, exacerbated by smoking, with a hormonal component.

However, Raynaud's syndrome, or secondary Raynaud's is associated with numerous environmental factors and diseases. Those most often associated include scleroderma, lupus, rheumatoid arthritis, eating disorders, atherosclerosis, Buerger's disease, and drugs such as beta-blockers, cytotoxins, cyclosporin, ergotamine, or sulfasalazine. Additionally, occupational hazards including exposure to vibrating equipment, vinyl chloride and cold as well as other comorbid conditions like hypothyroidism, cryoglobulinemia, cancer and reflex sympathetic dystrophy have also been associated with secondary Raynaud's phenomenon.

Risk factors
The exact cause of Raynaud's disease and Raynaud's syndrome is unknown. In this phenomenon, blood vessels in the digits overreact to cold temperatures or stress.

Risk factors of primary Raynaud's disease include sex, age, residing in colder climates and family history. Women tend to present with primary Raynaud's phenomenon more often than men. Also, individuals ages 15 to 25 present with primary Raynaud's disease more often than individuals in other age groups. Additionally, individuals that live in colder climates and with a family history of the phenomenon also present more frequently with primary Raynaud's disease.

The risk factors for secondary Raynaud's syndrome include patients with underlying comorbid conditions such as lupus and diabetes as well as individuals who operate machinery for their occupation.

Symptoms
Patients with either primary or secondary Raynaud's phenomenon present with painful, pale, discolored, and/or cold digits. Patients may also experience numbness or tingling as well as dull sensory perception in response to cold or stress.

Primary Raynaud's phenomenon, or Raynaud's disease, is considered systemic, whereas secondary Raynaud's phenomenon typically only presents in the extremities. Patients with secondary Raynaud's phenomenon also experience symptoms of the comorbid condition when experiencing Raynaud's symptoms. The symptoms of the phenomenon depend on the extent and degree of vasospasm the individual is experiencing.

For the most part, Raynaud's phenomenon mainly affects the digits, but can cause symptoms in other areas of the body including nose, nipples, lips, and ears. Also, the phenomenon may not always affect the same digits or areas of the body. The phenomenon can occur for short or long durations, ranging from minutes up to several hours.

<u>Diagnosis and screening</u>
Physical examination and diagnostic screening are typically used to diagnose both Raynaud's disease and syndrome, as no single test is available to diagnose these disorders.

Although clinical practitioners can easily diagnose Raynaud's phenomenon by the signs and symptoms patients present with (cold extremities with color changes onset by cold or stress), it remains difficult to determine if the phenomenon is primary or secondary. In order to distinguish between Raynaud's disease and Raynaud's syndrome, a nail fold capillaroscopy is typically performed. Distorted or fewer capillaries than normal suggests secondary Raynaud's. Diagnostic measurement of hand temperature gradients, digital artery pressure measurements, Doppler ultrasound, blood counts, and measurement of urea and electrolyte levels are other tools used to distinguish between primary and secondary forms of the phenomenon.

Additionally, blood tests to assess for secondary disorders like lupus or hypothyroidism are helpful.

Cardiomyopathy

Cardiomyopathy is defined as deterioration of myocardium function. The World Health Organization categorizes cardiomyopathy into 2 categories including extrinsic cardiomyopathy and intrinsic cardiomyopathy. Cardiomyopathies are considered extrinsic if their primary pathology is outside the myocardium. However, intrinsic cardiomyopathies are either secondary to genetic, infectious, or idiopathic.

Cardiomyopathy can also be classified as primary or secondary. Primary cardiomyopathy is idiopathic in nature, whereas secondary cardiomyopathies can be attributed to a specific cause such as high blood pressure, heart valve disease, or coronary heart disease.

More specific sub-types of cardiomyopathies include dilated cardiomyopathy, hypertrophic cardiomyopathy, restrictive cardiomyopathy, and arrhythmogenic right ventricular dysplasia.

Dilated cardiomyopathy is the most common type of cardiomyopathy. It presents most often in individuals ages 20 to 60 years, with the condition more common in men than women.

Hypertropic cardiomyopathy can occur at any age and occurs due to abnormal thickening of cardiac muscle. Hypertropic cardiomyopathy consists of 2 types of disease including obstructive and nonobstructive. Both types lead to thickening of cardiac muscle that, in turn, reduces the size of the left ventricle.

Restrictive cardiomyopathy tends to affect elderly patients. It occurs because the ventricles become thick due to abnormal tissue growth that replaces cardiac tissue, reducing blood flow and proper cardiac muscle function.

Arrhythmogenic right ventricular dysplasia is a rare cardiomyopathy that typically affects young adults. It is the leading cause of sudden death in young athletes. The disease presents due to formation of scar tissue in the right ventricle, which can lead to arrhythmias.

<u>Causes</u>
Factors that increase risk of cardiomyopathy include ischemic damage to the heart musculature from a heart attack, hypertension, gene mutation, and/or viral infection. However, in some cases, the actual cause of cardiomyopathy remains unknown.

In terms of the specific sub-types of cardiomyopathies, dilated cardiomyopathy can be inherited but also can be caused by coronary heart disease, heart attacks, infections, alcohol consumption, pregnancy complications, toxins, certain drugs such as amphetamines, or other disease such as diabetes or thyroid disease. Hypertropic cardiomyopathy can also be inherited, but can be caused by high blood pressure or natural aging. Restrictive cardiomyopathy can be caused by hemochromatosis, amyloidosis, sarcoidosis, and connective tissue disorders.

Risk factors

Natural aging is an independent risk factor for cardiomyopathy. However, certain types of cardiomyopathies are more prevalent in certain age and ethnic groups. Male gender and individuals of African American descent are at increased risk for dilated cardiomyopathy as compared to women and individuals of Caucasian descent. Also, young adults are more prone to arrhythmogenic right ventricular dysplasia as compared to elderly individuals.

Other risk factors include family history of cardiomyopathy, congestive heart failure, and sudden cardiac death. The presence of other comorbid conditions includes coronary heart disease, diabetes, metabolic disorders, alcohol abuse, and high blood pressure.

Symptoms

Typically, cardiomyopathies are asymptomatic until they inhibit blood flow or restrict cardiac muscle contraction. They also vary by type of cardiomyopathy. With progression of disease, symptoms include fatigue, weakness, shortness of breath with exertion, swelling of abdomen and extremities, dizziness, fainting, and palpitations. These symptoms tend to get worse as the degree and extent of disease progresses. However, the time to progression varies from patient to patient and ranges from sudden attack to a slow progression.

Diagnosis and screening

Physical examination and diagnostic screening tools are typically used to diagnose cardiomyopathies. However, cardiomyopathies are typically found when assessing other conditions or during routine examinations.

Hypertension is a risk factor for cardiomyopathy and can be diagnosed by measurement of blood pressure. Symptoms of high blood pressure include headaches, fatigue, dizziness, blurred vision, nausea and vomiting, facial flushing or tinnitus.

Cardiomyopathy diagnostic tools include chest x-ray to determine if heart is enlarged, echocardiogram to assess size and motion of the heart, electrocardiogram to determine the presence of electrical disturbances and blood tests to assess BNP levels. Thyroid levels and serum iron counts are also helpful. Clinical practitioners may also perform cardiac stress testing to assess cardiac muscle function as well as electrical activity when the heart is under physical stress. MRI and PET scans may also be used to evaluate cardiac structures, rhythm, and chemical activity in different areas of the heart.

Other more invasive diagnostic techniques include cardiac angiography and biopsy.

Congestive heart failure

Congestive heart failure is a condition where the heart is unable to pump adequate oxygenated blood throughout the body.

Congestive heart failure is caused by diseases that weaken or stiffen cardiac muscle. It can also be caused by diseases that increase oxygen demand, which the heart is unable to support.

The prevalence of congestive heart failure is approximately 5 million individuals in the United States, with half a million cases diagnosed each year and approximately 300,000 deaths per year. An important prognostic factor associated with congestive heart failure is the development of arrhythmias. Mortality due to congestive heart failure can be attributed to arrhythmias in 50% of patients and progressive heart failure in another 50% of patients.

Congestive heart failure is prevalent in individuals 65 years of age and older. It is also prevalent among African Americans, obese individuals and individuals with type II diabetes. Congestive heart failure is more prevalent among men than women.

Risk factors
Factors that can lead to congestive heart failure include heart muscle weakness, systolic dysfunction, heart valve disorders, viral infections, thyroid disorders, and arrhythmias. The most common causes of congestive heart failure include hypertension and coronary artery disease.

Other risk factors include a family history of congestive heart failure, presence of other comorbid conditions including previous heart attack, diabetes, metabolic disorders, and alcohol consumption.

Additional factors that can attribute to the progression of congestive heart failure include pharmacologic agents such as NSAIDs, corticosteroids, calcium channel blockers and diabetic agents.

Symptoms
Congestive heart failure can be asymptomatic until later stages of the disease. However, some patients may present with fatigue and muscle weakness during earlier stages of the disease.

Symptoms vary among patients and are based on end organ system involvement. With progression of disease, symptoms may include fatigue, weakness, shortness of breath after exertion, swelling of abdomen and extremities, dizziness, fainting, arrhythmias, increased urination, decreased appetite, nausea and palpitations.

These symptoms tend to get worse as the degree and extent of disease progresses. However, the time to progression varies from patient to patient and ranges from sudden onset to a slow progression.

Diagnosis and screening
Physical examination and diagnostic screening tools are typically used in addition to symptoms to screen for congestive heart failure. However, congestive heart failure is typically found when assessing other conditions or during routine examinations.

During physical examination, practicing clinicians aim to uncover excess fluid in the lungs, heart, liver or other end organ systems as well as estimate the level of cardiac function.

Congestive heart failure diagnostic tools include chest x-ray to determine if heart is enlarged, echocardiogram to assess size and motion of the heart, electrocardiogram to determine the presence of electrical disturbances and blood tests to assess BNP levels, thyroid levels and iron counts. Clinical practitioners may also perform cardiac stress testing to assess cardiac muscle function as well as electrical activity when the heart is under physical stress. MRI and PET scans may also be used to evaluate cardiac structures, rhythm, and chemical activity in different areas of the heart. Occasionally, a biopsy of the myocardium is necessary.

Cor Pulmonale

By definition, cor pulmonale is failure of the right heart not caused unrelated to left heart failure. Cor pulmonale is a disease that affects the structure and function of the right ventricle due to respiratory system abnormalities such as prolonged pulmonary hypertension. Pathophysiologic mechanisms that can lead to cor pulmonale include pulmonary vasoconstriction, compromise of vascular bed due to lung disease such as emphysema and interstitial lung disease, increased blood viscosity due to diseases like sickle cell anemia and primary pulmonary hypertension. The disease can present as a chronically evolving condition, but can also occur acutely due to pulmonary embolism or acute respiratory distress syndrome. In the United States, the prevalence of cor pulmonale associated with adult onset cardiac disease is approximately 6% to 7%. Nearly half of these cases are due to underlying chronic bronchitis, chronic obstructive pulmonary disease, or emphysema. Acute pulmonary embolism is the most common cause of death in patients with cor pulmonale. Of the 50,000 patients that die of acute pulmonary embolism in the United States, nearly half are associated with cor pulmonale. Of those patients with chronically evolving disease due to chronic obstructive pulmonary disease, 30% have a chance of surviving 5 years.

Causes
Cor pulmonale is caused by any condition that leads to prolonged pulmonary hypertension and can occur secondary to an array of cardiopulmonary diseases. Chronic pulmonary diseases that can put patients at a predisposition for cor pulmonale include COPD, obstructive sleep apnea, central sleep apnea, cystic fibrosis, primary pulmonary hypertension, pneumoconiosis, kyphoscoliosis, interstitial lung disease, chronic thromboembolic pulmonary disease, pulmonary vascular disease and pulmonary hypertension.

Acute causes of cor pulmonale include massive pulmonary embolization and exacerbation of chronic cor pulmonale.

Chronic causes of cor pulmonale include COPD, loss of lung tissue due to trauma or surgery, Pierre Robin sequence and end stage pneumoconiosis.

Cor pulmonale is caused by several mechanisms including pulmonary vasoconstriction, anatomic changes in vascularization, increased blood viscosity, and idiopathic or primary pulmonary hypertension.

Symptoms
The symptoms associated with Cor Pulmonale are typically nonspecific and can be associated with a variety of cardiopulmonary diseases. The symptoms of the disease also depend on whether the disease presents chronically or acutely due to pulmonary embolism or acute respiratory distress syndrome.

The symptoms of cor pulmonale include shortness of breath, coughing, wheezing, swelling of feet and ankles, fluid retention, exercise intolerance, tachypnea, hemoptysis, labored respiratory efforts with retractions of chest wall, hoarseness and chest pain or discomfort. Additionally, neurological symptoms may occur due to decreased cardiac output and hypoxemia.

<u>Screening and diagnosis</u>
Physical examination and diagnostic screening tools are typically used to diagnose cor pulmonale. Patients typically present with a bluish hue to their skin as well as distension of the neck veins caused by elevated right side heart pressures. Other indicators of the disease include abnormal fluid collection in abdomen, liver enlargement, increased chest diameter, prominent a or v waves, cyanosis, ankle and foot swelling as well as abnormal heart sounds.

Diagnostic tools used to diagnose the disease include echocardiogram, chest x-ray, CT scan, pulmonary angiography, magnetic resonance imaging, ECG-gated CT scanning, pulmonary function tests, ventilation/perfusion lung scans, arterial blood gas measurements, antibody testing and brain natriuretic peptide measurements. Additionally, more invasive diagnostic approaches include Swan-Ganz catheterization and lung biopsy.

Type I, II and Gestational Diabetes Mellitus

Type I diabetes occurs in approximately 10% of all cases of diabetes mellitus. The condition can affect both adults and children, but is referred to as juvenile diabetes because it typically affects adolescents. The incidence of type I diabetes is approximately 15 cases per 100,000 individuals annually.

Type II diabetes is the most common type of diabetes mellitus, approximately 90% of all cases of diabetes mellitus. Additionally, more than half of patients diagnosed with type II diabetes are obese. It is also more common in patients over 40 years of age, but can occur in young adults and adolescents. It is also more prevalent in Hispanics, Native Americans, African Americans, and Asians/Pacific Islanders than in Caucasians.

Gestational diabetes occurs in approximately 2% to 5% of all pregnancies and is treatable with careful supervision throughout pregnancy. Of those women affected with gestational diabetes, approximately 20% to 50% develop type II diabetes.

Diabetes mellitus is a condition resulting in high blood glucose level. The condition is caused by metabolic dysfunction due to either low levels of insulin or abnormal resistance to insulin combined with inadequate levels of insulin secretion.

Type I diabetes is also known as juvenile diabetes or insulin dependent diabetes. It is a chronic metabolic disorder that results in high blood glucose levels due to low levels of insulin. In type I diabetes, the pancreas does not produce enough insulin, resulting in high blood glucose levels.

Type II diabetes is also known as adult onset or noninsulin dependent diabetes. It is a chronic metabolic disorder that results in high blood glucose levels due to insulin resistance and/or low secretion of insulin. In type II diabetes, the body is resistance to insulin, which in turn results in high blood glucose levels. Early in the disease, insulin levels may actually be greater than normal, but eventually the beta cells in the pancreas "burn out" and insulin levels are lower than normal.

Gestational diabetes is not a chronic condition and typically occurs during pregnancy and resolves upon birth. The condition results in high blood glucose levels due to low insulin secretion and responsiveness.

Causes and risk factors

Individuals with type I diabetes typically have a genetic predisposition for the condition. Therefore, individuals with a parent or sibling with the disease have a higher risk for developing the condition. The causes and risk factors for type I diabetes are poorly understood, aside from some individuals having a predisposition for the disease.

It remains unclear why individuals develop type II diabetes, but the disease is associated with certain predisposing risk factors. Risk factors that increase the risk for developing type II diabetes include obesity, physical inactivity, family history, increasing age, prediabetes, and gestational diabetes. Also, individuals of African American, Hispanic, Native Americans, and Asian American descent are at higher risk for developing type II diabetes.

Medical conditions associated with a higher risk for developing type II diabetes include high blood pressure, elevated cholesterol levels, coronary artery disease, polycystic ovary syndrome, chronic pancreatitis, liver dysfunction, hemochromatosis, and cystic fibrosis.

Symptoms

The symptoms of type I diabetes include increased thirst, frequent urination, extreme hunger, weight loss, fatigue and blurred vision. Patients diagnosed with type I diabetes may also present with diabetic ketoacidosis, which may include altered mental status, coma, hyperventilation, and abdominal pain. The symptoms associated with type I diabetes tend to develop rapidly over a short period.

The symptoms of type II diabetes also include increased thirst, frequent urination, extreme hunger, weight loss, fatigue and blurred vision. The condition also includes slow healing sores or frequent infections. Also, patients diagnosed with type II diabetes may present in a hyperosmolar nonketotic state. The symptoms associated with type II diabetes develop over time and may be mistaken for other conditions or go unrecognized.

Diagnosis and screening

The diagnosis of both type I and type II diabetes is suggested by physical examination, patient symptoms, and diagnostic tools. Type I diabetes diagnosis is suggested by the sudden onset of symptoms. A fasting glucose greater than 126 mg/dL or random glucose greater than 200 mg/dL on 2 different occasions is diabetes. Age, family history, comorbidities, and demographics help suggest type I, II, or gestational diabetes. Additionally, C-peptide levels serve as a marker for insulin production. Elevated C-peptide suggests type II and low C-peptide suggests type I.

The diagnosis of type II diabetes is typically made during ordinary health examinations, but diagnosis can be made by detection of hyperglycemia during other examinations or based on the presence of secondary symptoms such as fatigue or vision changes. In many cases, type II diabetes is not diagnosed until the patient experiences a complications caused by the condition including heart attack, neuropathy, vision problems and/or foot ulcers. Diabetes screening tools include random blood glucose testing, fasting blood glucose testing, and more-formal blood glucose tolerance testing. Other lab studies include urine glucose and ketones as well as renal function tests. Blood tests include glycated hemoglobin, islet cell antibodies, thyroid function tests, antithyroid antibodies, lipid levels, and antigliadin antibodies.

Metabolic syndrome

Metabolic syndrome is defined as a group of risk factors that put individuals at risk for developing cardiovascular disease or other comorbid conditions such as diabetes. The risk of developing metabolic syndrome is closely linked to obesity, lack of physical activity, genetic factors, and poor diet.

Metabolic syndrome is also known as syndrome X, insulin resistance syndrome, dysmetabolic syndrome, hypertriglyceridemic waist and obesity syndrome.

The 5 risk factors associated with metabolic syndrome include a large waistline, higher than normal triglyceride levels, lower than normal high-density lipoprotein cholesterol, hypertension, and hyperglycemia. An increased number of risk factors raise an individual's risk of developing complications such as cardiovascular disease, diabetes, and/or stroke.

Approximately 47 million individuals have been diagnosed with metabolic syndrome in the United States. The incidence continues to increase annually, which can be attributed to increasing obesity rates within the United States.

The prevalence of metabolic syndrome in individuals greater than 20 years of age is more than 20%, increasing to over 40% in individuals greater than 60 years of age. Gender and ethnic descent affect the prevalence of metabolic syndrome. Mexican Americans have the highest rate of metabolic syndrome in the United States, followed by Caucasian Americans and African Americans.

The NCEP/ATP III (National Cholesterol Education Program/Adult Treatment Panel) defines metabolic syndrome as an individual with 3 or more of the following risk factors including waist circumference equal to or greater than 102 cm in men and 88 cm in women, triglyceride levels greater than 150 mg/dL, high-density lipid cholesterol less than 40 mg/dL in men and less than 50 mg/dL in women, blood pressure greater than or equal to 130/85 mmHg and fasting plasma glucose greater than 100 mg/dL.

The World Health Organization (WHO) defines metabolic syndrome as an individual with diabetes, impaired glucose tolerance (IGT), impaired fasting glucose (IFG) or insulin resistance, plus 2 or more of the following risk factors including body mass index greater than 30 kg/m^2 and/or waist-to-hip ratio greater than 0.9 in men and greater than 0.85 in women, triglyceride levels greater than 150 mg/dL and/or high-density lipid cholesterol less than 35 mg/dL in men and less than 39 mg/dL in women, blood pressure greater than or equal to 140/90 mmHG and urinary albumin excretion greater than equal to 20 µg/min or urinary albumin: creatinine ratio greater than or equal to 30 mg/g.

Causes and risk factors

The exact mechanisms that induce metabolic syndrome in some individuals remain unclear. The pathophysiology is very complex and poorly understood. However, several risk factors put some individuals at an increased risk of developing the condition. Risk factors associated with metabolic syndrome include obesity, lack of physical activity, dyslipidemia, history of familial diabetes, polycystic ovarian syndrome, insulin resistance, stress, aging, genetic factors and hormonal changes.

While genetic factors and aging cannot be addressed, individuals can prevent obesity by maintaining proper weight with diet and exercise as well as managing other comorbid conditions.

Patients diagnosed with metabolic syndrome also typically form blood clots and present with constant low-grade inflammation throughout the body. Additional conditions that have been associated with metabolic syndrome include fatty liver, polycystic ovary syndrome, gallstones, and sleep apnea.

<u>Symptoms</u>
The symptoms of metabolic syndrome present as a combination of other conditions. Therefore, the symptoms of metabolic syndrome are based on underlying conditions that define the condition such as hypertension, diabetes, or high cholesterol.

Other comorbid conditions associated with metabolic syndrome include elevated uric acid levels, fatty liver disease, polycystic ovary syndrome, hemochromatosis, and acanthosis nigricans.

<u>Screening and diagnosis</u>
Physical examination and diagnostic tools are used to diagnose metabolic syndrome. Patients with 3 or more of the following risk factors including abdominal obesity, higher than normal triglyceride levels, higher than normal high-density lipid cholesterol levels, hypertension, and hyperglycemia are diagnosed with metabolic syndrome. Patients with 1 or more than the above symptoms should seek medical attention to prevent other complications or comorbid conditions.

Patients with type II diabetes should be screened for metabolic syndrome as more than 80% of type II diabetes patients have comorbid metabolic syndrome and are at a higher risk for cardiovascular disease.

Endothelial dysfunction

Endothelial dysfunction is defined as abnormal functioning of the cells forming the endothelium, the innermost lining of blood vessels. It is characterized by reduced vasodilation, increased proinflammatory response and prothrombotic properties.

Patients with endothelial dysfunction typically present with an inability of arteries and veins to dilate properly or fully. Biochemical dysfunction of the endothelium leads to problems with coagulation, platelet adhesion, immune function and electrolyte balance.

Individuals diagnosed with endothelial dysfunction are at a higher risk for developing cardiovascular disease as well as having a heart attack or stroke due to presence of atherosclerosis. They are also at risk for developing the following comorbid complications, if not already present, including congestive heart failure, chronic renal failure, peripheral artery disease, and diabetes. The prognosis of endothelial dysfunction is dependent on the degree and extent of the disease as well as presence of other comorbid conditions.

Physical examination and comorbid conditions suggest the condition and diagnostic tools can be used to diagnose endothelial dysfunction. Patients with elevated risk for the disease including those with diabetes and other cardiovascular risk factors should be screened for the condition.

Diagnostic screening for endothelial dysfunction can be determined using the following methods: iontophoresis of acetylcholine, intra-arterial administration of vasoactive agents, localized heating of the skin and temporary arterial occlusion via inflating a blood pressure cuff to high pressures. Another more invasive approach is intracoronary catheterization, but it is not often performed due to increased risk of complications.

Hypertension

Hypertension is defined as high blood pressure chronically elevated at greater than or equal to 140/90 mmHg. Hypertension can be classified as primary hypertension or as result of a comorbid condition and referred to as secondary hypertension. Secondary hypertension can be attributed to kidney disease, metabolic disorders, or cancer. Primary hypertension occurs in 90% to 95% of individuals diagnosed with high blood pressure, as compared to secondary hypertension, which occurs in 2% to 10%.

The incidence and prevalence of hypertension increase with natural aging. In the United States, more than 40 million individuals have been estimated to have hypertension. In the United States, the prevalence of hypertension tends to be higher in Blacks and Hispanics as compared to Caucasians. Women under the age of 50 tend to have a lower risk of hypertension than men. However, women over the age of 50 have higher risk of hypertension than men.

Causes and risk factors

Primary hypertension can be attributed to a variety of causes including emotional stress, licorice toxicity, salt sensitivity, high renin levels, insulin resistance, sleep apnea, genetic factors, natural aging, and other factors. Individuals with a family member with primary hypertension are at an increased risk of developing the condition. Also, being of African American descent increases risk of hypertension compared to Caucasians.

Secondary hypertension can be attributed to renal disease, adrenal disease, Cushing syndrome, spinal misalignment, adrenal gland tumor, alcohol poisoning, anxiety, stress, pain, arteriosclerosis, obesity, pregnancy, hyperthyroidism, hypothyroidism, retroperitoneal fibrosis, oral contraceptives, antihypertensive medication withdrawal, and drugs such as NSAIDs.

The 2003 National Heart, Lung, and Blood Institute (NHLBI) guidelines divide blood pressure into 4 general categories for adults that include:
- The first category is "normal blood pressure," which includes individuals with a blood pressure below 120/80 mmHg.
- The secondary category is called "prehypertension" and includes individuals with a systolic blood pressure ranging from 120 to 139 and diastolic blood pressure ranging from 80 to 89. Without lifestyle modifications, prehypertension may worsen over time and should be monitored by a practicing clinician.
- The third category is referred to as "stage 1 hypertension" and includes individuals with systolic pressure ranging from 140 to 159 and/or a diastolic pressure ranging from 90 to 99.
- The fourth category is "stage 2 hypertension," which includes individuals with severe hypertension. Individuals who present with a systolic pressure above 160 and/or diastolic pressure above 100.

Diagnosis, screening and symptoms

Hypertension is typically diagnosed during routine physical examinations or when addressing other conditions or concerns. The only test used for diagnosis of hypertension is blood pressure measurement. However, blood pressure measurements need to be taken on a regular basis when persistent high blood pressure is a concern. Also, proper measurement is necessary for accurate diagnosis. If other cardiovascular complications are suspected, other testing including echocardiogram, urinalysis, CBC, serum electrolytes, serum creatine, serum glucose, and x-rays may be performed.

Most patients present with no symptoms, but some patients experience headaches, fatigue, dizziness, confusion, chest pain, irregular heartbeat, nosebleed, blurred vision, facial flushing, or tinnitus. Hypertension is sometimes misdiagnosed as stress and/or anxiety. Although stress and anxiety can contribute to elevated blood pressure, they cannot cause persistent hypertension.

Dyslipidemia

Dyslipidemia is a disorder of lipoprotein metabolism, including hyperlipidemia and hypolipidemia. Dyslipidemia can be classified as primary dyslipidemia or as result of a comorbid condition and referred to as secondary dyslipidemia. The condition is typically characterized by elevations in total cholesterol, low-density lipoprotein cholesterol, triglyceride levels, and a decrease in high-density cholesterol levels.

Primary dyslipidemia is more prevalent among adolescents and children than in adults. Secondary dyslipidemia is the main cause dyslipidemia in adults. African Americans and Hispanic Americans are at greater risk for the development of dyslipidemia and cardiovascular complications as compared to Caucasian Americans.

Causes and risk factors
The causes of dyslipidemia include genetic as well as environmental contributions.

In secondary dyslipidemia, increases in low-density lipoprotein levels can be caused by diabetes, hypothyroidism, nephrotic syndrome, obstructive liver disease, anabolic steroids, progestins, beta-adrenergic blockers, and thiazides. Increases in triglyceride levels can be caused by diabetes, hypothyroidism, obesity, renal insufficiency, beta-adrenergic blockers, bile acid binding resins, estrogens, and ticlopidine. Decreases in high-density lipoprotein levels can be caused by cigarette smoking, diabetes, hypertriglyceridemia, menopause, obesity, puberty, uremia, anabolic steroids, beta-adrenergic blockers, and progestins.

The risk factors associated with dyslipidemia that can lead to coronary heart disease include natural aging, male gender, family history of cardiovascular disease, cigarette smoking or tobacco use, hypertension and diabetes.

Diagnosis, screening and symptoms
The goal of dyslipidemia treatment is to control lipid levels, decreasing low-density lipoprotein levels and triglyceride levels and increasing high-density lipoprotein levels, as well as prevent the onset of cardiovascular diseases such as coronary artery disease, peripheral artery disease, heart attack and stroke. Treatment algorithms involve lifestyle modifications and pharmacologic management.

Individuals prescribed lifestyle modifications and pharmacologic drugs should be monitored by a clinical practitioner on a regular basis. Also, lipid levels should be checked on a periodic basis after starting treatment in case the dose needs to be titrated.

Myocardial infarction

Myocardial infarction is defined as the lack of blood flow to the heart caused by plaque rupture or blockage. Myocardial infarction is also known as heart attack or acute myocardial infarction.

In the United States, myocardial infarction and other cardiac ischemic conditions are the leading cause of mortality. Coronary heart disease is responsible for 1 in 5 deaths in the United States. Currently, the prevalence of coronary artery disease is over 7 million in men and over 6 million in women. More than 1 million individuals suffer an acute myocardial infarction per year, with nearly 40% dying because of the incident. Men are at a higher risk of myocardial infarction than women, especially with increasing age.

Causes and risk factors
Risk factors that can lead to myocardial infarction include a family history of vascular disease such as atherosclerosis, coronary artery disease and/or angina, previous heart attack or stroke, previous episodes of syncope or arrhythmias, natural aging, smoking or tobacco use, lack of physical activity, excessive alcohol consumption, abuse of drugs, elevated triglyceride levels, elevated low-density lipoprotein levels, decreased high-density lipoprotein levels, diabetes, hypertension, acute infections, obesity, chronic renal failure, stress, and anxiety.

Other contributing factors include socioeconomic factors such as lack of education and lower income that prevent individuals from seeking preventative care and/or routine management.

Symptoms
Symptoms associated with myocardial infarction include chest pain, pain radiating from the left side of the neck or arm, feeling of fullness or pressure in the chest, prolonged pain in upper abdomen, syncope, lightheadedness, dizziness, shortness of breath, nausea, vomiting, palpitations, sweating, weakness, fatigue, and anxiety. Some patients present with no symptoms, which is referred to as a silent heart attack. Also, men present with different symptoms than women in most cases. Women tend to present with shortness of breath, fatigue, and weakness.

The onset of symptoms typically occurs over a short period of time, worsening without intervention. However, nearly half of patients do not experience any symptoms such as chest pain or shortness of breath.

Diagnosis and screening
Physical examination, patient history, and diagnostic tools are used for diagnosis of myocardial infarction. Diagnostic tools include echocardiogram, electrocardiogram, chest x-ray, nuclear ventriculography, magnetic resonance imaging (MRI), and blood tests to detect elevation in cardiac markers. More invasive diagnostic tools used for diagnosis of myocardial infarction and atherosclerosis include angiography and angioplasty.

The World Health Organization criteria used to diagnose myocardial infarction include clinical history of ischemic type chest pain lasting more than 20 minutes, changes in electrocardiogram tracing and rise and fall of serum cardiac markers such as creatinine kinase-MB fraction and troponin I. Individuals that present with 2 or more of these criteria are typically diagnosed with having experienced a myocardial infarction.

Stroke

Stroke is defined as an acute condition where blood flow, and thus oxygen, to the brain is hindered or significantly reduced. There are 2 types of stroke including ischemic stroke and hemorrhagic stroke. Ischemic stroke is defined as a condition where blood flow to the brain is blocked because of blood clot formation or embolism. Approximately 80% to 85% of strokes are ischemic strokes, while 15% to 20% are hemorrhagic strokes. Another type of stroke is a transient ischemic attack, where blood flow to the brain is temporarily hindered.

In the United States, approximately 400,000 individuals are diagnosed with stroke per year, which is expected to increase on a yearly basis because of the aging of the U.S. population.

In the United States, stroke is the third leading cause of death annually following cancer and cardiovascular diseases. It is also the leading the cause of adult disability in the United States.

Ischemic and hemorrhagic stroke

Ischemic strokes include thrombotic strokes, which occur when a blood clot forms in arteries supplying the brain, and embolic stroke, which occurs when a blood clot (or other embolus, like a cholesterol plaque) formed in the cardiovascular system dislodges and blocks more distal arteries.

Hemorrhagic stroke occurs when a blood vessel ruptures and leaks into the brain. Hemorrhagic stroke includes intracerebral hemorrhage, which occurs when a blood vessel in the brain ruptures hindering blood flow and damaging tissue and subarachnoid hemorrhage, which occurs when a blood vessel lining the brain membrane bursts and leaks into the subarachnoid space.

Causes and risk factors

Patients at highest risk for an acute stroke are those individuals who have experienced a transient ischemic attack or experienced a previous stroke. Other risk factors include family history, natural aging, African American descent, hypertension, high cholesterol, cigarette smoking, diabetes, cardiovascular disease, alcoholism, illicit drug use, stress, anxiety, and elevated homocysteine levels.

Drugs may also increase an individual's risk of stroke including birth control pills and hormone replacement therapy. Furthermore, men are at a higher risk for stroke than women. The aged are especially at an increased risk with nearly 75% of strokes occurring individuals 65 years of age or older.

Symptoms

Patients experiencing an acute stroke typically present with sudden numbness or weakness of the arms, legs, and/or face, which occurs on 1 side of the individual's body. They also may experience confusion, slurred speech, difficulty speaking, vision loss, double vision, difficulty walking, dizziness, loss of balance, loss of coordination, pain, memory loss, problems with spatial orientation, perception loss, and severe headache of sudden onset.

Most patients who present with symptoms of stroke do not present with warning symptoms aside from the acute attack. However, in some cases, individuals may experience a transient ischemic attack with similar symptoms of an acute attack prior to experiencing an acute stroke.

<u>Diagnosis and screening</u>
Early recognition of signs and symptoms of stroke is very important for prevention of complications and death. Physical examination, patient feedback, and diagnostic tools are used to diagnose an acute stroke. Screening tools used to diagnose a stroke include carotid ultrasonography, arteriography, computerized tomography, magnetic resonance imaging, and echocardiography. Practicing clinicians may also perform blood work to assess other comorbid conditions that may have contributed to the stroke including lipids, glucose and homocysteine levels.

More invasive approaches such as angiography may be performed to assess the degree and extent of cardiovascular disease.

Peripheral arterial disease

Peripheral arterial disease is a condition in which blood flow is reduced to limbs and extremities. The prevalence of peripheral arterial disease increases with age, with individuals over the age of 55 having a prevalence of 10% to 25%. In the United States, approximately 10% to 20% of individuals 65 years or older are affected by peripheral arterial disease.

Most patients diagnosed with peripheral arterial disease are asymptomatic, with approximately 70% to 80% presenting with no symptoms upon diagnosis. However, the incidence of symptomatic peripheral arterial disease increases with age. Yet, the prevalence of symptomatic peripheral arterial disease varies based upon disease definition and age of patient population being evaluated.

<u>Causes and risks</u>
Atherosclerosis is the main cause of peripheral arterial disease. However, blood clots, injury to limbs, unusual anatomy of ligaments or muscles or infection may lead to peripheral arterial disease. Other diseases that can lead to onset of peripheral vascular disease include aortic aneurysms, Buerger's disease, pulmonary embolism, phlebitis, varicose veins, and Raynaud's syndrome.

Factors that increase an individual's risk for peripheral arterial disease include smoking, 50 years of age or older, diabetes, obesity, high blood pressure, high cholesterol or family history of cardiovascular diseases and/or atherosclerosis. Male individuals of African American descent as well as overweight individuals and those with a family history of cardiovascular disease are at a higher risk of peripheral vascular disease.

Other risk factors under clinical investigation include inflammatory mediators such as C-reactive protein, homocysteine, and fibrinogen.

<u>Symptoms</u>
More than half of individuals diagnosed with peripheral arterial disease do not present with symptoms. However, symptoms associated with peripheral arterial disease include leg numbness or weakness, cold legs and feet, sores or wounds on digits or extremities that will not heal, blue or pale hue to legs, feet, hands and/or arms, hair loss on feet and legs and changes in composition of nails.

Approximately one-third to one-half of individuals diagnosed with peripheral arterial disease present with intermittent claudication. Intermittent claudication is defined as muscle pain or cramping in appendages triggered by walking and physical activity. Individuals may also experience ischemic rest pain.

Diagnosis and screening

Early diagnosis of peripheral arterial disease is necessary for prevention of complications such as cardiovascular disease, heart attack, stroke, and sudden death. Physical examination and diagnostic screening tools are used to determine if a patient has peripheral arterial disease.

Upon physical examination, practicing clinicians use a stethoscope to determine the presence of bruits. They also look for evidence of poor wound healing, sores, color changes, temperature changes, and decreased blood pressure in limbs. Diagnostic screening tools include the ankle-brachial index and angiography. Additional tests include angiography, electrocardiogram, magnetic resonance angiography, blood tests, and ultrasound.

Inflammation

Inflammation is defined as a complex response of vascular tissues to irritants, pathogens, and/or damaged cells. It is a protective mechanism to remove harmful substances from the body and initiate the healing signal transduction cascade.

Inflammation can be classified as either acute or chronic. Acute inflammation is defined as the initial response by the body to irritants, pathogens, and/or damaged cells, recruiting neutrophils, monocytes, and macrophages from blood to affected tissue. Chronic inflammation is prolonged inflammation that is a process that recruits other cells such as monocytes, macrophages, lymphocytes, plasma cells, and fibroblasts involved in the pathogen removal and healing process.

Acute inflammation is caused by pathogens, irritants and/or damaged cells. The major cells involved in the acute inflammation process include neutrophils, monocytes, and macrophages. The primary mediators include vasoactive amines and eicosanoids. The onset of action of acute inflammation is immediate and lasts for approximately a few days. The initiation of acute inflammation leads to healing, abscess formation, and chronic inflammation stimulation.

Chronic inflammation is triggered by acute inflammation due to presence of pathogens, irritants and/or damaged cells and the body's reaction to these initial triggers. The presence of neutrophils, monocytes, and pathogens as well as other signaling transduction mechanisms trigger chronic inflammation. The major cells involved in the chronic inflammation process include monocytes, macrophages, lymphocytes, plasma cells, and fibroblasts. The primary mediators include cytokines, growth factors, reactive oxygen species, and hydrolytic enzymes. The onset of action of chronic inflammation is delayed and lasts for approximately several months or years. The initiation of chronic inflammation leads to tissue destruction and fibrosis.

Causes and risk factors

The causes of acute inflammation include presence of irritants, pathogens and/or damaged cells within the body. Acute inflammation is characterized by vascular changes including vasodilation, increased permeability, and/or reduced blood flow. The signaling cascades involved in acute inflammation include the complement system such as C3, C5a, membrane attack complex and thrombin, kinin system such as bradykinin, coagulation system such as thrombin and fibrinolysis system such as plasmin.

The cause of chronic inflammation is persistent acute inflammation due to bacterial infection, chemical exposure including silica exposure and/or autoimmune reactions as in rheumatoid arthritis, lupus, or psoriasis.

Symptoms

The symptoms of acute inflammation include swelling of joints and muscles, joint and muscle stiffness, redness, pain, heat and loss of function. Chronic inflammation is sometimes characterized by the same symptoms as acute inflammation. However, fever, chills, fatigue, low energy, headaches, appetite loss and muscle stiffness may characterize chronic inflammation.

Involvement of internal end organ systems may present with symptoms specific to that organ system. Involvement of the cardiovascular system may lead to chest pain, palpitations, hypertension, and/or high cholesterol. Involvement of the respiratory system may lead to asthma and/or allergic reactions. Involvement of the renal system may lead to kidney failure and/or infections. Involvement of the large intestines may lead to ulcerative colitis, Crohn disease, diverticulitis, and/or inflammatory bowel disease.

Diagnosis and screening

Inflammatory diseases are diagnosed after careful physical examination and use of diagnostic tools. Practicing clinicians will complete a physical examination and take an individual's medical history as well as family history of inflammatory disorders. They will examine painful joints, muscles and other organ systems. They will also examine and discuss the presence of other comorbid conditions.

Diagnostic screening tools used include x-rays, magnetic resonance imaging, CT scans, as well as other imagining techniques to assess impact on end organ systems including cardiovascular system, respiratory system, renal system and gastrointestinal system.

Pericarditis

Pericarditis is defined as inflammation of the pericardium, which is the thin membrane surrounding the heart muscle. Excess fluid can accumulate between the 2 layers of the membrane, impacting the proper function of the heart. There are 2 types of pericarditis including acute pericarditis and chronic pericarditis. Acute pericarditis is more prevalent than chronic pericarditis.

The condition is more prevalent among men than women between the ages of 20 to 50. Acute pericarditis episodes can last from 1 to 3 weeks, but additional episodes can occur in the future. Approximately 20% of individuals with pericarditis may have a reoccurrence within 1 month of the first episode.

Pericarditis occurs in approximately 15% of individuals that experienced an acute myocardial infarction/heart attack. Approximately 25% to 85% of cases present with no clear reason and are idiopathic in nature.

Causes and risk factors

The cause of pericarditis remains unclear. However, pericarditis can develop post heart attack or surgery. Other causes of pericarditis include systemic inflammatory disorders such as lupus and rheumatoid arthritis, trauma due to car accident, slip and fall or other traumatic events, comorbid conditions such as renal disease, bacterial infections such as tuberculosis, viral infections such as coxsackie virus or echo virus, fungal infections, myocardial infarction, uremia, aortic dissection, HIV/AIDS, malignancy metastasis, Dressler syndrome, hypothyroidism, renal disease, radiation and pharmacologic agents such as tetracyclines, isoniazid, cyclosporine, and hydralazine. In adolescents, pericarditis is most commonly caused by adenovirus or Coxsackie virus.

Symptoms

The most common symptoms associated with pericarditis include sharp chest pain behind the breast bone or left side of chest wall cavity, dull/sharp chest pain radiating to the back and relieved by sitting up forward and worsened by lying down, pressure or ache in chest wall, shortness of breath, difficulty breathing when lying down, anxiety, low grade fever, weakness, fatigue, ill feeling, dry cough, and abdominal or extremity swelling.

The symptoms of pericarditis are very similar to other cardiovascular diseases such as heart attack and congestive heart failure and respiratory conditions such as asthma, emphysema, pulmonary embolism, and chronic obstructive pulmonary disease.

Screening and diagnosis

Physical examination, medical history, and diagnostic tools are used to diagnose pericarditis. Practicing clinicians will evaluate the patient by listening to the individual's heart with a stethoscope and look for other comorbid conditions. Indicators of pericarditis upon physical examination include abnormal heart sounds such as muffling and friction rub, crackles in lungs and decreased breath sounds.

Diagnostic screening tools used to diagnose pericarditis include electrocardiogram, echocardiogram, chest x-ray, computerized tomography, and magnetic resonance imaging. Blood work may also be performed to rule out heart attack or congestive heart failure. Blood levels including complete blood count, C-reactive protein, and erythrocyte sedimentation rate may be evaluated.

Physical and diagnostic findings include friction rub, diffuse ST-elevation, and PR depression on electrocardiogram, enlarged heart, fluid surrounding pericardium, cardiac tamponade, and/or congestive heart failure on echocardiogram.

Vasculitis

Vasculitis is a condition that involves inflammation of blood vessels such as arteries, veins, and capillaries. Vasculitis causes thickening, weakening, narrowing, and scarring of the blood vessels leading to abnormal blood flow and cardiovascular complications and organ system damage. Vasculitis can be classified as primary vasculitis, having no known cause and secondary vasculitis, caused by another comorbid condition or pharmacologic approaches.

The incidence of Vasculitis in the general population is rare, even though there are various types of the condition and it can affect variety of end organ systems. Women, children, current or ex-smokers as well as individuals with chronic hepatitis B or hepatitis C are at increased risk for certain types of vasculitis. The course of disease is difficult to predict and can go into remission, recur or remain chronic.

Causes and risk factors

Various diseases and conditions can be classified as vasculitis or can lead to the condition. Some conditions that are commonly associated with vasculitis include Behçet syndrome, Buerger's syndrome, Churg-Strauss syndrome, cryoglobulinemia, giant cell arthritis, Henoch-Schönlein purpura, hypersensitivities, Kawasaki disease, microscopic polyangiitis, polyarteritis nodosa, polymyalgia rheumatica, rheumatoid conditions, lupus, Sjögren's syndrome, Takayasu's arteritis, and Wegener's granulomatosis. Pharmacologic approaches that can lead to vasculitis include antibiotics and diuretics.

Vasculitis can affect men, women, and children. Its cause remains unclear, but certain risk factors have been associated with the condition. Individuals most affected by vasculitis include current or ex-smokers, children, young women, middle-aged adults and individuals with chronic hepatitis B and/or hepatitis C.

<u>Symptoms</u>
The symptoms of vasculitis vary depending on which blood vessels and end organ systems are affected by the condition. The symptoms are also dependent on the extent and degree of vasculitis. Patients may experience few symptoms or have more extensive symptoms depending on the organ systems that are involved.

The most common symptoms among individuals diagnosed with vasculitis include weight loss, fever, general aches and pains, skin changes such as purple or red spots, shortness of breath, ulcers, abdominal pain, bloody stool, sinus infections, chronic middle ear infections, ulcers in nostrils, blurring or vision loss, headaches, confusion, changes in behavior, strokes, muscle and joint pain, loss of appetite, numbness, tingling, and weakness.

<u>Diagnosis and screening</u>
Physical examination, medical history, and diagnostic screening tools are used to diagnose vasculitis. However, the symptoms and physical findings of vasculitis resemble those of other conditions and can be difficult to diagnose.

Blood tests used for diagnosis of vasculitis and to rule out other conditions include erythrocyte sedimentation rate, C - reactive protein, anti-nuclear antibodies, complement levels, antineutrophil cytoplasmic antibody, and complete blood count such as red blood cells and platelets. A urinalysis may also be performed to detect any abnormalities such as increased protein in urine or presence of red blood cells.

Endocarditis

Endocarditis is defined as inflammation of the endocardium, which is the inner lining of the heart chambers and valves. Endocarditis can lead to cardiovascular disease, improper functioning of heart valves and chambers, as well as sudden death. The disease can be classified as infective or noninfective, but noninfective endocarditis is very rare and uncommon in clinical practice. Endocarditis is most common in individuals with damaged hearts either from heart attack or disease.

In the United States, the incidence of endocarditis is 1.4 to 4.2 cases per 100,000 individuals per year. Men are more prone to endocarditis than women. More than half of cases of endocarditis occur in individuals ages 50 years or older.

<u>Causes and risk factors</u>
The main cause of endocarditis is bacterial infection that resides in the endocardium. Bacteria entering the blood stream and attaching to the walls of the endocardium typically cause endocarditis. Other causes of endocarditis include common activities such as teeth brushing or chewing food, infection or other medication conditions such as skin sores, gum disease,

inflammatory bowel disease and sexually transmitted disease, insertion of contaminated catheters or needles and/or certain dental or respiratory tract procedures.

Individuals most at risk for developing endocarditis include those who have had a heart attack, have damaged heart valves or underlying heart abnormalities. Others at risk include those with artificial heart valves, congenital heart defect, and prior history of endocarditis. Also, individuals with healthy hearts but use illicit drugs with needles or are hospitalized with IV tubes may be at risk for endocarditis.

<u>Symptoms</u>
Endocarditis can be acute or develop over an extended period. The signs and symptoms of endocarditis are dependent on the underlying cause of the disease. The most common symptoms include fever, chills, heart murmur, fatigue, aching joints and muscles, swelling of feet, legs or abdomen, night sweats, shortness of breath, paleness, persistent cough, unexplained weight loss, blood in urine, chills, nail abnormalities, weakness and tenderness of spleen.

Other signs include red and tender spots under the skin of the fingers as well as purple or red spots on other areas of the skin such as whites of eyes or inside the mouth.

<u>Diagnosis and screening</u>
The diagnosis of endocarditis involves physical examination, medical history, and diagnostic screening tools. Upon physical examination, clinical practitioners will use a stethoscope to determine the presence of heart murmur or other arrhythmia problems. They will also look for enlarged end organ systems such as spleen. Other diagnostic testing involves blood tests such as complete blood count, culture and erythrocyte sedimentation rate, serology, chest x-ray, echocardiogram, electrocardiogram and transesophageal echocardiogram. More invasive approaches such as cardiac catheterization may be performed to determine the extent of heart valve damage.

Practicing clinicians look for signs of endocarditis in individuals with high-risk conditions such as congenital heart disease, intravenous drug use, recent dental work, and/or rheumatic fever.

Renovascular disease

Renovascular disease is a condition that involves narrowing and/or blockage of renal arteries or veins. There are 3 different types of renovascular disease. The 3 different types of renovascular disease include renal artery occlusion, renal vein thrombosis, and renal atheroembolism.

Renal artery occlusion occurs when 1 or both of the renal arteries become blocked. Renal vein thrombosis occurs when 1 or both of renal veins become blocked. Renal atheroembolism occurs due to the buildup of lipids in blood vessels leading to the renal capillaries. All 3 conditions can lead to chronic renal failure and death.

Renal artery occlusion

Renal artery occlusion is a condition that involves narrowing or blockage of 1 or both of the renal arteries. Alternative names used for renal artery occlusion include acute renal arterial thrombosis, renal artery embolism, acute renal artery occlusion, and renal artery stenosis.

Renal artery occlusion is the primary cause of hypertension in approximately 1% to 10% of the 50 million individuals diagnosed with hypertension in the United States. Renal artery occlusion is more prevalent among elderly individuals with atherosclerosis. The disease is more common in Caucasian Americans than African Americans.

<u>Causes and risk factors</u>
Renal artery occlusion can be caused by a variety of other comorbid conditions including atheroembolic renal disease, atherosclerosis, fibromuscular dysplasia of the renal wall, trauma to abdomen, back or side, emboli residing in renal arteries and scar formation in the renal artery.

Other risk factors include hypertension, aging, renal insufficiency, extrarenal atherosclerosis, diabetes, presence of other comorbid conditions such as cardiovascular disease or renal disease and smoking. Caucasian, elderly individuals with atherosclerosis are at highest risk for the development of renal artery occlusion.

<u>Symptoms</u>
Most individuals with renal artery occlusion typically present with no symptoms. The reason that patients present with few or no symptoms is that the second kidney takes over for the lack of functioning by the impaired kidney.

Diagnosis is typically made upon routine physical examination or when being examined for other cardiovascular or renal conditions. Some signs associated with renal artery occlusion include high blood pressure, history of high blood pressure and/or bruits of the kidneys.

<u>Diagnosis and screening</u>
Physical examination, medical history, and diagnostic tools are used to diagnose renal artery occlusion. The disease typically presents with few or no symptoms and is usually diagnosed upon routine physical examination or when being examined for other cardiovascular or renal conditions.

Practicing clinicians will use a stethoscope to listen for bruits of the kidney and check blood pressure to see if patient presents with high blood pressure. Other diagnostic tools used to diagnose renal artery occlusion include magnetic resonance imaging, computerized tomography, kidney ultrasound, radionucleotide conventional arteriography, contrast nephrotoxicity, renogram, renal perfusion scintiscan, urine concentration testing, urine specific gravity, and renal arteriography.

Blood work includes complete blood counts, serum creatinine levels, and serologic levels such as antinuclear antibodies, C3, C4 and antinuclear cytoplasmic antibodies.

Renal vein thrombosis

Renal vein thrombosis is a condition in which the veins leaving the kidney become occluded by thrombus. The condition leads to a reduction in blood drainage by the kidney, which can cause further complications.

Renal vein thrombosis is a rare condition that typically presents with other conditions including nephrotic syndrome, kidney cancer and/or other blood clotting disorders. Renal vein thrombosis occurs more often in adults than in infants, adolescents, or toddlers. However, it is typically more serious in infants, adolescents, or toddlers.

In the United States, the prevalence of renal vein thrombosis remains unknown. It is most commonly associated with nephrotic syndrome, but prevalence rates among these patients vary greatly, ranging from 5% to 60% on average.

<u>Causes and risks</u>
Renal vein thrombosis is uncommon and rare condition but can occur after trauma to the abdomen and/or back as well as due to scar formation, stricture, and/or tumor. It is also, more commonly, associated with nephrotic syndrome.

In infants, toddler and adolescents, renal vein thrombosis can occur due to severe dehydration, which is considered to be much more serious condition than when it occurs in adults. Other possible causes of renal vein thrombosis include blood clotting disorders such as hypercoagulability disorder, protein C or S deficiency, antiphospholipid antibody syndrome, pregnancy, post-renal transplant, Behçet syndrome, extrinsic compression such as lymph nodes, tumor, retroperitoneal fibrosis, or aortic aneurysm, sickle cell anemia, diabetes that affects the kidney, oral contraceptive use, illicit drug abuse, steroid use or thrombophlebitis migrans.

<u>Symptoms</u>
The symptoms of renal vein thrombosis are minimal, unless the vein becomes occluded suddenly. In patients who present with symptoms of renal vein thrombosis typically present with blood in urine or decreased urine volume upon excretion. Other signs of renal vein thrombosis include protein and/or red blood cells upon urinalysis.

Pulmonary embolism (from embolization of the thrombus) may be a sign that a patient has renal vein thrombosis. With pulmonary embolism, patients present with shortness of breath and chest pain made worse by breathing. Infants, toddlers, and adolescents typically present with lower back/abdominal pain, decreased urine excretion, fever, and blood in the urine.

<u>Diagnosis and screening</u>
Diagnosis of renal vein thrombosis is made by physical examination as well as the use of diagnostic imagining tools. Abdominal CT angiography scan is typically used to confirm the diagnosis of renal vein thrombosis, as physical examination does not always reveal renal vein thrombosis. Other diagnostic tools used for screening of renal vein thrombosis include abdominal MRI scan, X-ray, Doppler ultrasound, or abdominal ultrasound, which may reveal the occluded vein. Urinalysis may also be performed to detect increased protein levels and/or red blood cells. Blood tests may also indicate evidence of renal failure. Blood tests may involve lipid level testing, albumin levels and serum complement levels.

Renal biopsy may also be performed in patients who present with nephrotic syndrome as well.

Atheroembolic renal disease

Atheroembolic renal disease is a condition that involves lipid build-up and clot formation within the small arteries that serve the capillaries of the kidneys. The condition is also known as renal atheroembolism, cholesterol embolization syndrome or atherosclerotic disease. It is a condition that slowly progresses over time and can lead to severe complications such as heart attack, stroke, and brain damage. It is most commonly associated with atherosclerotic disease.

Approximately 25% of patients with renal failure due to atheroembolic renal disease recover renal function. The mortality rate among these patients is approximately 25% to 70%.

Causes and risk factors

Atheroembolic renal disease is strongly associated with atherosclerotic disease, which is very common disorder among patients with cardiovascular disease. The risk factors for atheroembolic renal disease are the same as for atherosclerotic disease.

Factors that can increase an individual's risk for atherosclerosis include high low-density lipoprotein cholesterol, low high-density lipoprotein, evaluated triglyceride levels, menopause, lack of physical activity, obesity, infection of the vascular smooth muscle cells, high blood pressure, history of smoking and diabetes.

Smoking not only predisposes individuals for atherosclerosis but it increases the progression of the disease. The progression of atherosclerosis itself also further increases the extent and degree of the condition, as further accumulation of lipids, cholesterol, and other substances stimulates the endothelium to produce substances that cause increased plaque build-up.

Symptoms

The symptoms of atheroembolic renal disease include foot pain and/or ulcers, discoloration of feet such as blue or purple feet or toes, claudication, pain in the abdomen, nausea, vomiting, pancreatitis, hepatitis, strokes, blindness, flank pain, blood in urine, decrease or no urine excretion and uncontrolled high blood pressure.

In some patients, renal failure may also occur, which would present with nausea, vomiting, bad taste in mouth, chest pain, high blood pressure, high cholesterol, weight loss, decreased or no urine excretion, swelling, decreased sensation, skin pigmentation changes, dry itchy skin, drowsiness, fatigue, confusion and/or lethargy.

Diagnosis and screening

Physical examination and diagnostic testing are used to diagnose atheroembolic renal disease. Practicing clinicians will look for signs of swelling of the ankles, wrists and/or parts of the body (signs of kidney failure), particles in blood vessels of the retina, abnormal blood flow from the heart, increased blood pressure, as well as skin ulcers on lower feet.

Diagnostic imaging tests used include abdominal CT scan, abdominal MRI, abdominal x-ray and kidney or abdominal ultrasound. Blood work performed may include chem.-7, chem.-20, complete blood count, serum complement levels, and serum lipid levels. More invasive diagnostic tools include kidney biopsy and renal arteriography. Urinalysis may also be performed to look for increases in protein excretion and/or red blood cells.

Marfan syndrome

Marfan syndrome is a connective tissue disorder, affecting the skeleton, lungs, eyes, heart, and major blood vessels. It is a genetic disorder that causes a reduction in fibrillin, leading to decrease in the elasticity and weakening of connective tissue.

Marfan syndrome affects men and women equally as well as individuals of all races and ethnic groups. In the United States, approximately 60,000 individuals have been diagnosed with Marfan syndrome. Most individuals with Marfan syndrome have a family history of disease. However, approximately 15% to 30% of individuals diagnosed with the disease have new genetic mutations.

Causes and risk factors

Marfan syndrome is a genetic disorder that results from a defect in the gene that enables the production of fibrillin. In this syndrome, the defect leads to lower production of fibrillin, which leads to weakened connective tissue in the skeletal system, aorta, and ligaments. The greatest risk factor for the condition is a parent with the disease.

Marfan syndrome is an autosomal dominant condition, which means that only one parent needs to have the gene for the condition to pass it on to off spring. Offspring have a 50% chance of inheriting the disease from one parent diagnosed with the condition.

Symptoms

Some patients with Marfan syndrome present with few or no symptoms. Also, patients typically present with varying symptoms dependent on the organ system affected. Symptoms can vary from very mild in some patients to severe in others. The degree and extent of symptoms also varies from patient to patient, which makes diagnosis difficult. However, most patients have common traits and characteristics such as being tall, thin with tapering fingers, chest wall abnormalities, high arched palate, long arms and legs, narrow face, loose joints, curvature of the spine, crowded teeth, flat feet, weakened part of aorta, heart murmur, nearsightedness, glaucoma, cataracts, detached retina, stretch marks, hernia, painful abdomen, weakened legs, collapsed lung, stiff air sacs, and snoring.

Diagnosis and screening

Physical examination and medical history are key in diagnosing Marfan syndrome. There are no key diagnostic tools solely used to confirm Marfan syndrome. However, patients with Marfan syndrome are typically tall, thin with tapering fingers, narrow face, loose joints, long arms and legs, curvature of the spine, chest wall abnormalities, and eye problems.

Therefore, diagnosis is made by a combination of clinical practitioners including cardiologists, ophthalmologist, orthopedic surgeon, and/or medical geneticist. Diagnostic tools used to diagnose Marfan syndrome include echocardiogram, chest X-ray, MRI and genetic testing. The Ghent criterion is typically used to make a diagnosis of Marfan syndrome.

Ghent criteria

Practicing clinicians use the Ghent criteria to diagnose patients with Marfan syndrome correctly, since the symptoms of the condition resemble those of other connective tissue disorders. The criteria are divided into 2 categories, major and minor. In patients with a family history of Marfan syndrome, they must have 1 major criterion in 1 organ system and involvement of another organ system to be diagnosed with the condition. If patients do not have a family history of the condition, then these individuals need to have 2 major criteria affecting different organs and the involvement of another organ system.

The major criteria for Marfan syndrome include an enlarged aorta, with or without aortic dissection; aortic dissection affecting ascending aorta; dislocation of the lens of an eye; dural ectasia; at least 4 skeletal problems such as chest deformities, long thin arms and legs, flat footedness and scoliosis; family history; and/or having an abnormal gene for Marfan syndrome. Minor criteria occur are symptoms and signs that occur in both patients with the disease as well as in the general population.

Atrial septal defect

Atrial septal defect is a congenital birth defect that involves an abnormality of the atrial chambers of the heart, which causes them not to close appropriately. Smaller defects may close on their own during infancy, toddler years, or early childhood. However, larger defects may cause problems later in life damaging the heart, lung, or other organ systems.

The disease is relatively uncommon and typically difficult to diagnose due to lack of symptoms. The risk of congenital heart disease in the general population is less than 1%. In children of parents with congenital heart disease, the risk of atrial septal defects increases to between 2% and 20%. The condition occurs equally in men and women as well as in race or ethnic descent.

<u>Causes and risk factors</u>
Atrial septal defect is a genetic condition that is congenital. It occurs during fetal circulation, which leads to the formation of a shunt, either left to right shunt or right to left shunt, depending on the nature of the condition. It can occur in combination with other genetic conditions such as Down syndrome. It can occur due to genetic inheritance or mutations during pregnancy or birth.

The following conditions during pregnancy may increase the risk of an offspring having a congenital heart defect such as atrial septal defects including rubella infection, poorly controlled diabetes, and illicit drug and/or alcohol abuse.

<u>Symptoms</u>
Individuals may present with few or no symptoms, making diagnosis rather difficult. However, symptoms may begin to present in infancy through childhood. Yet, some individuals may not present with symptoms until later in life due to presence of other comorbid conditions or progression of the defect. Individuals with small or minor defects may present with no symptoms or present with symptoms later in life.

Symptoms associated with atrial septal defect include frequent respiratory infections in children, difficulty breathing, shortness of breath with activity, fatigue, swelling of legs, feet, or abdomen, and heart palpitations in adults.

<u>Diagnosis and screening</u>
Physical examination and diagnostic tools are used to diagnose atrial septal defect, but diagnosis is difficult in patients who present with few or no symptoms. Practicing clinicians typically use a stethoscope to determine the presence of abnormal heart sounds. Murmur is a quiet ejection murmur heard at the left upper sternal border often with a split second heart sound. Murmur is not usually heard until after 1 year of age. Other diagnostic tools used to determine atrial septal defect include chest x-ray, echocardiography, Doppler ultrasound, transesophageal echocardiography, magnetic resonance imaging, pulse oximetry, and electrocardiogram. A more invasive approach such as cardiac catheterization may also be used.

Patients experiencing poor appetite, failure to gain weight, bluish discoloration of skin, shortness of breath, easy tiring, swelling of legs, abdomen or abdomen, and heart palpitations should seek medical attention.

Types of thromboembolism

The types of thromboembolism include pulmonary embolism and deep vein thrombosis. Pulmonary embolism is a condition that involves the blockage of arteries supplying the lungs. Typically, pulmonary embolism occurs due to the traveling of a blood clot to the lungs from another organ system. Deep venous thrombosis is a condition that involves the formation of blood clots in the veins deep within the body (usually the legs), which can dislodge and embolize into other organ systems such as the lungs, heart and brain. Of note, the superficial femoral vein in the leg is considered a "deep" vein.

In the United States, pulmonary embolism and deep venous thrombosis occur in approximately 2.5% to 5% of adults.

Pulmonary embolism

Pulmonary embolism is a condition that involves blockage of arteries that supplies the lungs. Typically, pulmonary embolism occurs due to the traveling of a blood clot to the lungs from another organ system.

In the United States, the incidence of pulmonary embolism is 0.9 cases per 100,000 population per year. The mortality rate associated with untreated pulmonary embolism in the United States averages between 18% and 30%. The mortality rate upon early diagnosis is approximately 8%.

Pregnant women in their third trimester are at high risk of pulmonary embolism as well as women undergoing treatment with hormone replacement therapy or oral contraceptives. The prevalence of pulmonary embolism increases with age.

Causes and risks
Risk factors for pulmonary embolism or clot formation include genetic predisposition, history of cardiovascular disease and/or family history of clot formation. Other factors that may lead to pulmonary embolism and clot formation include surgery such as hip and knee surgeries, long periods of inactivity such as prolonged bed rest or long plan or car trips, increased levels of clotting factors in the blood as associated with certain types of cancer, previous cardiovascular conditions such as heart attack or stroke, and injury to veins. The most common risk factor is the presence of deep venous thrombosis.

Additional factors that put you at high risk for pulmonary embolism include obesity, comorbid cardiovascular diseases such as high cholesterol and hypertension, pacemakers or venous catheters, pregnancy, childbirth, hormone replacement therapy and smoking.

Symptoms
The symptoms of pulmonary embolism vary depending on how much lung is involved, the size of the clot, the patient's comorbid conditions and general health. However, many patients with pulmonary embolism are asymptotic and diagnosed during routine physical examination or when being evaluated for other conditions.

Symptoms associated with pulmonary embolism include shortness of breath; chest pain that can radiate to an individual's arm, shoulder, neck, or jaw; chest wall tenderness; back pain; upper abdominal pain; painful respiration; cardiac arrhythmia; persistent cough with blood-streaked sputum; tachycardia; wheezing; leg swelling; clamminess; discoloration of skin including bluish-colored skin; excessive sweating; anxiety; weak pulse; lightheadedness; fainting; and/or fever.

<u>Diagnosis and screening</u>
Physical examination, medical history, and diagnostic tools are used to diagnose pulmonary embolism. However, the condition is difficult to diagnose because patients may present with varying symptoms and have other comorbid conditions such as respiratory or heart disease.

Diagnostic tools used to diagnose pulmonary embolism include chest x-ray, ventilation-perfusion scan, spiral computerized tomography scan, magnetic resonance imaging, ultrasound, and pulmonary angiogram. Blood tests may also be used to detect blood clots including D-dimer blood test. Other blood tests used to aid in the diagnosis of pulmonary embolism include complete blood count, lipid levels, and metabolic levels. More invasive approaches include venography. Of all these methods, most modern hospitals use computed tomography (CT) scans with intravenous (IV) contrast.

Deep venous thrombosis

Deep venous thrombosis is a condition that involves the formation of blood clots in the veins deep within the body, which can dislodge and embolize into other organ systems such as the lungs, heart, and brain. The condition mainly affects the lower legs and thigh. Deep venous thrombosis is also known as blood clots in the legs, venous thrombosis, and venous thrombus.

In the United States, the incidence of deep venous thrombosis is approximately 4.2 cases per 100,000 population per year. The incidence of deep venous thrombosis increases with age, with those over the age of 60 at higher risk.

<u>Causes and risk factors</u>
Risk factors for deep venous thrombosis includes prolonged sitting such as long car trips, plane trips or prolong bed rest as well as recent surgery, fractures, childbirth, and use of oral contraceptives and hormone replacement therapy. Malignancy and smoking are also important risk factors.

Individuals at higher risk for deep venous thrombosis include those with a history of deep venous thrombosis, inherited blood disorders, injury to deep vein from surgery or other trauma, slowed blood flow due to lack of physical activity, pregnancy, recent or ongoing cancer treatment, central venous catheter, obesity, and age over 60.

Deep venous thrombosis can be caused by damage to the vein's inner lining due to physical, chemical or biochemical factors such as surgery, injury, inflammation, or immune response. Other causes include hindered blood flow and more-viscous blood.

<u>Symptoms</u>
The symptoms of deep venous thrombosis include pain in 1 leg, tenderness in 1 leg, swelling of 1 leg, increased heat or warmth in 1 leg, and discoloration of skin color in 1 leg.

Individuals with deep venous thrombosis may also present with pulmonary embolism. Symptoms of pulmonary embolism include unexplained shortness of breath, pain with deep breathing, coughing up blood, and tachycardia.

A majority of patients diagnosed with deep venous thrombosis may also present with tendonitis, arterial insufficiency, arthritis, asymmetric peripheral edema, cellulites, hematoma, lymphedema, soft tissue injury, neurogenic pain, and postphlebitic syndrome.

Diagnosis and screening
Physical examination, medical history, and diagnostic testing are used to diagnose deep venous thrombosis. Upon physical examination, practicing clinicians may recommend a patient for further diagnostic testing when deep venous thrombosis is suspected.

Diagnostic testing tools include venography, Doppler ultrasound of leg in question, nuclear medicine imaging studies, magnetic resonance imaging, impedance plethysmography of leg, and D-dimer blood test. Other blood tests to evaluate the presence of blood clots include antithrombin III, protein C, protein S, factor V Leiden, prothrombin 2020a mutation, disseminated intravascular coagulation (DIC) test, and lupus anticoagulant and anticardiolipin antibodies.

Venous insufficiency

Venous insufficiency is a condition that involves abnormal blood flow through the veins, which can lead to complications such as heart failure and sudden death. Typically, the condition occurs when veins in the legs do not properly send blood back to the heart. Venous insufficiency can be associated with deep venous thrombosis, varicose veins and static dermatitis and ulcers.

The risk of venous insufficiency increases with age, with women over the age of 50 at highest risk for developing the condition. In the United States, the prevalence of venous insufficiency ranges from 7% to 60% on average.

Causes and risk factors
Patients diagnosed with venous insufficiency are also at risk for skin color changes around the ankles, redness of legs and ankles, thickening of skin on legs and ankles, and ulcers on the legs and ankles.

The most common risk factor for venous insufficiency is deep venous thrombosis. Other risk factors include natural aging, pregnancy, limited physical activity, smoking, sitting for long periods of time, obesity, phlebitis, family history, medical history of cardiovascular disease, and presence of other comorbid conditions. Blood pressure that is higher than normal in the leg can also lead to venous insufficiency.

Symptoms
The symptoms of venous insufficiency can vary based on the extent and degree of disease. However, some patients present with few or no symptoms. Also, symptoms may mimic other conditions and should be evaluated by a clinical practitioner to eliminate the presence of other comorbid conditions.

Common symptoms include throbbing, cramping, burning sensations, fatigue, ulcerations that do not heal, varicose veins, fluid retention and skin changes and discoloration in the legs. Other symptoms include pain that improves when raising the legs, but gets worse when standing as well as dull, aching, heaviness, and/or cramping in the legs. Varicose veins are complications that can lead to death if they rupture and bleed.

Diagnosis and screening
Physical examination, medical history, and diagnostic tools are used to diagnose venous insufficiency. Newer guidelines recommend the use of standard diagnostic tools. Practicing clinicians may use a clinical scoring system that rates signs and symptoms of venous insufficiency. The scoring system ranks 5 symptoms including pain, cramps, heaviness, pruritus, and paresthesia; and 6 signs including edema, hyperpigmentation, induration, venous ectasia, redness, pain and calf compression on a scale of 0 to 3, with 3 being most severe. Scores of 5 to 14 on 2 visits greater than 6 months apart indicate mild to moderate disease and scores greater than 15 indicate severe disease.

Valvular disease

Valvular disease is a condition that affects 1 of the 4 main cardiac valves including the aortic, tricuspid, mitral, and pulmonic valves.

Valvular stenosis is a condition that involves narrowing, stiffening, thickening, and/or blockage of 1 or more of the heart valves. Depending on the valve site, the condition can be referred to as aortic stenosis, tricuspid stenosis, mitral stenosis and/or pulmonic stenosis.

Valvular regurgitation is a condition that occurs when blood leaks back through the valve in the wrong direction due to improper closing of 1 or more of the cardiac valves. Depending on the valve site, the condition can be referred to as aortic regurgitation, tricuspid regurgitation, mitral regurgitation, and/or pulmonic regurgitation.

Valvular disease accounts for approximately 20,000 deaths in the United States annually. It is also considered a contributing factor to increased mortality in over 40,000 individuals annually. The majority of patients with valvular disease leading to death have aortic valve dysfunction, accounting for over 60% of cases, with over 10% having a contribution from mitral valve dysfunction. Deaths due to tricuspid and pulmonic valve dysfunctions are uncommon. Pregnant women with valvular disease are at higher risk for complications to the mother and fetus. Women aged 75 years or older are at an increased risk for developing atherosclerosis and potentially valvular disease than men of the same age group.

Causes and risk factors
The causes of valvular disease can be a combination of genetic and environmental factors. The most common cause of valvular disease is congenital defects and infections such as rheumatic fever and Marfan syndrome.

Diseases or other disorders that can lead to valvular disease include damage and scar tissue due to heart attack, endocarditis, other infections, high blood pressure, heart failure, and/or atherosclerosis. Other conditions that have been associated with valvular disease include systemic lupus erythematosus, cardiomyopathy, syphilis, hypertension, aneurysms, connective tissue disorders, carcinoid syndrome, metabolic disorders, diet medications, and radiation therapy.

Individuals at highest risk for developing valvular disease include those with comorbid cardiovascular diseases such as congestive heart failure, those older than 65 years of age, those with endocarditis and/or rheumatic fever.

Symptoms

The severity of symptoms associated with valvular disease depends on the extent and degree of the disease and the particular valves affected. However, patients with severe disease may present with few or no symptoms, while patients with more mild disease may have symptoms that are more extensive.

Gradual progression of valvular disease typically presents with fewer symptoms than sudden onset of valvular disease. Symptoms that can be associated with valvular disease include chest pain, palpitations, loss of breath, fatigue, fainting, swelling of ankles, feet or abdomen, weakness, dizziness and rapid weight gain.

Diagnosis and screening

The diagnosis of valvular disease can be difficult, especially when patients present with few or no symptoms. Most patients are diagnosed during routine physical examination or when examining the patient for other conditions.

Physical examination, medical history, and diagnostic tools are used to diagnose valvular disease. Practicing clinicians examine the patient for abnormal heart sounds such as murmur, evidence of heart enlargement and fluid build-up in the lungs.

Diagnostic tools used to screening for valvular disease include electrocardiogram, echocardiography, magnetic resonance imaging, and chest x-ray. Other diagnostic tests to rule out any other comorbid cardiovascular conditions include cardiac catheterization and cardiac stress testing.

Atresia and mitral valve prolapse

Atresia is a condition where 1 or more of the cardiac valves fail to develop properly and there is a small or no opening between the respective chambers. Depending on the valve site, the condition can be referred to as aortic atresia, tricuspid atresia, pulmonic atresia, and/or mitral atresia. Aortic atresia is often associated with a patent ductus arteriosus and, sometimes, coarctation of the aorta.

Mitral valve prolapse is a very common condition characterized by excessive retrograde movement of 1 or both mitral valve leaflets. It often is associated with regurgitation through the mitral valve due to anatomical defects in the valve flaps. It occurs in 1% to 2% of the population in the United States, affecting men and women equally. In most cases, the condition is considered benign with few or no symptoms. However, in some cases, it can lead to more-serious complications and various symptoms. Rarely, it is secondary to rheumatic carditis, Marfan syndrome, or ruptured chorda tendinea.

Cardiac vasospasm

Vasospasm is a condition that occurs when blood vessels spasm leading to vasoconstriction. The condition can cause ischemia, blood clot formation, hemorrhage, stroke, aneurysm, heart attack, and sudden death. The genetic and/or environmental factors that contribute to vasospasm remain vague and a combination of factors is usually the cause of vasospasm. Some patients present with few or no symptoms, while others present with more symptoms.

Cardiac vasospasm can be treated with lifestyle modifications, pharmacologic management and, in more severe cases, surgery. Pharmacologic approaches include nitrates such as nitroglycerin, isosorbide dinitrate and isosorbide mononitrate, and calcium channel blockers such as nifedipine, amlodipine, verapamil, and diltiazem.

Angina pectoris

Angina pectoris is a condition defined by chest pain and/or discomfort due to myocardial ischemia. The condition is reversible and dissipates over a short period. It can be associated with pain that radiates to the shoulders, neck, or jaw.

In the United States, the prevalence of angina pectoris is over 6 million individuals. The condition is more prevalent among women than men, with more than 4 million women being affected and over 2 million men affected. Individuals over the age of 50 are at an increased risk for angina pectoris, especially those individuals with other cardiovascular comorbid conditions.

Causes and risk factors
Angina pectoris is typically caused by the presence of atherosclerotic disease or blood clot formation in the coronaries. Other conditions contributing to angina pectoris include valvular disease, coronary artery spasm or abnormalities and other cardiovascular conditions. Angina pectoris is typically precipitated by cold, stress, exertion, or large meals.

Non-modifiable risk factors for angina pectoris include a medical history of cardiovascular disease, family history of heart disease, increasing age, female gender, and African American or Hispanic American descent. Modifiable risk factors include cigarette smoking, hypertension, elevated low-density lipoprotein levels, elevated triglycerides, low serum high-density lipoprotein, diabetes, previous stroke, alcohol or illicit drug abuse, obesity and/or physical inactivity.

Symptoms
Patient diagnosed with angina pectoris typically present with chest pain, vomiting, nausea, fatigue and other cardiovascular symptoms. The pain often radiates across the precordium, to the jaw, and to the shoulders. The degree and extent of symptoms depend on the condition, underlying cause of the condition, age of the patient and/or presence of other comorbid conditions.

Chronic stable angina pectoris typically presents with increased symptoms upon physical exertion and/or fatigue. Individuals with unstable angina pectoris typically present with similar symptoms but the symptoms are typically more severe, frequent, and /or prolonged.

Physical findings upon diagnosis include S4 heart sounds, cardiac murmur, dysrhythmia, tachycardia, hypertension, and/or hypotension.

Diagnosis and screening
Physical examination, medical history, and diagnostic tools are used to screen for angina pectoris. Practicing clinicians examine the patient for abnormal heart sounds, evidence of heart enlargement, presence of other cardiovascular comorbid conditions and/or fluid build-up in the lungs. Individuals suspected of angina pectoris or other comorbid conditions may be observed over a few days in a hospital setting to determine the reason for their chest pain and/or discomfort, specifically to rule out myocardial infarction.

Diagnostic tools used to diagnose angina pectoris include response to nitroglycerin and echocardiography. Other diagnostic tools used in the screening for angina pectoris to exclude other comorbid conditions include echocardiography, electrocardiogram, magnetic resonance imaging, ultrasound and chest x-ray. Other more invasive diagnostic approaches include cardiac catheterization and cardiac stress testing.

Atrial fibrillation

Atrial fibrillation is a dysfunctional cardiac arrhythmia. The condition is caused by absent p waves, irregular R-R intervals and f waves of variable shape and amplitude. Atrial fibrillation can occur as an acute condition or a chronic condition. Chronic atrial fibrillation is better tolerated than acute atrial fibrillation.

The incidence of atrial fibrillation increases with age and is the most common dysrhythmia. The condition occurs in approximately 20% to 30% of individuals undergoing coronary artery bypass surgery. In the general population, atrial fibrillation occurs in just under 10% of individuals over the age of 70. In the United States, the prevalence of atrial fibrillation is approximately 2 million.

Causes and risks
The key risk factors for atrial fibrillation include increasing age, heart disease, other chronic diseases such as thyroid dysfunction or lung disease, alcohol abuse and/or family history

Other risk factors associated with atrial fibrillation include pulmonary disease, valvular disease, congenital heart disease, coronary artery bypass surgery, congestive heart failure, atherosclerosis, myocardial infarction, rheumatic heart disease, and thyrotoxicosis.

Other possible causes of atrial fibrillation include high blood pressure, congenital heart defects, hyperthyroidism, metabolic imbalance, exposure to stimulants such as caffeine, illicit drugs, alcohol or tobacco, sick sinus syndrome, emphysema, lung disease, previous heart surgery, viral infections, stress due to pneumonia or other illnesses, and/or sleep apnea.

Symptoms
Many individuals with atrial fibrillation do not have any symptoms of disease but are diagnosed during routine physical examination or when being assessed for another ailment or condition. However, some patients present with more-extensive symptoms. Symptoms may also vary from patient to patient. In addition, the severity of symptoms and impact on quality of life parameters may vary from patient to patient.

Symptoms associated with atrial fibrillation include fatigue, dizziness, weakness, physical activity intolerance, hypotension, inability to perform daily living activities, cardiac palpitations, shortness of breath, fainting, confusion, chest pain, and lightheadedness.

Diagnosis and screening
Symptoms of atrial fibrillation vary, and therefore, patients may not present with symptoms upon diagnosis. Physical examination, medical history, and diagnostic tools are used to screen for atrial fibrillation. Upon physical examination, practicing clinicians will look for rapid or irregular heart rate, varying intensity and frequency of S1 and hypotension. Diagnostic screening tools used to confirm diagnosis of atrial fibrillation and likely etiologies include echocardiogram, electrocardiogram, Holter monitor, event recorder, chest x-ray, magnetic resonance imaging, and thyroid function tests.

Also, blood work may be completed to access other contributing factors including thyroid function tests, electrolyte levels, and metabolic function tests.

Arrhythmia

Arrhythmia is defined as a condition that involves dysregulation of cardiac electrical activity. Arrhythmia can cause a slowing, speeding up, or irregular heartbeat. Tachycardia is a condition that occurs when an arrhythmia is faster than normal, whereas bradycardia is a condition that occurs when an arrhythmia beats slower than normal.

There are many types of arrhythmias including premature beats, supraventricular arrhythmias, ventricular arrhythmias, and bradyarrhythmias. Premature beats can originate in both atria and the ventricles. Supraventricular arrhythmias originate in the atria and include atrial fibrillation, atrial flutter, and Wolf-Parkinson-White syndrome. Arrhythmias that originate in the ventricles include ventricular tachycardia, ventricular fibrillation, and long QT syndrome. Bradycardias occur when the heart rate is below 60 beats per minute and can be categorized as sick sinus or conduction block.

Causes and risk factors

Both genetic and environmental factors can contribute to the development of arrhythmias. However, sometimes the cause of an arrhythmia may remain unknown. Factors that increase an individual's risk for developing arrhythmias include age; family history; medical history of cardiovascular conditions such as congestive heart failure, rheumatic heart disease, coronary artery disease, or previous heart surgery; thyroid dysfunction, including hyperthyroidism and hypothyroidism; drugs containing pseudoephedrine or other stimulants; alcohol or illicit drug abuse; high blood pressure; obesity; diabetes; stress; excessive exercise; obstructive sleep apnea; electrolyte imbalance; and/or stimulant use such as caffeine or tobacco.

Symptoms

Some patients who are diagnosed with an arrhythmia present with few or no symptoms. However, many patients present with symptoms upon diagnosis. Yet, these symptoms vary from patient to patient and in terms of severity. Cardiovascular comorbid conditions may also impact the symptoms that patients diagnosed with arrhythmias present with.

Symptoms commonly associated with different types of arrhythmias include cardiac palpitations, slow heartbeat/heart rate, irregular heartbeat, skipped heartbeats, feeling of pauses between heartbeats, anxiety, weakness, dizziness, lightheadedness, fainting, sweating, shortness of breath, chest pain, inability to perform activities of daily living, confusion, fatigue, physical activity intolerance, and hypotension.

Diagnosis and screening

Diagnosis of arrhythmias can be difficult if patients present with few or no symptoms. Physical examination, medical history, and diagnostic tools are used to screen to atrial fibrillation. Upon physical examination, practicing clinicians will look for rapid or irregular heart rate of varying heart rate and/or hypotension.

Diagnostic screening tools used to confirm diagnosis of an arrhythmia primarily include electrocardiogram, Holter monitor, and event recorders. Of note, echocardiography chest x-ray, magnetic resonance imaging, and thyroid function tests will help elucidate the underlying cause. Also, blood work may be completed to assess other contributing factors including thyroid function tests, electrolyte levels, and metabolic function tests. More invasive diagnostic tools used include stress test, tilt table test, and/or electrophysiologic testing.

Atrial flutter

Atrial flutter is a condition that is similar to atrial fibrillation. However, the condition presents with a more organized and less chaotic abnormal heartbeat, compared with atrial fibrillation. Yet, atrial flutter may develop into atrial fibrillation, and the reverse is possible.

In atrial flutter, the atrial rhythm is regular and the ventricular rhythm may be regular or irregular. In atrial fibrillation, the atrial rhythm is irregular, so the ventricular rhythm is also irregular.

The symptoms, diagnosis, risk factors, and complications of atrial flutter are similar to atrial fibrillation. However, atrial flutter is as not life threatening as atrial fibrillation. Also, patients diagnosed with atrial flutter respond better to catheter ablation than patients diagnosed with atrial fibrillation. Both conditions are more common in elderly patients.

Causes and risk factors
The causes and risk factors for atrial flutter are similar to that of atrial fibrillation. Both genetic and environment factors can lead to the onset of atrial flutter.

The most common causes include rheumatic heart disease, high blood pressure, coronary artery disease, alcohol or illicit drug abuse, hyperthyroidism, hypothyroidism, pulmonary disease, valvular disease, congenital heart disease, coronary artery bypass surgery, congestive heart failure, atherosclerosis, myocardial infarction, rheumatic heart disease, metabolic imbalance, exposure to stimulants such as caffeine or tobacco, sick sinus syndrome, emphysema, lung disease, previous heart surgery, viral infections, stress due to pneumonia or other illnesses, and/or sleep apnea.

Symptoms
Some patients diagnosed with an atrial flutter present with few or no symptoms. However, many patients present with a variety of symptoms upon diagnosis. Yet, these symptoms vary from patient to patient and in terms of severity. Cardiovascular comorbid conditions may also affect the symptoms that are presented in patients diagnosed with atrial flutter.

Symptoms commonly associated with atrial flutter include cardiac palpitations, irregular heartbeat, anxiety, weakness, dizziness, lightheadedness, fainting, sweating, shortness of breath, chest pain, inability to perform activities of daily living, confusion, fatigue, physical activity intolerance, and hypotension.

Diagnosis and screening
The diagnosis of atrial flutter can be difficult if patients present with few or no symptoms. Physical examination, medical history, and diagnostic tools are used to screen to atrial fibrillation. Upon physical examination, practicing clinicians will look for rapid or irregular heart rate and/or hypotension.

Diagnostic screening tools used to confirm diagnosis and cause of atrial flutter include echocardiogram, electrocardiogram, Holter monitor, event recorder, chest x-ray, magnetic resonance imaging, and thyroid function tests. Also, blood work may be completed to assess other contributing factors including thyroid function tests, electrolyte levels and metabolic function tests. More invasive diagnostic tools used include stress test, tilt table test, and/or electrophysiologic testing.

Wolff-Parkinson-White syndrome

Wolf-Parkinson-White syndrome develops because of the formation of extra electrical circuits within the heart. The condition leads to rapid heart rate and abnormal electrocardiogram.

In the United States, Wolf-Parkinson-White syndrome occurs in less than 0.2% of the general population. Most patients diagnosed with the syndrome have no evidence of other cardiovascular comorbid conditions. Wolf-Parkinson-White syndrome is the most common cause of tachycardia in young children, toddlers, and infants. The syndrome is more common in men than women, with 60% to 70% of cases in men. However, the syndrome can occur in individuals of all ages and ethnic/racial descents. The highest incidence occurs in individuals between the ages of 30 and 40.

Causes and risks
Wolf-Parkinson-White syndrome is a syndrome, and by definition, an identifiable external cause is not known. It is caused by an accessory pathway in the cardiac conduction system that causes arrhythmias in some individuals. The condition is congenital, and thus, there are no risk factors.

Symptoms
The symptoms of Wolff-Parkinson-White syndrome include rapid heart rate and abnormal electrocardiogram. Patients diagnosed with the condition may have a few episode of increased heart rate, while others may present with more consistent episodes of increased heart rate, as much a few times per week. Symptoms may also vary from patient to patient and may vary in terms of severity. Cardiovascular comorbid conditions may further affect the symptoms that present in patients who are diagnosed with the syndrome.

The most common symptoms associated with the syndrome include cardiac palpitations, lightheadedness, fainting, confusion, dizziness, shortness of breath, chest pain, chest tightness, fluttering in chest, anxiety, sweating, inability to perform activities of daily living, fatigue, physical activity intolerance, and hypotension. Wolff-Parkinson-White is one of the most common causes of tachycardia in infants and children.

Diagnosis and screening
Physical examination, medical history, and diagnostic tools are used to screen for Wolff-Parkinson-White syndrome. Upon physical examination, practicing clinicians will look for rapid or irregular heart rate of varying heart rate and/or hypotension.

Diagnostic screening tools used to confirm diagnosis of Wolff-Parkinson-White syndrome include electrocardiogram, Holter monitor, event recorders, and electrophysiologic testing and mapping.

Ventricular fibrillation

Ventricular fibrillation is a very serious condition caused by uncoordinated contractions of cardiac muscle in the ventricles of the heart. In this condition, the contractions of the atria and ventricles are uncoordinated. If not addressed promptly, the condition can lead to heart failure and sudden death.

In the United States, approximately 300,000 individuals are diagnosed with ventricular fibrillation. The condition is more common in men than women. Individuals of African American descent are also at a higher risk for ventricular fibrillation. The condition rarely occurs in infants under the age of 6 months and in adults ages 45 to 75 years old.

Causes and risk factors

The main cause of ventricular fibrillation is myocardial infarction, but the condition can result from other cardiovascular comorbid conditions and/or when the heart does not get enough oxygen. Other conditions that can lead to ventricular fibrillation include congenital heart disease, coronary artery disease, shock, electrical shock, drowning, very low levels of potassium, electrocution accidents, injury to heart, cardiomyopathies, congestive heart failure, heart surgery, administration of drugs that affect electrical currents such as sodium blockers, and/or ischemia.

Additional risk factors include family history of cardiovascular disease, medical history of cardiovascular conditions, hypertension, high cholesterol, diabetes, smoking, and/or alcohol or illicit drug abuse.

Symptoms

Ventricular fibrillation is a serious condition that, if not attended to promptly, may result in sudden death or congestive heart failure. The symptoms associated with the condition can resemble that of other cardiovascular conditions and can vary from patient to patient. Individuals with an acute ventricular fibrillation episode typically present by fainting or suddenly collapsing and/or becoming unconscious. They also typically present with very rapid or undetectable heart rate.

Symptoms that typically occur before an individual having an acute ventricular fibrillation episode faints or becomes unconscious include chest pain, seizures, dizziness, nausea, vomiting, rapid heartbeat, shortness of breath, confusion, and weakness.

Diagnosis and screening

Ventricular fibrillation is an emergency condition that requires immediate attention to prevent serious complications such as congestive heart failure and sudden death. Physical examination, medical history, and diagnostic tools are used to screen for ventricular fibrillation. Upon physical examination, practicing clinicians will look for rapid or irregular heart rate of, hypertension, or hypotension. The patient may also present with a very low or no heart rate and a cardiac monitor will demonstrate a disorganized heart rate.

Diagnostic screening tests used to confirm diagnosis of ventricular fibrillation include electrocardiogram, cardiac monitor, Holter monitor, and event recorder.

Ventricular tachycardia

Ventricular tachycardia is a condition that is initiated in the ventricle and results in a very rapid or irregular heartbeat. The condition is triggered by 3 or more consecutive premature ventricular heartbeats. Ventricular tachycardia can result in heartbeats ranging from 160 to 240 beats per minute. The condition can be classified as nonsustained or sustained.

In the United States, ventricular tachycardia occurs in approximately 2 out of 10,000 individuals. The incidence of ventricular tachycardia in the United States remains unknown due to overlap with ventricular fibrillation. Ventricular tachycardia is more prevalent among men than women, but varies with the risk factors for atherosclerosis. The incidence of ventricular tachycardia increases with natural aging and with prevalence of coronary artery disease.

<u>Causes and risk factors</u>
The most common cause of ventricular tachycardia is the presence of coronary artery disease. Ventricular tachycardia can result from the presence of other comorbid cardiovascular conditions or in the absence of any other cardiac diseases. It can also occur as a result of myocardial infarction, congestive heart failure, cardiomyopathy, cardiac valvular disease, myocarditis, ischemia, electrolyte abnormalities, high potassium levels, high magnesium levels, adrenergic stimulation, and post–cardiovascular surgery.

Additional risk factors include family history of cardiovascular disease, medical history of cardiovascular conditions, hypertension, high cholesterol, diabetes, smoking, and/or alcohol or illicit drug abuse.

<u>Symptoms</u>
The symptoms of ventricular tachycardia can vary depending on the degree and extent of disease. Some patients present with severe symptoms that require emergency treatment. However, other patients may present with few or no symptoms, which may or may not require medical intervention. In addition, symptoms may start and stop suddenly. Ventricular tachycardia is most commonly associated with coronary artery disease and can present with a nonsustained or sustained rapid heart rate.

The most common symptoms individuals with ventricular tachycardia present with include heart palpitations, rapid heartbeat, lightheadedness, dizziness, confusion, weakness, fatigue, fainting, shortness of breath, and chest discomfort.

<u>Diagnosis and screening</u>
Physical examination, medical history, and diagnostic tools are used to diagnose ventricular tachycardia. Upon physical examination, practicing clinicians will look for rapid or irregular heart rate and changes in blood pressure. The patient may also present with a very low or no heart rate and normal or low blood pressure. Individuals with ventricular tachycardia may present with fainting or in an unconscious state.

Diagnostic tools used to screen for ventricular tachycardia and assess for causes include electrocardiogram, echocardiogram, Holter monitor, intracardiac electrophysiology studies, event recorder, chest x-ray, magnetic resonance imaging, and thyroid function tests. Also, blood work may be completed to access other contributing factors including thyroid function tests, electrolyte levels, and metabolic function tests.

Intermittent claudication

Intermittent claudication is a condition that arises from peripheral arterial disease. Approximately one-third to one-half of individuals diagnosed with peripheral arterial disease present with intermittent claudication. The condition occurs after physical exertion and consists of pain during physical activity, which resolves once the activity is stopped. The pain most commonly occurs in the calves, thighs, and/or buttocks.

The condition is defined as muscle pain or cramping in appendages triggered by walking and physical activity. Individuals may also experience ischemic rest pain. The condition results from inadequate oxygen supply to the legs because of impeded blood flow.

Intermittent claudication occurs more commonly in men than women. It also occurs more often in individuals with a history of smoking, cardiovascular comorbid conditions, diabetes, and high blood pressure. The estimated prevalence of intermittent claudication is approximately 4.5 million individuals. It has been estimated that 60% to 70% of individuals with intermittent claudication have persistent symptoms, 20% to 25% symptoms get worse, and 10% require surgical intervention. The rate of amputation is approximately 1% to 2% per year.

Causes and risk factors
Intermittent claudication is most commonly associated with peripheral arterial disease. Both genetic and environmental factors can contribute to the onset of intermittent claudication.

The risk factors and causes for intermittent claudication are very similar to peripheral arterial disease as the former is a symptom of the latter. Conditions that can lead to intermittent claudication include blood clots, injury to limbs, and unusual anatomy of ligaments or muscles or infection. Other diseases that can lead to onset of peripheral vascular disease include aortic aneurysms, Buerger's disease, pulmonary embolism, phlebitis, varicose veins, and Raynaud's syndrome.

Factors that increase an individual's risk for peripheral arterial disease and intermittent claudication include smoking, 50 years of age or older, diabetes, obesity, high blood pressure, high cholesterol or family history of cardiovascular diseases and/or arthrosclerosis. Male individuals of African American descent as well as overweight individuals and those with a family history of cardiovascular disease are at a higher risk of peripheral vascular disease and intermittent claudication.

Symptoms
The main symptoms of intermittent claudication include pain in a functional muscle group located in the legs such as calf, buttock, and thigh, pain after strenuous activity such as brisk walking or physical activity, and reduction of pain once physical activity is stopped.

The symptoms of intermittent claudication are associated with other symptoms of peripheral arterial disease including leg numbness or weakness, cold legs and feet, sores or wounds on digits or extremities that will not heal, blue or pale hue to legs, feet, hands and/or arms, hair loss on feet and legs, and changes in composition of nails.

Diagnosis and screening
The symptoms of individuals with intermittent claudication may vary. Therefore, practicing clinicians should assess the patient's medical history, presence of comorbid conditions and examine the patient. Physical examination, medical history, and diagnostic screening tools are used to determine if a patient has intermittent claudication.

Upon physical examination, practicing clinicians use a stethoscope to determine the presence of bruits. They also look for evidence of poor wound healing, sores, color changes, muscle pain or cramping upon physical activity, temperature changes and decreased blood pressure in limbs. Diagnostic screening tools include the ankle-brachial index and angiography. Additional tests include electrocardiogram, magnetic resonance angiography, blood tests, and ultrasound.

Hypotension

Hypotension is defined as low pressure, particularly lower than 90/60 mmHg. However, what practicing clinicians consider low blood pressure varies from patient to patient because some individuals have naturally low blood pressure with no symptoms. Also, patients with comorbid conditions like hepatic disease (cirrhosis) may have lower than normal blood pressure at baseline.

Drops in blood pressure of more than 20 mmHg are more of a concern from a patient's normal blood pressure, as it can cause symptoms of dizziness, fainting and decreased mental capacity. It can also be an indicator of a more serious underlying condition such as uncontrolled bleeding, severe infections, and/or allergic reactions

Orthostatic hypotension or postural hypotension is defined as low blood pressure upon standing. In this condition, an individual's blood pressure drops when going from a sitting to standing position, leading to dizziness, lightheadedness, blurred vision, and fainting or syncope. The causes of orthostatic hypotension include dehydration, prolonged bed rest, pregnancy, diabetes, heart problems, burns, excessive heat exposure, large varicose veins, and certain neurological disorders. Drugs that can lead to orthostatic hypotension include diuretics, beta-blockers, calcium channel blockers, angiotensin-converting enzyme inhibitors, and antidepressants.

The condition is more common in older individuals, with 20% of cases occurring in individuals aged 65 or older.

Postprandial hypotension is a condition that involves a sudden drop in blood pressure after eating. It typically affects elderly individuals with other cardiovascular comorbid condition or neurological disorders. Symptoms of the condition include dizziness, fatigue, syncope or fainting, mental confusion, and/or lightheadedness. Postprandial hypotension is more common among individuals with high blood pressure or autonomic nervous system disorders. Lifestyle modifications such as eating smaller meals low in carbohydrates more often may reduce symptoms. Also, lowering the dose of blood pressure medications may decrease the onset of postprandial hypotension.

Shy-Drager syndrome, also known as multiple system atrophy with orthostatic hypotension, is a rare disease that causes progressive damage to the autonomic nervous system. Deterioration of the autonomic nervous system leads to improper functioning of blood pressure, heart rate, breathing, and digestion. The main characteristic of Shy-Drager syndrome is severe hypotension when standing and severe hypertension when lying down. Other symptoms of the disease include muscle tremors, slowed movement, problems with coordination and speech, and incontinence. The disease is progressive, with few treatment approaches, and usually leads to death within 7 to 10 years from time of diagnosis.

Neurally mediated hypotension is a condition that causes a drop in blood pressure after standing for long periods. The symptoms associated with neurally mediated hypotension include dizziness, lightheadedness, heart palpitations, sweating, nausea, confusion, and fainting or syncope. The condition tends to affect younger adults and is caused by a malfunction between the brain and cardiovascular system, which causes blood pooling in the legs and feet leading to sudden blood pressure drops. Lifestyle modifications including the vagal maneuver, increased sodium intake and use of graduated compression stocking may improve symptoms. Pharmacologic agents such as beta-blockers, alpha-adrenergic inhibitors, and agents that maintain salt in the kidneys can improve symptoms.

Causes and risk factors

The causes and risk factors associated with hypotension vary from individual to individual. Athletes and individuals who exercise regularly tend to have lower blood pressure than unfit and/or obese individuals. The main risk factors and causes of hypotension, as outlined by the American Heart Association, include pregnancy; certain pharmacologic agents such as diuretics, beta-blockers, Parkinson disease drugs, tricyclic antidepressants, sildenafil particularly in combination with nitroglycerine, narcotics and alcohol; cardiac conditions such as bradycardia, cardiac valvular disease, myocardial infarction and congestive heart failure, endocrine problems such as hypothyroidism, hyperthyroidism, Addison disease, hypoglycemia and diabetes; blood loss as from major surgery or severe injury; severe infection; allergic reaction; and nutritional deficiencies such as lack of vitamins B-12 and folate; natural aging; and dehydration.

Symptoms

The symptoms of hypotension vary from patient to patient and depend on the extent and degree of the condition. It also depends on the patient's overall health and presence of other comorbid conditions. Also, some individuals experience more severe symptoms than another, even if their blood pressure is relatively normal. However, patients with relatively low blood pressure may experience few or no symptoms.

Symptoms associated with hypotension include dizziness, lightheadedness, fainting or syncope, lack of concentration or decrease mental capacity, weakness, fatigue, blurred vision, nausea, cold, clammy and/or pale skin, rapid or shallow breathing, depression, and/or thirst.

Diagnosis and screening

Physical examination, medical history, and diagnostic tools are used to diagnose hypotension and determine which type of hypotension a patient presents with. The goal is to determine the underlying cause of hypotension in order to treat the symptoms of hypotension or treat the underlying cause to improve an individual's blood pressure.

Diagnostic tools used to assess hypotension include blood tests such as red blood cell counts and blood glucose levels, electrocardiogram, echocardiogram, stress test, Valsalva maneuver, and/or tilt-table test.

Compartment syndrome

Compartment syndrome is a condition that involves the compression of nerves and blood vessels within an enclosed space, which leads to decreased blood flow as well as muscle and nerve damage. Compartment syndrome can be acute or chronic depending on the underlying cause. Chronic compartment syndrome can be caused by repetitive activities that lead to swelling such as running or excessive physical activity.

The incidence of compartment syndrome in the United States is relatively low, averaging up to 12%. The mortality rate depends on the time of diagnosis and treatment of the condition. The condition is more common in men than women.

Causes and risk factors

Risk factors and causes of compartment syndrome include swelling due to high-energy trauma from a car accident or surgery, tight bandages or casts with significant swelling. In addition, a variety of physical injuries can lead to compartment syndrome. Compartment syndrome can be caused by increased pressure, swelling and/or decreased compartment size. Increased swelling or fluid buildup can be caused by intensive muscle use, daily physical exertion, burns, intraarterial injection, envenomation, decreased serum osmolarity, infiltrated infusion, and hemorrhage. Decreased compartment size can be caused by military anti-shock trousers, burns, tight bandages, and/or casts. The abdomen can also be a site of compartment syndrome if excessive swelling.

<u>Symptoms</u>
The main symptom associated with compartment syndrome is severe pain that does not respond to elevation or pain medication. However, in more severe cases, patients may present with decreased sensation, weakness, and paleness of the skin. The degree and extent of symptoms depend on the severity of compartment syndrome and whether or not it is a chronically occurring.

Typically, patients diagnosed with compartment syndrome present with severe pain when a muscle running through a compartment is passively moved or squeezed, such as toe, foot, or leg. The skin covering the compartment being affected will be shiny and swollen.

<u>Diagnosis and screening</u>
Diagnosis of compartment syndrome involves physical examination, medical history, and diagnostic screening tools. A practicing clinician will examine a patient for any swollen toes, legs, or feet. They will also move or squeeze muscle groups potentially affected to see if the patient expresses severe pain.

The diagnosis is made by directly measuring the pressure in the compartment with a needle and pressure meter, which is called the compartment pressure measurement. If the compartment pressure is greater than 45 mmHg or the diastolic blood pressure is within 30 mmHg, then a diagnosis of compartment syndrome is made. Other diagnostic screening tools used include blood tests such as complete metabolic profile, complete blood count, creatine phosphokinase and urine myoglobin, serum myoglobin, toxicity screen, and prothrombin and activated partial thromboplastin time. Urinalysis may also be performed as well as use of imaging tools such as radiography and ultrasonogram.

If chronic compartment syndrome is suspected, then direct blood pressure measurement needs to be determined post–physical exertional activity.

Pulmonary edema

Pulmonary edema is a condition that involves increased blood pressure in the blood vessels of the lungs forcing fluid into the air sacs, which prevents the absorption of oxygen. The elevated pulmonary capillary pressures lead to increased fluid in the interstitial compartment and alveoli. Decreased cardiac output, inadequate tissue perfusion, and acute pulmonary congestion are characteristic of the condition.

Acute pulmonary edema is a serious condition that requires prompt medical attention. However, if treated aggressively and immediately, prognosis is generally good. Yet, delayed intervention can lead to severe complications including death. In the acute care setting, the mortality rate associated with pulmonary edema is as high as 15% to 20%, on average.

<u>Causes and risk factors</u>
The causes and risk factors for pulmonary edema are generally environmental and can be exacerbated by the presence of other comorbid conditions. The causes and risk factors for

pulmonary edema include coronary artery disease, congestive heart failure, myocardial infarction, cardiomyopathy, cardiac valve dysfunction, and high blood pressure.

Noncardiac causes and risk factors for pulmonary edema include lung infections, exposure to certain toxins such as chlorine, ammonia and nitrogen dioxide, kidney disease, smoke inhalation, adverse drug reaction to drugs such as illicit drugs and chemotherapy drugs, acute respiratory syndrome, and high altitudes.

Symptoms
The symptoms of pulmonary edema can vary from patient to patient. The symptoms are also dependant on the degree and extent of the condition as well as a patient's overall general health and presence of other comorbid conditions. However, the most common symptoms associated with pulmonary edema include extreme shortness of breath or difficulty breathing, a feeling of suffocating or drowning, wheezing or gasping for breath, anxiety, restlessness, a sense of apprehension, a cough that produces frothy sputum that may be tinged with blood, excessive sweating, grunting or gurgling sounds when breathing, restlessness, anxiety, nasal flaring, inability to speak, decreased awareness, pale skin, and chest pain.

Symptoms that may develop more gradually include difficulty breathing while lying down, awakening at night out of breath, increased shortness of breath, and significant weight gain.

Diagnosis and screening
Physical examination, medical history, and diagnostic screening tools are used to diagnose pulmonary edema. Acute pulmonary edema requires prompt medical attention for prevention of severe complications. Patients with pulmonary edema typically present with rapid breathing, increased heart rate, crackles in lungs, and pale or blue skin.

Diagnostic tools used for screening of pulmonary edema include blood tests such as arterial blood gas concentrations, chest x-ray, electrocardiogram, echocardiogram, and transesophageal echocardiography. A more invasive diagnostic approach used to diagnose pulmonary edema when diagnosis is unclear is pulmonary artery catheterization.

First-degree atrioventricular block

First-degree atrioventricular block is defined as a delay in conduction of impulses from the sinoatrial (SA) node to the atrioventricular (AV) node. The condition is typically asymptomatic and undiagnosed. It can occur in individuals of all ages. The disease is typically benign and not associated with an increase in morbidity and mortality.

In the United States, the prevalence of first-degree atrioventricular block varies up to 1.6%. Higher prevalence in younger adults occurs in athletes and medical school students. The condition is more prevalent in African Americans than Caucasian Americans. The condition also increases with natural aging and more prevalent among elderly patients with other cardiovascular comorbid conditions.

Causes and risk factors
Other comorbid conditions that can lead to first-degree atrioventricular block include cardiac ischemia, myocardial infarction, congestive heart failure, coronary artery disease, scarring of atrial tissue in internodal pathways, infiltration by amyloid, sarcoid, Lyme carditis, endocarditis,

degenerative diseases, rheumatic cardiac disease, electrolyte imbalances, atrial stretch, increased vagal tone, and inflammatory diseases.

Pharmacologic agents that can lead to first-degree atrioventricular block include digoxin, calcium channel blockers such as nifedipine, amlodipine, verapamil and diltiazem, and beta-blockers.

The condition is characterized by prolonged PR interval (greater than 200 msec), which can also occur as a normal variant in some individuals.

Symptoms
Individuals who present with first-degree atrioventricular block have few or no symptoms and typically are not at risk of developing other comorbid conditions. Diagnosis is typically made during routine physical examination or when being examined for another compliant. In patients with first-degree atrioventricular block, heart rate and rhythm are typically normal, and there may be nothing wrong with the heart. However, some patients may present with fainting and syncope, bradycardia, left ventricular systolic dysfunction, as well as comorbid congestive heart failure.

Many well-trained athletes may present with first-degree atrioventricular block but do not present with symptoms.

Diagnosis and screening
Physical examination, patient history, and diagnostic screening tools are used to diagnose first-degree atrioventricular block. The condition is often hard to diagnose, as patients typically present with few or no symptoms. Many individuals go undiagnosed due to lack of symptoms. Additionally, some individuals have prolonged PR interval due to a normal variant that is typically asymptomatic.

The condition is often diagnosed during routine electrocardiogram screening and is found incidentally. Diagnosis is made by a PR interval greater than 200 msec.

Second-degree atrioventricular block type I

Second-degree atrioventricular block type I, also known as Wenckebach or Mobitz I, is also an asymptomatic dysrhythmia. The condition typically occurs in adults post myocardial infarction or with inferior wall ischemia. It is usually caused by disease of the atrioventricular node.

A small percentage of second-degree atrioventricular block type I occurs due to underlying structural disease. Second-degree atrioventricular block type I is the most common type of second-degree atrioventricular block. The condition occurs in adults and equally both in men and women. There is no correlation between ethnicity and/or race and second-degree atrioventricular block type I.

Second-degree atrioventricular block type I

Second-degree atrioventricular block type I, also known as Wenckebach or Mobitz I, is also an asymptomatic dysrhythmia. The condition typically occurs in adults as post–myocardial infarction or with inferior wall ischemia.

Causes and risk factors

Second-degree atrioventricular block type I can occur due to the presence of structural heart disease. However, structural heart disease does not have to be present for the disease to occur. The condition may also occur due to a normal variant or autosomal dominant trait, making the individual genetically predisposed.

Pharmacologic agents that slow conduction through the atrioventricular node have been shown to cause second-degree atrioventricular block type I. These agents include cardioactive drugs such as digoxin, beta-blockers, calcium channel blockers, and certain antiarrhythmia drugs such as sodium channel blockers (procainamide).

Other disorders that can lead to second-degree atrioventricular block type I include inflammatory diseases such as endocarditis, myocarditis, Lyme disease, and acute rheumatic fever, infiltrative diseases such as amyloidosis, hemochromatosis, and sarcoidosis, metabolic disorders such as hyperkalemia, hypermagnesemia, and Addison disease, and vascular diseases such as ankylosing spondylitis, dermatomyositis, rheumatoid arthritis, scleroderma, lupus, and Reiter syndrome. Also, acute myocardial infarction has been associated with second-degree atrioventricular block type I.

Symptoms

Individuals who present with second-degree atrioventricular block type I have few or no symptoms and typically are not at risk of developing other comorbid conditions. Diagnosis is typically made during routine physical examination or when being examined for another compliant. In patients with second-degree atrioventricular block type I, heart rate, and atrial rhythm are typically abnormal due atrioventricular node dysfunction. However, some patients may present with lightheadedness, dizziness, decreased cardiac output, activity intolerance, shortness of breath, chest pain, hypotension, bradycardia, heart failure, stroke, and syncope.

Yet, symptoms in patients diagnosed with second-degree atrioventricular block type I can vary greatly depending on the overall health and physical conditioning of the patient as well as presence of other comorbid conditions.

Diagnosis and screening

Physical examination, patient history, and diagnostic screening tools are used to diagnose second-degree atrioventricular block type I. The condition is often hard to diagnose, as patients typically present with few or no symptoms. Many individuals go undiagnosed due to lack of symptoms.

The condition is diagnosed on electrocardiogram by progressive lengthening of PR interval followed by a p wave without an associated QRS complex. Holter monitor or event recorder can be used to diagnose outpatients. Laboratory tests including serum electrolyte and magnesium levels, serum digoxin levels, and thyroid function tests may be used to find the cause. Other imagining tests may be performed depending on the patient's symptoms and presence of comorbid cardiovascular conditions. Diagnostic electrophysiologic testing may be necessary to determine the site of block and need for a pacemaker.

Second-degree atrioventricular block type II

Second-degree atrioventricular block type II, also known as Mobitz II, is an intermittent failure of conduction of impulses below the AV node. The condition is often associated with HIS-Purkinje system cardiac disease, which can lead to complications such as complete heart block or ventricular asystole. It occurs most often in adults and is associated with a high mortality rate, as the condition can progress rapidly to a complete heart block.

The condition is highly associated with infra- and intranodal blocks, which indicate the location of the blocks. A small percentage of second-degree atrioventricular block type II occurs due to underlying structural disease. The condition occurs in adults and equally both in men and women. There is no correlation between ethnicity and/or race and second-degree atrioventricular block type II. The condition is less common than second-degree atrioventricular block type I. Second-degree atrioventricular block type II is associated with a high mortality rate when it occurs with comorbid anterior wall myocardial infarction.

Causes and risk factors
Second-degree atrioventricular block type II can occur due to presence of structural heart disease. However, structural heart disease does not have to be present for the disease to occur. The condition may also occur due to normal variant or autosomal dominant trait, making the individual genetically predisposed.

Pharmacologic agents that slow conduction through the AV node have been shown to cause second-degree atrioventricular block type II. These agents include cardioactive drugs such as digoxin, beta-blockers, calcium channel blockers, and certain antiarrhythmia drugs such as sodium channel blockers (procainamide).

Other disorders that can lead to second-degree atrioventricular block type II include inflammatory diseases such as endocarditis, myocarditis, Lyme disease and acute rheumatic fever; infiltrative diseases such as amyloidosis, hemochromatosis, and sarcoidosis; metabolic disorders such as hyperkalemia, hypermagnesemia, and Addison disease; and vascular diseases such as ankylosing spondylitis, dermatomyositis, rheumatoid arthritis, scleroderma, lupus, and Reiter syndrome. Also, acute myocardial infarction, congestive heart failure, coronary artery disease, and primary diseases have been associated with second-degree atrioventricular block type II.

Symptoms
Some patients may present with lightheadedness, dizziness, decreased cardiac output, activity intolerance, shortness of breath, chest pain, hypotension, bradycardia, diaphoresis, pauses in pulse, heart failure, stroke, and/or syncope or fainting.

Yet, symptoms in patients diagnosed with second-degree atrioventricular block type I can vary greatly depending on the overall health and physical conditioning of the patient as well as presence of other comorbid conditions.

Diagnosis and screening
Physical examination, patient history, and diagnostic screening tools are used to diagnose second-degree atrioventricular block type II. The condition is typically associated with significant underlying conduction system conditions. Patients often present with hypotension, diaphoresis, and pauses in pulse caused by decreased cardiac output.

The condition is diagnosed by electrocardiogram, Holter monitor, or event recorder. Not every p wave has an associated QRS complex (1:3, etc) and there is NO progressive prolongation of PR interval. Lab tests and echocardiography may be necessary to elucidate further the underlying cause. Also, diagnostic electrophysiologic testing may be necessary to determine the site of the block and need for a pacemaker.

Third-degree atrioventricular block

Third-degree atrioventricular block, also known as complete heart block, involves complete dissociation of impulses between the atria and ventricles. The condition is not well tolerated and most common in adults, but can occur in adolescents with congenital heart disease. The condition can occur intermittently or consistently depending on the underlying cause of the condition.

In the United States, the prevalence of third-degree atrioventricular block is approximately 0.02%. The incidence of third-degree atrioventricular block increases with age, but may occur in infants or adolescents due to congenital complete heart block.

Causes and risk factors
The most common causes of third-degree atrioventricular block include drugs that target the atrioventricular node such as beta-blockers, calcium channel blockers, quinidine, and procainamide; degenerative diseases such as Lenègre disease and Lev disease; infectious causes such as Lyme disease, rheumatic fever, myocarditis, and Chagas disease; rheumatic diseases such as ankylosing spondylitis, Reiter syndrome, relapsing polychondritis, rheumatoid arthritis, and scleroderma; infiltrative processes such as amyloidosis, sarcoidosis, tumors, Hodgkin disease, and multiple myeloma; neuromuscular disorders such as Becker muscular dystrophy and myotonic muscular dystrophy; ischemia or infarction; and metabolic causes such as hypoxia and hyperkalemia.

Symptoms
Most patients diagnosed with third-degree atrioventricular block present with symptoms. However, some patients present with few or no symptoms. Additionally, third-degree atrioventricular block may be an underlying condition in patients who present with sudden cardiac death.

The symptoms associated with third-degree atrioventricular block include fainting or syncope, near-syncope, lightheadedness, fatigue, dyspnea, and chest pain. Patients diagnosed with third-degree atrioventricular block typically present with a series of P-waves and QRS complexes that do not relate to one another. Additionally, atrial heart rate is normal but ventricular heart rate is abnormal.

Diagnosis and screening
Physical examination, medical history, and diagnostic screening tools are used to diagnose third-degree atrioventricular block. Electrocardiogram (ECG), Holter monitor, and event recorders are used to diagnose. On the ECG, there is no association between p waves and QRS complexes. Further tests including echocardiography and lab tests may be necessary to elucidate fully the source of the block.

Cardiogenic shock

Cardiogenic shock is a condition characterized by inadequate perfusion from cardiac dysfunction. It is an emergency situation and requires immediate treatment. Cardiogenic shock is the most common cause of mortality in patients who experience a myocardial infarction.

In the United States, cardiogenic shock occurs in approximately 8.6% of patients experiencing ST-segment elevation myocardial infarction, with about 29% of those presenting to the hospital already in shock. Cardiogenic shock occurs in a smaller percentage of patients with non-ST segment elevation myocardial infarction, occurring in approximately 2% of patients. The condition is the leading cause of mortality in patients experiencing myocardial infarction.

Morality rates vary from 1 race to another, with Hispanics at highest risk, followed by African Americans and then Caucasians and Asians. Women comprise 42% of all patients with cardiogenic shock.

<u>Causes and risk factors</u>
The most common cause of cardiogenic shock is myocardial infarction. However, not every patient who experiences a myocardial infarction goes into cardiogenic shock. The individuals at highest risk for cardiogenic shock include patients who have experience a myocardial infarction, older age, history of congestive heart failure, diabetes, dysrhythmia, and/or coronary artery disease.

Common causes of cardiogenic shock include ventricular septal rupture, papillary muscle infarction or rupture, myocarditis, endocarditis, arrhythmias, pericardial tamponade, and pulmonary embolism.

Other causes of cardiogenic shock include beta-blocker overdose, calcium channel blocker overdose, myocardial contusion, respiratory acidosis, hypocalcemia, hypophosphatemia, ventricular hypertrophy, restrictive cardiomyopathies, aortic stenosis, hypertrophic cardiomyopathy, dynamic outflow obstruction, aortic coarctation, malignant hypertension, mitral stenosis, endocarditis, mitral or aortic regurgitation, atrial myxoma, tamponade, and cardiotoxic drugs such as doxorubicin.

<u>Symptoms</u>
The symptoms associated with cardiogenic shock vary depending on the patient and presence of underlying comorbid conditions. Younger patients in good health tend to present with fewer symptoms than older patients with other comorbid cardiovascular conditions.

The common symptoms associated with cardiogenic shock include confusion, lack of alertness, loss of consciousness, palpitations, sweating, fainting or syncope, pale skin, weak pulse, rapid breathing, shortness of breath, decreased or no urine output, cold hands and/or feet, anxiety, nervousness, weakness, lethargy, fatigue, loss of ability to concentrate, decreased mental status, restlessness, agitation, coma, dizziness, and lightheadedness.

<u>Diagnosis and screening</u>
Physical examination, medical history, and diagnostic screening tools are used to diagnose cardiogenic shock. The condition is treated on an emergency basis and requires prompt attention and is typically diagnosed in the emergency room setting. It is typically diagnosed when a patient has been admitted to the emergency room for a myocardial infarction.

Diagnostic screening tools used to diagnose cardiogenic shock include blood pressure monitoring, electrocardiogram, echocardiogram, chest x-ray, and coronary angiography. Laboratory blood tests that may be performed include arterial blood gas measurement, electrolyte levels, cardiac enzyme levels, renal function, liver function, lactate levels, and thyroid function tests.

Planning, Implementation, and Outcome Evaluation

CHEST and AHA guidelines for anticoagulation administration

CHEST guidelines promote the use of a systematic protocol for anticoagulation therapy including daily international normalized ratio prothrombin time (INR-PT/INR) monitoring to evaluate dosing levels. Optimal therapeutic INR range while on anticoagulants should be tightly controlled between 2.0 and 3.0. This method requires a high level of accountability in coordinating care and communication with treatment team members as well as the patient regarding test results and rationale behind current dosing levels. The patient should be continuously instructed regarding self-management skills in anticipation for self care. Anticoagulant therapy is contraindicated in the critically ill patient with active—or a high risk for—bleeding. These recommendations are also sanctioned by the American Heart Association.

AHA practice guidelines regarding chronic heart failure

AHA identifies heart disease by four stages: A, B, C and D. Stage A (patients at high risk but without established heart disease) and stage B (patients with measurable damage to the heart who are still currently without symptoms) are the stages where progression to further disease is still preventable. Care is focused on education and prevention measures. ACE inhibitors may be added to the care of patients in stage B.

Stage C (patients with heart disease and symptom complaints) would increase pharmaceutical treatments to also include diuretics. Dietary intervention might include low-salt diets and/or restricted fluid intake.

Stage D (patients who have escalated to end-stage heart disease and require extreme medical measures or end-of-life care) may require surgical interventions on a case-by-case basis, including valve surgery, ventricular assist device (VAD) or transplant. Most patients at this stage do not qualify for such interventions and will enter into care focused on end-of-life comfort.

Risk factors and treatment recommendations for peripheral artery disease (PAD) as endorsed by the PAD coalition and AHA

Patients with the greatest risk for PAD include individuals with diabetes, abnormal extremity pulses, known cardiac disease, high cholesterol, high blood levels of homocysteine, high blood pressure, impaired wound healing on extremities, age over 70 or a history of smoking. The presence of PAD in turn increases the patient's risk for myocardial infarction and stroke.

Treatment includes smoking cessation and other risk management. Further interventions might include physical or exercise rehabilitation, medication (including thrombolytics, vasodilators and medications to treat related risk factors) and surgical interventions including stents or amputation in extreme cases.

Treatment priorities for aortic regurgitation

Aortic regurgitation is a condition created by valve inadequacy affecting the flow of blood from the aorta into the left ventricle and causes audible variances (murmur) in the heartbeat. Common causes include rheumatic heart disease and bacterial endocarditis. Whenever possible, treatment for aortic regurgitation is focused on surgical repair of the defective valve.

Monitor heart rate, oxygen saturation levels and administer medications such as inotropes, vasodilators, glycosides and antibiotics to promote stabilization while preparing for surgery. If surgical intervention is not possible begin chronic and/or end-of-life treatment plans.

Alternative therapies for cardiovascular patients

Alternative therapies are sought by approximately 36% of all cardiovascular patients. Those seeking out complementary therapies are generally younger patients, those of female gender or Asian descent, and those with higher education and income than the general population.

These individuals most often utilize herbal remedies such as echinacea, garlic, ginseng, ginkgo biloba and glucosamine to treat conditions unrelated to their cardiovascular disease.

Herbs are closely followed by physical interventions such as meditation, relaxation and deep breathing to improve mind-body connections and promote cardiac wellness and recovery. Interventions such as meditation and tai chi may be safely and effectively recommended for stress reduction. At this time, not enough research supports positive cardiovascular health changes associated with acupuncture or chelation (removal of heavy metals).

Regardless of the type of therapy used, the majority of those seeking complementary or alternative treatments report that they found the treatments helpful.

Physical signs and symptoms that suggest congestive heart failure

Key identifiers for many cardiovascular disorders are the presence of cyanosis (peripheral and central) and pallor. This, combined with shortness of breath related to position (supine) and exertion, fatigue, fluid retention and swelling, changes in heart rate, weight gain and wheezing and/or productive cough (white or pink fluid) all suggest the presence of congestive heart failure (CHF).

Treatment priorities include oxygenation and fluid reduction with diuretics. Other priorities, depending on individual patient needs, might include anxiety reduction and blood pressure reduction.

Coexisting cardiovascular risk factors associated with renovascular disease

A history of hypertension is positively related to the development of renal disease. In turn, the presence of renovascular disease and its progression to end-stage renal disease (ESRD) and chronic renal failure can often lead to the development of heart failure, hypertrophic cardiomyopathy, and coronary atherosclerosis. The presence of renovascular disease complicates the risk factors of surgical interventions that might be considered for the treatment of cardiovascular disease. Highest nursing concerns will often focus on blood pressure, electrolyte and fluid balances. Medications used to treat cardiac conditions often need to be adjusted and more closely monitored to accommodate for the reduced kidney function.

Angina pectoris vs. myocardial infarction

Angina pectoris often serves as a warning sign for myocardial infarction.

Angina is chest pain occurring from reduced blood flow to the myocardium. This pain is described as squeezing, burning or pressure and is focused on the chest cavity. It is intermittent, often correlating with increased activity and dissipating with rest and/or the use of nitroglycerine.

Myocardial infarction occurs when the lack of oxygen perfusion to the heart causes myocardial tissue death. This pain is more extreme, often referred to as crushing, and extends beyond the chest to radiate out toward the back, shoulder, neck and jaw. Rest and nitroglycerin will have no effect on this type of pain. Initial treatments will include oxygen and morphine sulfate for pain control.

Angina may be diagnosed with an exercise stress test. In the face of an MI, an electrocardiogram will show ST changes and laboratory results will show elevated troponin and creatinine levels.

Common types of congenital heart disease found in an adult patient

Atrial septal defects: The most common congenital deformity is created from the incomplete closure of the patent foramen ovale after birth, leaving a small opening that increases the risk of the patient forming emboli that may lead to cerebrovascular incidents or peripheral artery blockage. This deformity may be repaired with a transseptal patch or left untreated if it is small enough. Patients with septal defects are generally only treated for embolisms if they become symptomatic.

Marfan syndrome: A genetic connective tissue disorder that affects cardiac tissue, causing deformity of the valves and/or weakness of vessels that can cause aortic aneurysm. Physical signs might include unusually elongated limbs and a deformity of the chest area (either appearing sunken in or protruding outward).

Evidence-based interventions that could be performed on the patient experiencing paroxysmal supraventricular tachycardia (PSVT)

PSVT refers to occasional, intermittent rapid heart rate which lasts from a few minutes to several hours. This most often occurs in younger patients and can be brought on by alcohol, caffeine, smoking, illicit drug use or digitalis toxicity. Intervention of any kind might not be needed unless the patient is presenting symptoms such as anxiety, dizziness, shortness of breath, an uncomfortable feeling of chest tightness, racing heart or fainting. Emergency treatment options might include the Valsalva maneuver (instructing the patient to bear down as if having a bowel movement), splashing the face with ice water, IV adenosine or cardioversion. Long-term stability may be maintained by oral medications such as propafenone, flecainide, moricizine, sotalol, and amiodarone; the use of a pacemaker; or, more often, radiofrequency catheter ablation.

Role of a case manager

The American Nurses Credentialing Center defines a nursing case manager as someone who provides a dynamic, orderly, efficient and cooperative approach to client care that improves healthcare continuity and provides the patient with quality care options. The case manager is responsible for coordinating efforts between multiple care professions to make sure the patient's needs are met in a timely, efficient and cost-effective manner. He/she ensures that health education needs are met to allow for informed care decisions while acting as a patient advocate and facilitator of effective healthcare relationships between patient, family and significant others as well as the healthcare team.

Priority nursing diagnoses and best practices for management of hypertension (HTN)

Potential nursing diagnoses for hypertension might include decreased cardiac output, pain (headache), activity intolerance, ineffective coping and knowledge deficits. Nursing care priorities should first focus on blood pressure (and related pain) control with medication. Initial treatment choices would include a combination of a thiazide diuretic and ACE inhibitor, beta-blocker or calcium-channel blocker.

Further interventions should focus on careful monitoring to reduce risk of HTN-related cardiovascular emergencies; educational interventions to promote lifestyle changes including smoking cessation, diet and exercise; and being a patient advocate to support patient decisions regarding care.

Priority nursing diagnoses and the best practices for chronic heart failure (CHF)

Potential nursing diagnoses for CHF include decreased cardiac output, excess fluid volume, activity intolerance, deficient knowledge, risk for impaired gas exchange and impaired skin integrity.

Medical treatment is a careful balancing act between medications, lifestyle adaptations and surgical interventions.

Medication choices might include angiotensin-converting enzyme (ACE) inhibitors to lower blood pressure and improve blood flow. Other options might include angiotensin II receptor blockers and beta-blockers. Diuretics may be used to try and maintain proper fluid balances and improve lung perfusion. If diuretics are used, carefully monitor the patient's electrolytes as well as blood pressure.

Other areas to monitor include oxygen saturation levels and activity tolerance. Education efforts and long-term planning might include energy conservation, diet and cardiac rehabilitation to increase activity tolerance levels.

Surgical procedures might include coronary bypass to relieve severely blocked arteries, heart valve surgery, pacemaker placement, implantable cardioverter-defibrillators (ICD) or ventricular assist devices (pumps).

Nursing diagnoses for common arrhythmias

Arrhythmias include any malfunction of the normal beating of the heart. This can include beating too fast, too slow, or beating irregularly. An arrhythmia may be constantly present when not controlled or appear sporadically due to known or unknown causes. Nursing diagnoses might include decreased cardiac output, deficient knowledge, and in the case of digitalis, toxicity poisoning. Treatment for an arrhythmia may only occur in the symptomatic patient; this treatment might include cardiac monitoring, medication, cardioversion or use of a pacemaker.

Assessment findings and treatment priorities for pulmonary embolism

Pulmonary embolism is the second leading cause of sudden death. Immediate recognition and treatment for pulmonary embolism is crucial to the patient's chances of survival. Symptoms can be vague and nonspecific but might include chest pain, dyspnea, tachypnea, cough, abnormal lung sounds, low blood pressure or even just a sense of impending doom or nonspecific agitation. Pulmonary angiography or CT angiography is used to make a positive diagnosis. Priority care is given to basic life functions, including monitoring oxygen saturation levels and administering oxygen as needed. Anticoagulants and thrombolytics may be used to dissolve the clot, or it may need to be surgically removed. Nitroglycerin, ACE inhibitors and loop diuretics may also be administered. A vein filter may also be inserted to prevent further clots from reaching the lungs.

Aneurysm treatment

Treatment recommendations for aneurysms are based on the size and location of the aneurysm. Typically, aneurysms found early can be treated with aggressive risk factor modification including cessation of smoking, lowering cholesterol, treating hypertension, diet, exercise, and treatment with anti-platelet agents. However, surgery is often necessary if an aneurysm is large and at risk for rupture.

Once an aneurysm has ruptured, the goals of treatment are to surgically stop the bleeding, reestablish blood flow to prevent permanent end organ damage as well as to reduce the risk of recurrence. Although repair of a ruptured aneurysm is possible, the likelihood of survival in patients with ruptured cerebral, abdominal, or thoracic aneurysms remains low.

Treatment of aneurysms involves management with pharmacologic agents such as anti-hypertensive, anti-coagulant, anti-arrhythmia agents targeted at decreasing blood pressure, and/or heart rate. By decreasing blood pressure and heart rate, practicing clinicians can manage the patient's risk of stroke, heart attack, and death.

The guidelines used for the treatment of aneurysms depend on the size of the aneurysm and the types of symptoms the patient is experiencing.

For patients with an abdominal or thoracic aortic aneurysm with a diameter less than 3 cm without symptoms, follow-up screening should be conducted within 5 to 10 years. For patients with an aorta of 3 to 4 cm in diameter, follow-up screening should be performed on a yearly basis.

For patients with a diameter of greater than 4 cm, careful follow-up needs to be performed on a bi-yearly basis. If a patient presents with an aorta with a diameter greater than 5 cm, surgery is recommended, which would include abdominal or open chest repair or endovascular repair.

Treatment of cerebral aneurysms is dependent on the size and location of the aneurysm in the brain. If the aneurysm is small and not causing symptoms, follow-up screening is recommended. However, surgery is recommended for large, symptomatic aneurysms due to their risk of rupture and stroke. Currently there are 2 surgical approaches for brain aneurysms including surgical clipping or endovascular coiling. If an aneurysm is infected, pharmacologic treatment is necessary.

For thoracic or abdominal aneurysms less than 5 cm in diameter and not causing symptoms, pharmacologic approaches are typically used in combination with continuous monitoring. Surgical or interventional repair are options reserved for large unruptured aneurysms where the risk of rupture exceeds the risk of surgery.

Peripheral aneurysms in the extremities are typically asymptomatic and do not require treatment due to their low risk of rupture. Treatment of peripheral aneurysms depends on the presence of symptoms, the location of the aneurysm, and whether the blood flow through the artery is blocked.

Prevention of aneurysms

Few options are available for the prevention of aneurysms, but individuals should maintain proper blood pressure control, avoid smoking and stimulant drugs, avoid straining, use caution with aspirin use, exercise regularly, and maintain proper cholesterol levels.

Factors that put individuals at higher risk for aneurysms that cannot always be prevented or controlled include family history of aneurysms, hypertension or high cholesterol, natural aging, and diabetes. Secondary types of hypertension that could put an individual at high risk for aneurysms include renal disease, pheochromocytoma, Cushing syndrome, thyroid or pituitary dysfunction, and/or pregnancy.

Pharmaceutical approaches to atherosclerosis treatment

Treatment recommendations for atherosclerosis are based on the size and location of the plaque. Typically, plaques found early can be treated successfully with pharmacologic approaches. Pharmacologic agents are typically used first line to decrease blood viscosity, and reduce the risk of detachment or plaque size.

Pharmacologic agents used for the treatment of the disease include cholesterol-lowering medications such as statins. Anti-platelet medications are also used such as aspirin, ticlopidine, and clopidogrel. In situations where the atherosclerotic plaque is unstable, anticoagulants like heparin and warfarin are used. Concomitant risk factors are also treated including antihypertensives (beta-blockers, calcium channel blockers, angiotensin-converting enzyme [ACE] inhibitors) for hypertension, anti-diabetic medications for diabetes, and pharmacological agents for smoking cessation.

Lifestyle modifications and surgical approaches to atherosclerosis treatment

Lifestyle modifications include physical exercise, healthy diet, dietary supplementation, smoking cessation and treatment of comorbid conditions.

However, surgery may be performed if a plaque is large, inhibiting blood flow, and/or at risk for embolizing. Surgery or other procedures are used for individuals that present with more severe symptoms such as end organ dysfunction. Surgical approaches include angioplasty, endarterectomy, thrombolytic therapy, and bypass surgery. These approaches are used to physically expand narrowed arteries or create new additional blood supply connections.

Prevention of atherosclerosis

Preventing the onset of atherosclerotic plaque formation and/or progression of atherosclerosis includes stress reduction, smoking cessation, maintaining a diet low in saturated fats and sodium, physical exercise, as well as maintaining proper body mass index, blood pressure, blood sugar, and cholesterol levels. Patients should also reduce their homocysteine levels.

Patients with multiple risk factors should consult a practicing clinician to reduce prophylactically the risk of developing cardiovascular disease or experiencing heart attack and/or stroke.

Factors that put individuals at higher risk for plaque formation that cannot always be prevented or controlled include family history and natural aging.

Treatment and prevention of Buerger's disease

The main treatment for patients with Buerger's disease is smoking cessation, which will halt progression of the disease. Individuals who continue to smoke with Buerger's disease will likely have their digits amputated. Patients who need help to quit smoking should consult with their practicing clinician for alternatives like nicotine gum or patches.

Other options for the treatment of Buerger's disease include anti-coagulation agents or anti-platelet agents to improve blood flow, surgery to cut nerves in infected painful areas, as well as digit amputation due to extensive infection or gangrene. Experimental therapies with prostaglandins and thrombolytics have been used experimentally with some success.

Patients with Buerger's disease should dress any cuts or scrapes in the affected areas to prevent infection. Any cuts or scrapes that do not heal properly or in a timely manner should be addressed by a clinical practitioner.

The cause of Buerger's disease remains unclear, but has been strongly linked to cigarette smoking and tobacco use. Therefore, smoking cessation is essential to preventing the onset and progression of the disease. Overall, the underlying mechanism of Buerger's disease is immunologic, but remains unknown.

Buerger's disease is typically not life threatening, but the death rate is higher in patients that continue to smoke and due to other comorbid conditions such as emphysema or cancer. The disease is associated with amputation in up to 36% of patients. Major amputations are nearly twice as common in patients who continue to smoke.

Treatment and prevention of Raynaud's phenomenon

Treatment of Raynaud's phenomenon involves self-care for patients with mild forms of the phenomenon including keeping hands and feet warm and avoiding trauma to digits. However, in more moderate to severe cases, pharmacologic management to reduce degree and extent of condition as well as to prevent tissue damage and treat any underlying causes of the condition can be used.

Pharmacologic agents used in the treatment of Raynaud's phenomenon include calcium channel blockers to dilate blood vessels, alpha-blockers to counteract the constriction of blood vessels as well as vasodilators to dilate and relax blood vessels.

Patients diagnosed with Raynaud's phenomenon should avoid over the counter agents such as cold remedies that contain pseudoephedrine, beta-blockers, and oral contraceptives due to impact on blood circulation. They should also avoid stress and occupational hazards, such as tools that vibrate the hands.

Other options for patients with severe primary or secondary Raynaud's phenomenon include nerve surgery to reduce frequency and duration of symptoms, chemical injection to block sympathetic nerves affected and/or amputation due to the development of infection or gangrene.

Patients diagnosed with the condition should dress warmly in cold climates, take precautions outdoors, and consider moving to a warmer climate.

Self-care approaches that can reduce the degree and frequency of Raynaud's phenomenon include smoking cessation, physical activity, stress management, avoidance of vasoconstrictors such as caffeine, maintain hands and feet carefully avoid stress triggers and occupational hazards.

In order to avoid complications, individuals having a Raynaud's attack should move to a warmer area, wiggle fingers and toes to stimulate blood circulation, place hands/feet behind knee caps, under armpits, under warm water and/or massage hands and feet. Also, relaxation techniques such as cognitive behavior therapy, biofeedback, breathing techniques or meditation may also improve Raynaud's symptoms when stress triggers the attack.

Cardiomyopathy treatment and prevention

Treatment of cardiomyopathy depends on the type, extent, and degree of disease. Patients with mild disease may only require lifestyle modifications and short-term pharmacologic treatment, whereas patients with more moderate-severe disease may require pharmacologic management and/or surgery. Lifestyle modifications include smoking cessation, diet low in saturated fats and sodium, physical activity, alcohol and drug cessation, weight loss in overweight individuals, resting, reducing stress, and treating underlying comorbidities such as diabetes and high blood pressure. The goals of cardiomyopathy management include treatment of comorbid conditions such as diabetes and congestive heart failure, control symptoms, prevent disease progression, and reduce associated risks and complications. Pharmacologic agents used for the treatment of cardiomyopathy include diuretics, ACE inhibitors, beta-blockers, calcium channel blockers, anticoagulants, antiarrhythmia agents, antibiotics and corticosteroids. Surgical approaches include septal myectomy, surgically implanted devices such as left ventricular devices or implantable cardioverter defibrillators and heart transplant. Another nonsurgical approach used by clinical practitioners is alcohol septal ablation, which uses ethanol to shrink thickened tissue in the myocardium.

Dilated cardiomyopathies can be treated with a combination of pharmacologic agents and/or surgical approaches. Pharmacologic agents used for treatment of this condition include angiotensin-converting enzyme (ACE) inhibitors, angiotensin-receptor blockers, and beta-blockers. For more serious cases of dilated cardiomyopathies, implantable cardioverter defibrillators (ICDs) or pacemakers may be implanted to coordinate the contractions between the left and right ventricles and reduce the chance of sudden cardiac death.

Hypertrophic cardiomyopathy can also be treated with a combination of pharmacologic agents and/or surgical approaches. Pharmacologic agents include beta-blockers and calcium channel blockers. Other surgical options include implantation of ICDs or pacemakers and septal myectomy. Alcohol ablation is another option for patients not candidates for surgery.

Restrictive cardiomyopathy treatment involves symptom management. Self-care is recommended in which patients monitor sodium and water intake. Pharmacologic agents may also be recommended including diuretics, antihypertensive agents, and antiarrhythmia agents.

Cardiomyopathy can be prevented by managing comorbidities and environmental factors. Although patients with familial cardiomyopathy cannot prevent onset of disease, they can reduce extent and degree of disease through self-care and proper disease management. In order to prevent onset of cardiomyopathy and decrease disease progression, individuals should avoid alcohol and drug consumption, avoid smoking, maintain proper blood pressure, eat diet low in saturated fats and sodium and maintain an active lifestyle.

Patients should also undergo regular examinations by their clinical practitioner, follow practitioner's advice regarding cardiomyopathy management and adhere to pharmacologic treatment regimens.

Congestive heart failure treatment and prevention

Treatment of congestive heart failure depends on the extent and degree of disease. Patients with mild disease may only require lifestyle modifications and short-term pharmacologic treatment, whereas patients with more moderate-severe disease may require pharmacologic management and/or surgery. Lifestyle modifications include smoking cessation, diet low in saturated fats and sodium, reduced fluid intake, physical activity depending on patient's health, alcohol and drug cessation, weight loss in overweight individuals, resting, reducing stress, treating underlying comorbidities such as diabetes and high blood pressure.

The goals of treatment include controlling excess fluid accumulation, improving cardiac function and reducing cardiac workload.

Treatment guidelines recommend that patients with congestive heart failure should not intake more than 2000 mg of sodium per day. Patients need to aggressively monitor their body weight, as rapid weight gain could be due to fluid accumulation. Therefore, if patients experience weight gain of more than 2 to 3 lbs over 2 to 3 days, they should contact their clinical practitioner immediately.

Pharmacologic agents used for the treatment of congestive heart failure include diuretics, ACE inhibitors, digoxin, beta-blockers, calcium channel blockers, anticoagulants, antiarrhythmia agents, antibiotics, and corticosteroids.

Surgical approaches include coronary artery surgery or catheter procedures, such as angioplasty or intracoronary stenting, to restore blood flow. Other options include heart transplantation, left ventricular assist devices, and pacemakers.

Congestive heart failure can be prevented by managing comorbidities and environmental factors. Although patients with familial congestive heart failure cannot prevent onset of disease, they can reduce extent and degree of disease through self-care and proper disease management.

In order to prevent onset of congestive heart failure or decrease disease progression, individuals should avoid alcohol and drug consumption, avoid smoking, maintain proper blood pressure, eat a diet low in saturated fats and sodium, reduce fluid intake, treat other comorbidities and maintain an active lifestyle.

Patients should also undergo regular examinations by their clinical practitioner, follow the practitioner's advice regarding congestive heart failure management, and adhere to pharmacologic treatment regimens.

Teatment and prevention of cor pulmonale

Current treatments reduce symptoms and complications of disease, which are geared toward addressing the underlying cause of the disease. The type of treatment depends on whether cor pulmonale occurs acutely or evolves chronically.

The use of pharmaceutical agents such as vasodilators (nifedipine and other calcium channel blockers), diuretics (furosemide), anticoagulants (warfarin), cardiac glycosides (digoxin), methylxanthines (theophylline), and endothelin receptor antagonists (bosentan) can be used for treatment of Cor Pulmonale.

In some patients, the disease can progress rapidly, while in others the disease can become chronically maintained. Surgery is an option for advanced cases where heart defects are the source of failure. Also, in more severe cases, heart and/or lung transplantation may be recommended.

Supplemental oxygen may also be prescribed to increase blood oxygen levels.

Prevention of cor pulmonale includes avoidance of environmental factors that can lead to chronic pulmonary hypertension such as cigarette smoking, tobacco use, and inhalation of toxic fumes, chemicals and/or smoke. A pulmonary specialist should monitor patients with cardiopulmonary disease in order to prevent the onset of cor pulmonale. Adolescents with serious heart murmurs caused by various cardiac defects should be monitored and treated throughout their lifespan in order to prevent onset of cor pulmonale.

Supplemental oxygen may prevent further worsening of cor pulmonale and underlying disease progression. Oxygen supplementation also improves survival, decreases symptom burden, and improves patient quality of life.

Treatment approaches for type I and type II diabetes

Treatment of both type I and type II diabetes involves management of short-term and long-term complications. Proper lifestyle modifications as well as pharmaceutical management need to be maintained in an effort to prevent long-term complications such as coronary artery disease, peripheral vascular disease, and vision problems. Patients also need to monitor their blood sugar levels on a daily basis and comply with treatment recommendations.

Patients need to make lifestyle modifications including diet, exercise and smoking cession. Pharmacologic management, including proper insulin or oral diabetic agent usage, is also necessary.

Lifestyle modifications and pharmaceutical treatment of type II diabetes

For type II diabetes, patients need to maintain a healthy diet, exercise, and comply with oral pharmacologic agents and insulin regimens. In some cases, type II diabetes can be cured with gastric bypass surgery in obese patients.

Pharmaceutical agents used for treatment of type II diabetes include sulfonylurea agents such as glipizide, glyburide, and glimepiride; meglitinides such as repaglinide; biguanides such as metformin; thiazolidinediones such as pioglitazone and rosiglitazone; dipeptidyl inhibitors such as sitagliptin; incretin mimetics such as exenatide; amylin analogs such as pramlintide acetate; and alpha glucosidase inhibitors such as acarbose and miglitol.

Lifestyle modifications and pharmaceutical treatment

Type I diabetes
For type I diabetes, patients need to maintain a consistent healthy weight and exercise routine as well as maintain compliance with insulin use. Blood sugar monitoring is of extreme importance to avoid the extreme highs and lows, both of which can be life threatening. They also need to avoid smoking and/or tobacco use to decrease risk of cardiovascular complications.

Type I diabetes pharmacologic approaches include antidiabetic agents such as insulin lispro, insulin NPH, protamine zinc, insulin aspart, insulin glargine and insulin glulisine. There is no cure for type I diabetes and management of the disease requires chronic care. However, pancreatic transplantation, islet cell transplantation and stem cell transplantation are possible cures for type I diabetes, but are currently investigational and not always successful.

Type II diabetes
Onset of type I and type II diabetes can be attributed to both genetic as well as environmental factors. Therefore, certain steps can be taken to control environmental triggers, but nothing can be done to prevent the genetic contribution. However, type I diabetes is typically not preventable, as the disease is associated with a larger genetic contribution.

Prevention of type II diabetes involves maintaining a healthy diet rich in proteins, fruits, and vegetables and low in saturated fats, increasing physical activity with 2 1/2 hours of exercise per week, management of other comorbid conditions, and maintaining proper body fat and weight for an individual's height.

Other preventative measures for type I and type II diabetes are under investigation and not recommended by the American Diabetes Association, such as copper supplementation and niacin.

Treatment and prevention of metabolic syndrome

Currently, there are no set guidelines for the management of metabolic syndrome. However, the overall goal is to reduce an individual's risk of developing cardiovascular disease and development of type II diabetes. It is recommended to encourage patients to maintain proper diet and exercise, avoid smoking and tobacco use, lose excess weight, maintain proper lipid levels, maintain proper blood pressure levels, maintain proper glucose levels, and maintain proper albumin excretion and creatinine levels.

Pharmacologic agents used to treat metabolic syndrome include lipid-lowering agents, antihypertensives, anticoagulants and diabetic agents such as oral agents and insulin.

Certain risk factors such as having a genetic predisposition for metabolic syndrome and natural aging are unpreventable. To prevent the onset, individuals need to maintain proper diet and exercise, avoid smoking and tobacco use, lose excess weight, maintain proper lipid levels, maintain proper blood pressure levels, maintain proper sugar levels, and maintain proper albumin excretion and creatinine levels.

Metabolic syndrome is a chronic condition that needs to be managed by lifestyle modifications and pharmacologic management of comorbid conditions. Patients should carefully watch their waistline measurement and calculate their body mass index in order to prevent abdominal obesity.

Treatment of endothelial dysfunction

Comorbid conditions that can lead to the development of endothelial dysfunction include septic shock, hypertension, hypercholesterolemia, congestive heart failure, peripheral artery disease, chronic renal failure, diabetes, and insulin resistance. Another factor that can increase the risk of developing endothelial dysfunction is smoking and/or tobacco use.

Treatment of endothelial dysfunction involves dietary changes and increased physical activity. Pharmacologic agents such as anticoagulants, antihypertensive agents and lipid-lowering agents may be used to treat comorbid conditions and reduce an individual's risk for developing cardiovascular disease.

Treatment and prevention of hypertension

The treatment of hypertension involves lifestyle modification and pharmacologic management. Lifestyle modifications include weight loss, diet low in saturated fats and sodium, physical activity, smoking cessation, limiting tobacco use and stress reduction.

The goals of pharmacologic management include reduction of blood pressure in order to prevent onset of comorbid conditions and/or complications. Pharmacologic agents include diuretics such as hydrochlorothiazide, spironolactone, amiloride and furosemide; alpha-1-adrenergic blockers including prazosin; beta-adrenergic blockers such as atenolol; alpha/beta-adrenergic blockers such as labetalol; peripheral vasodilators such as hydralazine; calcium channel blockers such as diltiazem; angiotensin-converting enzyme inhibitors such as captopril; angiotensin II receptor antagonists such as losartan; aldosterone antagonists such as eplerenone; alpha-adrenergic agonists such as methyldopa; and renin inhibitors such as aliskiren.

Patients with diabetes and/or renal disease should be treated with pharmacologic approaches at a blood pressure of 130/80 mmHg or below due to increased risk of cardiovascular events.

Certain risk factors such as having a genetic predisposition for hypertension and natural aging are not preventable. However, certain aspects of hypertension can help reduce the onset of the condition by having individuals maintain a diet low in sodium and saturated fats, increase potassium intake, increase exercise and physical activity, avoid smoking and tobacco use, lose excess weight, maintain proper lipid levels, maintain proper sugar levels and maintain proper albumin excretion and creatinine levels.

Treatment of comorbid conditions is necessary to prevent the onset of secondary hypertension. Also, individuals being prescribed oral contraceptives, NSAIDs or other pharmacologic agents that can elevate blood pressure should monitor their blood pressure on a daily basis if at risk for hypertension or cardiovascular complications.

Pharmacologic agents

Elevated triglyceride (TG) levels and decreased high-density lipoprotein (HDL) cholesterol levels in dyslipidemia management

Pharmacologic agents used for the treatment of elevated triglyceride levels include fibrates such as gemfibrozil, ciprofibrate, clofibrate, fenofibrate and bezafibrate; nicotinic acid such as niacin; and statins such as fluvastatin, lovastatin, simvastatin, pravastatin, atorvastatin and rosuvastatin. Another approach that has been demonstrated to be effective in lowering triglyceride levels includes high doses of omega-3 fatty acids.

Elevated low-density lipoprotein (LDL) levels

Pharmacologic agents used for treatment depend on the type of lipid abnormality, even though multiple lipid abnormalities may present together. The goal of low-density lipoprotein levels is 100 mg/dL or below, but recent evidence suggests lower target of 70 mg/dL. Lipid-lowering approaches available include statins such as fluvastatin, lovastatin, simvastatin, pravastatin, atorvastatin, and rosuvastatin; nicotinic acid such as niacin; bile acid sequestrants such as cholestyramine, colestipol, and colesevelam; fibrates such as gemfibrozil, ciprofibrate, clofibrate, fenofibrate, and bezafibrate; cholesterol absorption agents such as ezetimibe; and combination agents such as extended release niacin/lovastatin.

Treatment of dyslipidemia

Individuals are typically diagnosed with dyslipidemia during routine physical examinations or when seeking medical attention for other complaints. Xanthelasma, or yellow streaks on the eyelids, and xanthomas, yellow nodules on tendons, can be suggestive. Diagnostic testing involves measurement of fasting serum lipid levels including low-density lipoprotein levels, high-density lipoprotein levels and triglyceride levels. Diagnostic tests for secondary causes of dyslipidemia should be performed including fasting serum glucose level, liver enzymes, creatinine levels, thyroid-stimulating hormone, and urinalysis.

Dyslipidemia does not typically present with any specific symptoms unless associated with comorbid cardiovascular disease including coronary artery disease or peripheral artery disease. Increased low-density lipoprotein levels may cause symptoms including vision problems and joint problems. Individuals with elevated triglyceride levels may also present with vision and joint problems as well.

Complications, prognosis, and prevention of dyslipidemia

The main complication associated with dyslipidemia is cardiovascular disease complications such as heart attack, stroke, and sudden death. However, aggressive treatment with lipid-lowering agents such as statins has been shown to reduce plaque formation and onset of cardiovascular disease.

Certain risk factors, such as having a genetic predisposition for dyslipidemia and natural aging, are not preventable. However, certain complications of dyslipidemia can be prevented by having individuals maintain a diet low in sodium and saturated fats, increase potassium intake, increase exercise and physical activity, avoid smoking and tobacco use, lose excess weight, maintain proper lipid levels, and maintain proper glucose levels.

Treatment and prevention of myocardial infarction

In individuals who experience an acute myocardial infarction, practicing clinicians should initiate oxygen, aspirin and sub lingual glyceryl trinitrate therapies to prevent further myocardium damage and/or complications. Invasive approaches for the treatment of myocardial infarction and underlying comorbid conditions include thrombolysis, percutaneous coronary intervention, angioplasty and stent insertion. In more severe cases, with invasive plaque formation or multiple blockages, cardiopulmonary bypass surgery may be performed.

Upon myocardial infarction diagnosis, pharmacologic agents prescribed include antithrombotic agents such as aspirin; blood thinners such as heparin and enoxaparin; vasodilators such as nitroglycerin; beta-adrenergic blockers such as metoprolol and esmolol; thrombolytic agents such as alteplase, anistreplase and tenecteplase; platelet aggregation inhibitors such as clopidogrel, eptifibatide and tirofiban; analgesics such as morphine sulfate; and angiotensin-converting enzyme inhibitors such as captopril.

Post myocardial infarction, patients are recommended to make lifestyle modifications including a diet with low fat and low sodium foods, increased physical activity, smoking and alcohol cessation as well as stress reduction. It is also recommended to comply with pharmacologic treatment regimens despite their complexity.

Lifestyle modifications and pharmacologic management can prevent the onset of myocardial infarction as well as recurrent myocardial infarction in patients with a previous occurrence. Patients should maintain a diet low in sodium and saturated fats, increase potassium intake, increase exercise and physical activity, avoid smoking and tobacco use, lose excess weight, maintain proper lipid levels, and control diabetes if present.

Patients with previous myocardial infarction who comply with lifestyle modification and pharmacologic management are at a much lower risk for recurrent disease. Pharmacologic agents used to prevent recurrent myocardial infarction include antiplatelet agents such as aspirin or clopidogrel, beta-blockers such as metoprolol or carvedilol, ACE inhibitor agents and statin therapy. Other approaches include aldosterone antagonists such as eplerenone and omega-3 fatty acids.

Treatment and prevention of stroke

An acute stroke is a medical emergency and requires immediate medical attention. Individuals experiencing an ischemic stroke should seek medical attention within 3 hours of onset to receive anti-coagulant and/or thrombolytic approaches to restore blood flow. Other surgical approaches include carotid endarterectomy, angioplasty, and catheter embolectomy. Pharmacologic approaches used post stroke include anti-platelet agents and anti-coagulants.

Surgical approaches are typically used to treat hemorrhagic stroke including aneurysm coiling, coiling, and arteriovenous malformation (AVM) removal.

Pharmacologic agents used to treat stroke include fibrinolytic agents such as alteplase and anti-platelet agents such as aspirin and ticlopidine.

Please note that acute lowering of blood pressure during a stroke is NOT part of the treatment as it is important to maintain perfusion pressure to the brain.

Preventive measures that individuals can take to reduce the risk of stroke include maintaining proper lipid levels, blood pressure, healthy weight, healthy diet low in sodium and saturated fats, avoiding smoking, controlling diabetes, exercising regularly, managing stress and anxiety, reducing alcohol consumption, and avoiding illicit drug use.

The American Heart Association recommends that individuals over the age of 20 undergo risk factor screening, which includes blood pressure measurement, body mass index, waist circumference and cholesterol and glucose monitoring at least every 2 to 5 years.

Prevention involves primary, secondary, and tertiary prevention. Primary prevention involves reduction of risk factors such as smoking cessation and other behavioral measures. Secondary prevention involves reduction of risk factors in individuals at an increased risk for stroke. Tertiary prevention involves reduction of risk factors in individuals who have already experienced a transient ischemic attack or an acute stroke.

Treatment and prevention of peripheral arterial disease

Treatment of peripheral arterial disease involves lifestyle modifications and pharmacologic management. Lifestyle changes including smoking cessation, increased physical activity, and dietary changes, may improve symptoms and complications of peripheral arterial disease.

Pharmacologic agents used in peripheral arterial disease and comorbid conditions include anti-platelet agents, lipid-lowering agents, anti-hypertensive agents, diabetes agents, anti-thrombolytic agents, and symptom-relief medications. The goal of treatment is to prevent the onset of complications.

Surgical approaches used for patients with peripheral arterial disease and intermittent claudication include angioplasty. Other surgical approaches used for peripheral arterial disease include transcatheter intervention and peripheral vascular bypass.

Lifestyle modifications and pharmacologic management prevent the onset of arteriosclerosis and peripheral arterial disease. Patients should maintain a diet low in sodium and saturated fats, increase potassium intake, increase exercise and physical activity, avoid smoking and tobacco use, lose excess weight, avoidance of illicit drug use, maintain proper lipid levels, maintain proper sugar levels and control complications of diabetes.

Patients with peripheral arterial disease should practice good foot hygiene to prevent the onset of complications such as infections and gangrene. Patients should wash their feet daily and moisturize them, wear thick socks and comfortable shoes, promptly treat fungal infections, trim toe nails, avoid walking barefoot and immediately have sores and open wounds treated.

Treatment of inflammatory disease

The treatment of inflammation and inflammatory disease depends on the organ systems being affected. Treatment options include lifestyle modifications such as diet, exercise and rehabilitation, pharmacologic approaches and surgery. The type of treatment approach depends on patient's health status, age, extent and degree of disease, presence of other comorbid conditions, medical history, and type of pharmacologic agents already being prescribed.

Pharmacologic agents used include analgesics, anti-inflammatory agents such as nonsteroidal anti-inflammatory agents, corticosteroids, anti-malarial agents such as hydroxychloroquine and other agents including methotrexate, sulfoalanine, leflunomide, anti-tumor necrosis factor medications, cyclophosphamide and mycophenolate. Other pharmacologic agents may be used to treat specific inflammatory conditions affecting specific organ systems.

Prevention of cardiovascular disease with inflammatory biomarkers

Inflammation is an important mechanism present in cardiovascular diseases such as atherosclerosis. In cardiovascular disease, acute phase inflammation occurs in the presence of C - reactive protein. Therefore, screening patients for the presence of C - reactive protein may be a proactive approach to reducing the risk of congestive heart failure, heart attack, and stroke. C-reactive protein may also be a good biomarker in predicting recurrent disease in patients with previous heart attack, stroke, and/or persistent cardiovascular disease. Recent data has demonstrated that the higher the C - reactive protein levels, the higher the risk of heart attack and/or stroke.

Atherosclerosis is actually an inflammatory response to development of lipids in arteries, with every step of atherosclerotic disease responding to inflammatory signaling mechanisms.

Treatment and prevention of pericarditis

Treatment goals
Treatment of pericarditis involves lifestyle modifications, pharmacologic approaches, and surgery. Treatment depends on the extent and degree of pericarditis as well as the patient's overall health, age, diet, physical activity, and/or presence of other comorbid conditions. In some more mild cases, pericarditis may resolve itself on its own without medical intervention. However, in cases that are more moderate to severe, pharmacologic agents and/or surgical approaches may be used based on the underlying cause of the condition.

Lifestyle modifications may include reduction of physical activity as well as increased rest and relaxation until condition resolves.

Pharmacologic agents and surgical approaches used to treat pericarditis
Pharmacologic agents include anti-inflammatory agents such as nonsteroidal anti-inflammatory agents, narcotics such as morphine, or colchicine, diuretics, antifungals, antibiotics, aspirin, and corticosteroids.

Surgical approaches may be used in severe cases of pericarditis including pericardiocentesis, pericardiotomy, and pericardiectomy. Pericardiocentesis is a procedure that uses a catheter to remove excess fluid from the pericardium. Pericardiectomy involves removal of the entire pericardium. This procedure is typically reserved for patients with constrictive pericarditis.

Prevention of pericarditis

Acute and chronic pericarditis are typically not preventable, but diseases associated with pericarditis are preventable. For example, decreasing the risk of myocardial infarction or regular dialysis in patients with diabetes to avoid uremia will decrease the risk of pericarditis.

Early intervention with pericarditis may prevent onset of complications such as pericardial effusion, arrhythmias, constrictive pericarditis and cardiac tamponade as well as decrease risk for reoccurrence of the condition.

Treatment and prevention of vasculitis

Treatment of vasculitis involves lifestyle modifications, pharmacologic approaches, and surgery. The goal of treatment is to address the underlying cause of the condition and organ systems involved. Early intervention prevents onset of complications.

Pharmacologic approaches include corticosteroids such as prednisone, prednisolone, and methylprednisolone to reduce inflammation; cytotoxic drugs such as azathioprine and cyclophosphamide to suppress inflammation; and nonsteroidal anti-inflammatory agents such as aspirin and ibuprofen to treat mild symptoms. Other pharmacologic approaches used for treatment of vasculitis include anticoagulants such as heparin and enoxaparin; immunodulators such as immune globulin; antibiotics such as trimethoprim-sulfamethoxazole; and stronger anti-inflammatory agents such as methotrexate.

Pharmacologic agents under clinical investigation for the treatment of vasculitis include mycophenolate mofetil, tumor necrosis factor inhibitors, and rituximab.

Typically, vasculitis cannot be prevented but early treatment and maintenance of good health promote better outcomes in patients diagnosed with the condition. Also, compliance with treatment recommendations may prevent reoccurrence and/or delay vasculitis onset if detected early.

In the United States, immunization of hepatitis B is standard of care, which may help to prevent onset of vasculitis. Avoiding IV drug use and unprotected sex decreases the risk of hepatitis C and HIV, thus decreasing the risk of vasculitis.

General preventive measures that individuals can take to reduce the risk of vasculitis and disease complications include maintaining proper lipid levels, blood pressure, healthy weight, healthy diet low in sodium and saturated fats, avoiding smoking, controlling diabetes, obtaining adequate vitamin D and calcium, exercising regularly, managing stress and anxiety, reducing alcohol consumption, and avoiding illicit drug use.

Treatment and prevention of endocarditis

The treatment of endocarditis involves the treatment of the underlying condition leading to endocarditis as well as prevention of further progression of the disease. The main goal is to prevent additional complications associated with endocarditis such as heart attack, stroke, and sudden death.

Pharmacologic agents such as intravenous antibiotics including penicillin, gentamicin, vancomycin, rifampin, and linezolid are used to fight infection and nonsteroidal anti-inflammatory agents to

- 73 -

reduce fever, inflammation and associated pain. Most patients are hospitalized initially to receive intravenous antibiotics but will continue oral antibiotics for up to 6 weeks.

Heart valve replacement surgery may be an option for patients experiencing strokes due to the condition, patients with congestive heart failure and evidence of end organ system damage.

Patients at higher risk for endocarditis including those with artificial heart valves, previous endocarditis infection, congenital heart defects, and heart transplant are recommended preventative antibiotics before certain medical and dental procedures.

New 2007 guidelines recommend that patients at high risk for endocarditis undergoing certain dental procedures and procedures involving respiratory tract, infected tissue should be prescribed preventative antibiotics.

Individuals diagnosed with endocarditis should maintain good dental hygiene by brushing teeth, flossing and maintaining gums. They should also avoid procedures that may lead to skin infections including body piercing and tattoos. General preventive measures that individuals can take to reduce the risk of endocarditis and disease complications include maintaining proper lipid levels, blood pressure, healthy weight, healthy diet low in sodium and saturated fats, avoiding smoking, controlling diabetes, exercising regularly, managing stress and anxiety, reducing alcohol consumption, and avoiding illicit drug use, especially intravenous drugs.

Treatment and prevention of renal artery occlusion

The treatment of renal artery occlusion depends on the extent and degree of the condition as well as other organ systems involved. In more severe cases, where patients present with renal failure, surgical intervention may be necessary. Another alternative surgical approach is balloon angioplasty or stenting of renal arteries being affected.

Revascularization is an option in patients with bilateral stenosis, stenosis in a solitary functioning kidney and unilateral stenosis with renal insufficiency. Revascularization is also recommended in patients with normal renal function if their degree of stenosis is more than 80% and if the degree of stenosis is 50% to 80% with activation of intrarenal arterial occlusion. In patients who do not meet these criteria, guidelines recommend practicing clinicians to monitor patients over a 6-month period and then reevaluate.

Pharmacologic agents used to treat associated conditions with renal artery occlusion include angiotensin-converting enzyme inhibitors such as captopril and enalapril, angiotensin II receptor antagonists such as losartan and HMG-coenzyme A reductase inhibitors such as atorvastatin.

Smoking cessation can prevent the onset of renal artery occlusion. General preventive measures that individuals can take to reduce the risk of renal artery occlusion and disease complications include maintaining proper lipid levels, blood pressure, healthy weight, healthy diet low in sodium and saturated fats, avoiding smoking, controlling diabetes, exercising regularly, managing stress and anxiety, reducing alcohol consumption, and avoiding illicit drug use.

In an effort to prevent further progression of renal arterial occlusion, practicing clinicians need to follow patients closely monitoring serum creatine levels, blood pressure levels, serum potassium levels, and complete blood counts. Follow-up ultrasound should also be performed and compared to baseline to determine progression.

Treatment and prevention of renal vein thrombosis

Treatment of renal vein thrombosis involves lifestyle modifications, pharmacologic approaches, and possibly surgery to remove occlusion. However, surgery to remove the occluding factor is rarely performed. Lifestyle modifications include bed rest and/or limited activity for a short period to reduce embolization and new clot formation. Anti-coagulation therapy is the standard pharmacologic approach for management. However, fibrinolytic agents may also be used to dissolve the blood clot.

Pharmacologic agents used to treat renal vein thrombosis include angiotensin-converting enzyme inhibitors such as benazepril, captopril, enalapril, fosinopril, moexipril, perindopril and lisinopril and angiotensin receptor blockers such as candesartan, eprosartan, irbesartan, losartan, telmisartan, and valsartan.

The goal of treatment is to decrease risk of new clot formation, prevent progression of current clots, as well as prevent embolization of formed clots to other organ systems including heart, lungs, and/or brain.

Prevention of renal vein thrombosis is difficult, as it is a rare condition. However, adults can avoid trauma to the abdomen or back, make sure they are properly hydrated and maintain good lifestyle habits.

Infants, toddlers and adolescents with the flu, out in very hot weather or exposed to other factors that can cause severe dehydration, should take preventative measures to avoid dehydration and potential for renal vein thrombosis.

General preventive measures that individuals can take to reduce the risk of renal vein thrombosis and disease complications include maintaining proper lipid levels, blood pressure, healthy weight, healthy diet low in sodium and saturated fats, avoiding smoking, controlling diabetes, exercising regularly, managing stress and anxiety, reducing alcohol consumption, and avoiding illicit drug use.

Treatment and prevention of atheroembolic renal disease

Treatment of atheroembolic renal disease is similar to atherosclerotic treatment. Pharmacologic agents used for the treatment of the disease include cholesterol medications such as statins; anti-platelet medications such as aspirin, ticlopidine, and clopidogrel; anti-coagulants such as heparin and warfarin; anti-hypertensive agents such as ACE inhibitors, beta-blockers, or calcium channel blockers; and other classes of agents for concomitant or predisposing conditions such as diabetes. Patients at high risk for atherosclerosis may also be treated prophylactically with low dose aspirin and/or statins.

Lifestyle modifications are also recommended, which include maintaining proper lipid levels, blood pressure, glucose levels, healthy weight, healthy diet low in sodium and saturated fats, avoiding smoking, controlling diabetes, exercising regularly, managing stress and anxiety, reducing alcohol consumption, and avoiding illicit drug use. Lifestyle modifications can help prevent the progression of disease and initial onset of atheroembolic renal disease and/or atherosclerosis. However, pharmacologic management has not been demonstrated to improve patient outcomes or prevent onset of disease.

General preventive measures that individuals can take to reduce the risk of atheroembolic renal disease and disease complications include maintaining proper lipid levels, blood pressure, glucose levels, healthy weight, healthy diet low in sodium and saturated fats, avoiding smoking, controlling diabetes, exercising regularly, managing stress and anxiety, reducing alcohol consumption, and avoiding illicit drug use.

Treatment and prevention of Marfan syndrome

There are no treatments currently available to treat Marfan syndrome directly. However, practicing clinicians can address complications of the condition such as cardiovascular, skeletal, and eye complications.

Pharmacologic agents used to treat Marfan syndrome with cardiovascular complications include antihypertensive agents such as beta-blockers, calcium channel blocker, angiotensin-converting enzyme inhibitors, or angiotensin receptor inhibitors. Surgical approaches include aorta composite graft repair or an aortic valve sparing technique. The extent of surgery depends on how much of the aorta is involved.

For skeletal complications, a back brace may be used to treat scoliosis. Other options for scoliosis include surgery to correct the curvature of the spine as well as posterior spinal fusion. Surgery may also be an option for children with a concave chest that affects their breathing capabilities.

For eye complications such as dislocated lens, patients may wear glasses or undergo intraocular lens implant surgery. Glaucoma is not curable but can be treated with eye drops, oral agents, and surgical approaches. Patients with cataracts can undergo surgery to correct the problem.

Pharmacologic agents used for the treatment of Marfan syndrome include beta-adrenergic inhibiting agents such as atenolol and calcium channel blockers such as verapamil hydrochloride. Other antihypertensive agents may be used in combination or as second-line therapy in patients who either fail first-line approaches or who cannot tolerate adverse events. Other pharmacologic approaches can be used to treat other complications of the condition including agents directed toward the skeletal system and other cardiovascular agents. However, pharmacologic agents will not cure the Marfan syndrome but will treat the complications of the syndrome. Yet, progression of complications may continue even with pharmacologic management. Therefore, lifestyle modifications and surgery may be other options.

Pregnancy is not recommended for women with Marfan syndrome due to risk of aortic dissection and rupture. Also, women can pass the disease to their offspring; therefore, not having children is the only way to prevent passing the disease onto offspring.

General preventive measures that individuals can take to reduce the risk of Marfan syndrome and disease complications include maintaining proper lipid levels, blood pressure, glucose levels, healthy weight, healthy diet low in sodium and saturated fats, avoiding smoking, controlling diabetes, managing stress and anxiety, reducing alcohol consumption, and avoiding illicit drug use. Physical activity is recommended based on the type of organ systems affected by Marfan syndrome.

Treatment and prevention of atrial septal defect

In patients with atrial septal defects with few or no symptoms, treatment may not be required, especially in patients with a small defect. However, in patients with larger defects, surgical closure is recommended. Devices such as the Amplatzer device may be used to close the defect using catheterization. Minimally invasive surgical approaches may be used to prevent use of blood or blood products in certain patients.

In some cases, especially in very young patients or elderly patients, prophylactic antibiotics may be administered prior to surgery to prevent onset of infective endocarditis post surgery. Also, postsurgical care to prevent onset of infective endocarditis may also be recommended. Pharmacologic management does not fix the defect, but can be used to alleviate some of the symptoms associated with the condition. Pharmacologic agents that may be recommended include beta-blockers such as metoprolol, propranolol, and digoxin, diuretics such as furosemide, and anti-coagulants such as warfarin, and anti-platelet agents such as aspirin.

Since atrial septal defects are inherited, they cannot be prevented. However, addressing the defect earlier on in the progression of the condition may prevent complications associated with the condition. Yet, the only way to prevent potential transmission of atrial septal defects is not to have children. However, in some cases, the disease arises from new genetic mutations during pregnancy.

Treatment and prevention of pulmonary embolism

Treatment of pulmonary embolism involves lifestyle modifications, pharmacologic management and, in more severe cases, surgery. Immediate treatment with anti-coagulation therapy is necessary for patients with suspected pulmonary embolism, as treatment decreases mortality risk.

Fibrinolytic therapy is recommended for patients who are hemodynamically unstable, right heart strain, exhausted cardiopulmonary reserves, and those at risk for pulmonary embolism reoccurrence. Long-term anti-coagulation therapy is considered for patients diagnosed with pulmonary embolism to prevent reoccurrence.

Pharmacologic agents used for pulmonary embolism include fibrinolytics such as reteplase, alteplase, and urokinase and anticoagulants such as enoxaparin, tinzaparin, unfractionated heparin, and warfarin.

Pulmonary embolism may occur post-surgically or as a result of other cardiovascular conditions. Therefore, hospitals take a prophylactic approach to prevent pulmonary embolism. Preventative strategies include heparin or warfarin therapy, use of graduated compression stockings, use of pneumatic compression, and increased physical activity.

Preventative measures individuals at high risk can take while traveling include increasing physical activity, exercising while seated by flexing and extending legs, using compression stockings, staying well hydrated, and using anti-coagulants for long trips.

General preventive measures that individuals can take to reduce the risk of pulmonary embolism and disease complications include maintaining proper lipid levels, blood pressure, glucose levels, healthy weight, healthy diet low in sodium and saturated fats, avoiding smoking, exercising regularly, controlling diabetes, managing stress and anxiety, reducing alcohol consumption, and avoiding illicit drug use.

Treatment and prevention of deep venous thrombosis

The goals of treatment of deep venous thrombosis are to prevent pulmonary embolism and other complications associated with the condition. Treatment also aims to prevent the reoccurrence of formation of additional blood clots. Treatment involves lifestyle management, pharmacologic therapy, and, in more severe cases, surgical approaches. Pharmacologic management involves the use of anticoagulation therapy such as warfarin and/or heparin. Other pharmacologic approaches include antithrombotic agents and thrombolytics. Additional types of treatment include vena cava filter and graduated compression stockings.

Pharmacologic agents for deep venous thrombosis include anticoagulation therapy such as fondaparinux sodium, dalteparin, warfarin, enoxaparin, and tinzaparin and thrombolytics such as tenecteplase, urokinase, streptokinase, and alteplase.

Preventative strategies for deep venous thrombosis and risk of pulmonary embolism include heparin or warfarin therapy, use of graduated compression stockings, use of pneumatic compression, and increased physical activity.

Preventative measures individuals at high risk can take while traveling include increasing physical activity, exercising while seated by flexing and extending legs, using compression stockings, staying well hydrated, and using anti-coagulants for long trips.

Treatment and prevention of venous insufficiency

The goal of treatment of venous insufficiency is to alleviate symptoms and address the underlying cause of the condition.

Treatment of venous insufficiency involves lifestyle modifications, pharmacologic management and, in some very severe cases, surgery. However, lifestyle modifications including bed rest to reduce leg swelling, avoiding prolonged periods of standing or sitting as well as the use of graduated compression stockings are the most common and effective approaches. Other more invasive approaches include valvuloplasty, radiofrequency ablation, vein stripping with ligation, sclerotherapy, skin grafting, and endovenous laser therapy.

Pharmacologic agents used to treat venous insufficiency include sclerosing agents such as sodium tetradecyl sulfate, antibiotics for infection and corticosteroids for associated inflammation.

Mild skin infections can be treated with antibiotics and/or steroids. Skin ulcerations can be treated with ointments, antibiotics, steroids and, in more severe cases, surgery.

Individuals with a family history of venous insufficiency should discuss prevention options with their practicing clinician. Also, individuals who are on their feet for long periods of the day with other cardiovascular comorbid conditions should consider the use of compression stockings.

General preventive measures that individuals can take to reduce the risk of venous insufficiency and disease complications include maintaining proper lipid levels, blood pressure, glucose levels, healthy weight, healthy diet low in sodium and saturated fats, avoiding smoking, controlling diabetes, managing stress and anxiety, reducing alcohol consumption, and avoiding illicit drug use.

Treatment and prevention of valvular disease

Lifestyle modifications, pharmacologic management, and surgery are approaches used to treat valvular disease. The goal of treatment is to reverse the underlying cause of the disease and/or alleviate symptoms in more mild cases. Treatment of valvular disease depends on the degree and extent of disease as well as the presence of other comorbid condition and the individual's overall health.

Pharmacologic treatment does not cure the condition, but does relieve the symptoms of the disease and prevent further complications. Pharmacologic approaches used for valvular disease include vasodilators such as ACE inhibitors, anti-arrhythmic agents, antibiotics, anticoagulants such as Coumadin, diuretics such as furosemide and hydrochlorothiazide, and inotrope.

Surgical approaches include percutaneous balloon valvuloplasty, valvulotomy, cardiac valve repair or replacement and minimally invasive heart surgery.

Congenital defects and infections such as rheumatic fever are the most common causes of valvular disease. Therefore, prompt treatment of streptococcal throat infections is necessary to prevent rheumatic fever. Also, addressing cardiovascular comorbid conditions and receiving proper treatment post myocardial infarction may prevent the onset of valvular disease. Also, proper treatment of connective tissue disease is important as is avoiding risk factors for endocarditis like IV drug use.

General preventive measures that individuals can take to reduce the risk of valvular disease and disease complications include maintaining proper lipid levels, blood pressure, glucose levels, healthy weight, healthy diet low in sodium and saturated fats, avoiding smoking, controlling diabetes, managing stress and anxiety, reducing alcohol consumption, and avoiding illicit drug use.

Treatment and prevention of angina pectoris

Treatment of angina pectoris involves lifestyle modifications, pharmacologic management, and surgery depending on the underlying causes of the condition. The type of treatment used depends on the extent and degree of the underlying cause of angina pectoris.

Pharmacologic management of angina pectoris involves use of antiplatelet agents such as aspirin, anticoagulants like heparin, beta-adrenergic blockers, lipid-lowering agents, nitrates such as nitroglycerin, isosorbide dinitrate and isosorbide mononitrate, and calcium channel blockers such as nifedipine, amlodipine, verapamil, and diltiazem.

Lifestyle modifications include weight loss for obese patients, reduction of saturated fats and sodium in diet, increase in physical activity, cessation of smoking, stress reduction and management, and cessation of alcohol and illicit drug use.

Addressing cardiovascular comorbid conditions and receiving proper treatment post myocardial infarction may prevent the onset of angina pectoris. Also, individuals with a family history of cardiovascular disease and/or a medical history of heart disease should monitor symptoms closely.

General preventive measures that individuals can take to reduce the risk of angina pectoris and disease complications include maintaining proper lipid levels, blood pressure, glucose levels, healthy weight, healthy diet low in sodium and saturated fats, avoiding smoking, controlling diabetes, managing stress and anxiety, reducing alcohol consumption, and avoiding illicit drug use.

Treatment and prevention of atrial fibrillation

The goals of treatment of atrial fibrillation include controlling heart rate, restoring sinus rhythm, controlling ventricular response, preventing complications such as thromboembolism and other cardiovascular complications. Treatment approaches include lifestyle modifications, pharmaceutical management, and use of assistance devices. Electrical conduction management of the heart can be maintained with synchronized electrical cardioversion and permanent atrial pacemaker. Pharmacologic management of atrial fibrillation involves the use of use of beta-adrenergic blockers; digitalis antiplatelet agents like aspirin; anticoagulants such as Coumadin and heparin; antidysrhythmia agents; and calcium channel blockers such as nifedipine, amlodipine, verapamil, and diltiazem. Other pharmacologic agents used to treat comorbid cardiovascular conditions include lipid-lowering agents and nitrates such as nitroglycerin, isosorbide dinitrate, and isosorbide mononitrate. Note that rate control (beta-blockers, etc) with anticoagulation is equivalent to rhythm control with respect to mortality. More invasive approaches include AV node ablation, radiofrequency catheter ablation, and surgical maze procedure.

Addressing cardiovascular comorbid conditions and receiving proper treatment post–myocardial infarction may prevent the onset of atrial fibrillation. Also, individuals with a family history of cardiovascular disease and/or a medical history of heart disease should pay careful attention to their symptoms.

General preventive measures that individuals can take to reduce the risk of atrial fibrillation and disease complications include maintaining proper lipid levels, blood pressure, glucose levels, healthy weight, healthy diet low in sodium and saturated fats, avoiding smoking, controlling diabetes, managing stress and anxiety, reducing alcohol consumption, and avoiding illicit drug use. Also, to make sure respiratory comorbidities like chronic obstructive pulmonary disease (COPD) are under good control, as this is a common source of atrial fibrillation in the elderly.

Treatment and prevention of arrhythmias

The treatment of arrhythmia depends on the type of arrhythmia including bradycardias, supraventricular tachycardias and ventricular tachycardias. In addressing bradycardias, practicing clinicians will assess whether an underlying condition such as thyroid dysfunction is present and treat the underlying cause to correct the problem. Another approach with undetermined bradycardias or necessary medications includes the use of a pacemaker.

In addressing tachycardias originating either in the atria or ventricles, treatment may involve the use of vagal maneuvers such as straining or coughing, anti-arrhythmic agents, cardioversion, and cardiac ablation. Implantable devices such as a pacemaker or implantable cardiac defibrillator may also be used. In more severe cases, surgery may be performed, which involves the maze procedure, ventricular aneurysm surgery, or coronary bypass surgery.

Patients diagnosed with an arrhythmia will be recommended to make lifestyle changes that include maintaining a healthy diet low in saturated fats and sodium, increase physical activity, quit smoking, reduce caffeine and alcohol intake, reduce stress, and avoid stimulants. Vagal maneuvers such as gagging, holding breath, and coughing may be recommended as well.

Addressing cardiovascular comorbid conditions and receiving proper treatment post–myocardial infarction may prevent the onset of arrhythmias. Also, individuals with a family history of cardiovascular disease and/or a medical history of heart disease should pay careful attention to signs and symptoms of disease.

General preventive measures that individuals can take to reduce the risk of arrhythmias and disease complications include maintaining proper lipid levels, blood pressure, glucose levels, healthy weight, healthy diet low in sodium and saturated fats, avoiding smoking, controlling diabetes, managing stress and anxiety, reducing alcohol consumption, and avoiding illicit drug use.

Treatment and prevention of atrial flutter

Lifestyle modifications, pharmacologic management and invasive approaches are used to treat atrial flutter depending on the impact on quality of life and presence of other comorbid conditions. Treatment involves slowing the heart rate and restoring cardiac rhythm as well as prevention of blood clot formation.

Pharmacologic approaches used for the treatment of atrial flutter include calcium channel blockers such as diltiazem and verapamil; beta-blockers such as metoprolol and esmolol; class I anti-arrhythmics such as procainamide and quinidine; class III anti-arrhythmics such as amiodarone, dofetilide, and ibutilide; and cardiac glycosides such as digitalis.

More invasive approaches include cardioversion and catheter ablation. Patients diagnosed with atrial flutter respond better to catheter ablation than patients diagnosed with atrial fibrillation.

Patients diagnosed with atrial flutter will be recommended to make lifestyle changes that include maintaining a healthy diet low in saturated fats and sodium, increasing physical activity, quitting smoking, reducing caffeine and alcohol intake, reducing stress, and avoiding stimulants.

Addressing cardiovascular and respiratory comorbid conditions and receiving proper treatment post myocardial infarction may prevent the onset of atrial flutter or atrial fibrillation. Also, individuals with a family history of cardiovascular disease and/or a medical history of heart disease should pay careful attention to the signs and symptoms of disease.

General preventive measures that individuals can take to reduce the risk of atrial flutter and disease complications include maintenance of proper lipid levels, blood pressure, glucose levels, healthy weight, healthy diet low in sodium and saturated fats, management of stress and anxiety, reduction of alcohol consumption, and avoidance of illicit drug use.

Treatment and prevention of Wolff-Parkinson-White syndrome

Lifestyle modifications, pharmacologic management, and surgery are options for treatment of Wolff-Parkinson-White syndrome. The goal of treatment is to reduce tachycardia and restore normal heart rhythm.

Pharmacologic approaches used to treat Wolff-Parkinson-White syndrome include anti-arrhythmic agents such as adenosine and procainamide.

The most effective and curative approach for the treatment of Wolff-Parkinson-White syndrome is radiofrequency catheter ablation. However, surgical destruction of the accessory pathway may be performed and be effective, but radiofrequency catheter ablation is typically the most safe and efficacious curative approach.

Patients diagnosed with Wolff-Parkinson-White syndrome will be recommended to make lifestyle changes that include maintaining a healthy diet low in saturated fats and sodium, increasing physical activity, quitting smoking, reducing caffeine and alcohol intake, reducing stress, and avoiding stimulants. Other vagal maneuvers may be recommended to reduce a patient's heart rate including coughing and bearing down as during a bowel movement.

Wolff-Parkinson White syndrome is not preventable, but not all patients develop symptoms. Addressing cardiovascular comorbid conditions and receiving proper treatment post myocardial infarction may prevent the onset of complications associated with Wolff-Parkinson-White syndrome. Also, addressing modifiable risk factors and addressing other cardiovascular comorbid conditions promptly will reduce the likelihood of complications associated with the syndrome.

General preventive measures that individuals can take to reduce the risk of disease complications include maintaining proper lipid levels, blood pressure, glucose levels, healthy weight, healthy diet low in sodium and saturated fats, exercising regularly, avoiding smoking, controlling diabetes, managing stress and anxiety, reducing alcohol consumption, and avoiding illicit drug use.

Treatment and prevention of ventricular fibrillation

Ventricular fibrillation is a serious medical condition that should be treated as a medical emergency. If an individual is suspected of having an acute ventricular fibrillation episode, then a practicing clinician may perform cardiopulmonary resuscitation and will shock the heart using an external defibrillator. The goal of treatment is to restore normal heart rhythm to reestablish proper cardiac output and blood oxygenation. The shock is given as soon as possible and, if a defibrillator is available, even before cardiopulmonary resuscitation (CPR).

Pharmacologic agents will also be administered to control the individual's heart rate and function. Pharmacologic agents used to treat ventricular fibrillation include vasopressors or sympathomimetics such as epinephrine, antidysrhythmia agents such as lidocaine, amiodarone, bretylium tosylate, and procainamide, and electrolytes such as magnesium sulfate, sodium bicarbonate, and calcium chloride. A more invasive approach includes the use of an implantable cardiac defibrillator post an acute ventricular fibrillation episode to prevent sudden cardiac death.

Addressing cardiovascular comorbid conditions and receiving proper treatment postventricular fibrillation may prevent the onset of complications associated with the condition. Also, addressing modifiable risk factors and addressing other cardiovascular comorbid conditions promptly will reduce the likelihood of complications associated with the condition.

General preventive measures that individuals can take to reduce the risk of ventricular fibrillation and complications associated with the condition include exercising regularly, maintaining proper lipid levels, blood pressure, glucose levels, healthy weight, healthy diet low in sodium and saturated fats, avoiding smoking, controlling diabetes, managing stress and anxiety, reducing alcohol consumption, and avoiding illicit drug use.

Treatment and prevention of ventricular tachycardia

Treatment of ventricular tachycardia depends on the degree and extent of the condition. It also varies on the individual patient, patient's general health and presence of other comorbid conditions. In some individuals, emergency management is necessary, and in others, no treatment is required. Treatment involves lifestyle modifications, pharmacologic management and. in more severe cases, surgical approaches.

If an individual has acute ventricular tachycardia and is pulseless or symptomatic, defibrillation is necessary. Cardiopulmonary resuscitation (CPR) is also often necessary. The goal of treatment is to restore normal heart rhythm to reestablish proper cardiac output and blood oxygenation.

Pharmacologic management of ventricular tachycardia involves treatment with antiarrhythmia agents such as lidocaine, procainamide, amiodarone, sotalol, mexiletine, acebutolol, atenolol, metoprolol, flecainide, propafenone, and quinidine.

Addressing cardiovascular comorbid conditions and receiving proper treatment post ventricular tachycardia may prevent the onset of complications associated with the condition. Also, addressing modifiable risk factors and addressing other cardiovascular comorbid conditions promptly will reduce the likelihood of complications associated with the condition.

General preventive measures that individuals can take to reduce the risk of ventricular tachycardia and complications associated with the condition include maintaining proper lipid levels, blood pressure, glucose levels, healthy weight, healthy diet low in sodium and saturated fats, exercising regularly, avoiding smoking, controlling diabetes, managing stress and anxiety, reducing alcohol consumption, and avoiding illicit drug use.

Treatment and prevention of intermittent claudication

Lifestyle modifications, pharmacologic management and, in more severe cases, surgical intervention are used for the treatment of intermittent claudication.

Lifestyle modifications include treatment of other comorbid cardiovascular disease, management of hypertension and high cholesterol, maintenance of proper glucose levels, increased physical activity, compliance with diabetes treatment, cessation of smoking, and/or avoidance of alcohol or illicit drug use.

Pharmacologic agents used to treat intermittent claudication include pentoxifylline and cilostazol, which act by dilating blood vessels, increasing blood flow to the extremities and reducing clot formation. Surgical approaches used for patients with peripheral arterial disease and intermittent claudication include angioplasty and cardiopulmonary bypass surgery. Other surgical approaches used for peripheral arterial disease and intermittent claudication include transcatheter intervention and peripheral vascular bypass.

Lifestyle modifications and pharmacologic management prevent the onset of arteriosclerosis, peripheral arterial disease, and intermittent claudication. Patients should maintain a diet low in sodium and saturated fats, increase potassium intake, increase exercise and physical activity, avoid smoking and tobacco use, lose excess weight, avoid beta-blockers and illicit drug use, maintain proper lipid levels, maintain proper glucose levels, and maintain proper albumin excretion and creatinine levels.

Patients with peripheral arterial disease and intermittent claudication should maintain their feet to prevent the onset of complications such as infections and gangrene. Patients should wash their feet daily and moisturize them, wear thick socks and comfortable shoes, promptly treat fungal infections, trim toe nails, avoid walking barefoot, and immediately have sores and open wounds treated.

Treatment and prevention of hypotension

If blood pressure drop is acute and life threatening, pressors (norepinephrine) may be necessary. Treatment of the underlying cause is of primary concern, such as antibiotics for infection or defibrillation for arrhythmia. Lifestyle modifications and pharmacologic management are used to treat chronic hypotension. The type of treatment depends on the degree and extent of hypotension as well as the underlying cause of the condition. Treatment varies by the symptoms that the patient presents.

Lifestyle modifications include dietary changes like increased salt intake if no other comorbid cardiovascular conditions are present and increased fluid intake, and use of graduated compression stockings. Other modifications include avoiding alcohol and illicit drug use, avoid smoking, avoid prolonged heat exposure, maintain a healthy diet, and eating small meals every few hours.

Pharmacologic agents used to treat hypotension include fludrocortisone, pyridostigmine, nonsteroidal anti-inflammatory drugs, erythropoietin, and/or caffeine.

Lifestyle modifications and pharmacologic management prevent the onset of hypotension. Patients should maintain a diet high in sodium if they do not have any other cardiovascular comorbidities, increase potassium intake, increase exercise and physical activity, avoid smoking and tobacco use, lose excess weight, avoid alcohol and illicit drug use, maintain proper lipid levels, maintain proper glucose levels, and maintain proper albumin excretion and creatinine levels.

The following lifestyle modifications may prevent serious complications associated with hypotension: getting up slowly after sitting in patients with orthostatic hypotension, avoid standing for long periods of time in patients with neurally mediated hypotension, eat small low carbohydrate meals, drink plenty of fluids, avoid alcohol and tobacco use, increase salt intake if no other cardiovascular comorbid conditions exist, use graduated compression stockings, and maintain daily physical activity.

Treatment and prevention of compartment syndrome

Although lifestyle modifications and pharmacologic management may be effective for compartment syndrome, surgical intervention is the most effective approach to management of acute and chronic disease. The pressure and swelling in the compartment can be relieved by a long incision in the fascia of the compartment. The incision is typically left open for 48 to 72 hours post–initial surgery and then a second surgery is performed to close the incision. With larger incisions, skin grafts may be used to close the incision.

If a tight cast or bandage causes the problem, then the bandage and/or cast will be loosened to relieve the syndrome.

Although little can be done to prevent the onset of compartment syndrome, patient education and increased awareness in individuals with a history of the condition or who exert themselves physically on a regular basis are important for prompt diagnosis and treatment.

Patients should also maintain a diet low in sodium and saturated fats, increase potassium intake, increase exercise and physical activity, avoid smoking and tobacco use, lose excess weight, avoid beta-blockers and illicit drug use, maintain proper lipid levels, maintain proper glucose levels, and maintain proper albumin excretion and creatinine levels.

Treatment and prevention of pulmonary edema

Lifestyle modifications, pharmacologic management, and, in more severe cases, ventilatory support, are used to treat pulmonary edema. In acute pulmonary edema, oxygen is immediately administered to prevent tissue damage.

Pharmacologic management depends on the underlying cause of pulmonary edema and the presence of other cardiovascular comorbid conditions. Pharmacologic agents used to treat pulmonary edema include preload reducers such as nitroglycerin, diuretics such as furosemide, morphine, afterload reducers such as nitroprusside, enalapril, and captopril, aspirin, and blood-pressure agents.

In treating patients with high altitude–induced pulmonary edema, patients should decrease a few thousand feet and carry oxygen with them. Pharmacologic management with acetazolamide may be beneficial.

Although little can be done to prevent the onset of pulmonary edema, patient education and increased awareness in individuals with a history of the condition or have other comorbid cardiovascular or respiratory risk factors is important for prompt diagnosis and treatment.

Patients should also maintain a diet low in sodium and saturated fats, increase potassium intake, increase exercise and physical activity, avoid smoking and tobacco use, get enough folic acid, manage stress, lose excess weight, avoid beta-blockers and illicit drug use, maintain proper lipid levels, maintain proper glucose levels, and maintain proper albumin excretion and creatinine levels.

If traveling or climbing at high altitudes, individuals should acclimate themselves slowly but ascending no more than 1,000 to 2,000 feet per day once an individual has reached 8,000 feet. Patients at risk for high altitude induced pulmonary edema should also make sure to drink plenty of fluids and bring oxygen with them.

Treatment and prevention of 1st degree atrioventricular block

Lifestyle modifications and pharmacologic management may be used to treat first-degree atrioventricular block, but most patients diagnosed with the condition do not require treatment. Patients with asymptomatic first-degree atrioventricular block do not require treatment. However, patients who present with symptoms should discontinue medication that could be contributing to the atrioventricular block or seek electrophysiological consultation.

Pharmacologic agents that may be used to treat first-degree atrioventricular block include parasympathetic blockers such as atropine and sympathomimetics such as isoproterenol. Patients undergoing pharmacologic management should be monitored to make sure their condition does not progress to a higher degree of atrioventricular block.

For patients who present with severe bradycardia, syncope, and left ventricular systolic dysfunction, a pacemaker may be required.

Typically, first-degree atrioventricular blocks are not preventable unless induced by pharmacologic drugs; then the drug can be stopped or titrated down. However, it remains unclear if a particular drug will induce a first-degree atrioventricular block, as it depends on the patient. Yet, certain drugs have been known to cause the condition.

In order to prevent progression to higher degrees of atrioventricular block, patients should be monitored by their practicing clinician, especially patients with concomitant bundle-brachial blocks.

Patients should also maintain a diet low in sodium and saturated fats, increase potassium intake, increase exercise and physical activity, avoid smoking and tobacco use, get enough folic acid, manage stress, lose excess weight, avoid beta-blockers and illicit drug use, maintain proper lipid levels, maintain proper glucose levels, and maintain proper albumin excretion and creatinine levels.

Treatment and prevention of second-degree atrioventricular block type I

The treatment of second-degree atrioventricular block type I depends on the presence or absence of symptoms. Treatment also varies on the extent and degree of the condition and the presence of other comorbid cardiovascular conditions. In patients diagnosed with second-degree atrioventricular block type I with few or no symptoms, treatment may not be necessary. However, asymptomatic patients that present with intra- or infra bundle blocks may require a pacemaker. Also, patients that present with bradycardia, heart failure, myocardial infarction, and asystole greater than or equal to 3 seconds, a pacemaker may be required. Additionally, patients that present with comorbid Lyme disease, drug toxicity, and hypoxia associated with sleep apnea may require treatment and modifications of drug dosing and/or lifestyle changes.

Anticholinergic agents such as atropine sulfate may be used to treat the condition but pacemaker placement is considered standard of care when necessary.

Typically, second-degree atrioventricular blocks type I are not preventable unless induced by pharmacologic drugs and then the drug can be stopped or titrated down.

In order to prevent progression to higher degrees of atrioventricular block, patients should be monitored by their practicing clinician, especially patients with concomitant bundle-branch blocks.

Patients should also maintain a diet low in sodium and saturated fats, increase potassium intake, increase exercise and physical activity, avoid smoking and tobacco use, get enough folic acid, manage stress, lose excess weight, avoid beta-blockers and illicit drug use, maintain proper lipid levels, maintain proper glucose levels, and maintain proper albumin excretion and creatinine levels.

Treatment and prevention of second-degree atrioventricular block type II

Treatment of second-degree atrioventricular block type II varies on the extent and degree of the condition and the presence of other comorbid cardiovascular conditions. The goal of treatment is to restore sinus rhythm or maintain cardiac output.

Patients that present with bradycardia, heart failure, myocardial infarction, wide QRS complexes, and asystole greater than or equal to 3 seconds, a pacemaker may be required. Additionally, patients that present with comorbid Lyme disease, drug toxicity, and hypoxia associated with sleep apnea may require treatment and modifications of drug dosing and/or lifestyle.

Anticholinergic agents such as atropine sulfate may be used to treat the condition but pacemaker placement is considered standard of care. Also, in patients with extensive symptoms, isoproterenol and dopamine may be used to achieve hemodynamic stability until a pacemaker can be placed.

Typically, second-degree atrioventricular type II blocks are not preventable unless induced by pharmacologic drugs and then the drug can be stopped or titrated down. In order to prevent progression to higher degrees of atrioventricular block, patients should be monitored by their practicing clinician, especially patients with concomitant bundle-branch blocks.

Furthermore, family members and/or caregivers should be taught cardiopulmonary resuscitation (CPR) and how to contact emergency medical services in the event of cardiac arrest. Pacemaker education is necessary to make sure that patients do not have a problem with the battery or the device.

Patients should also maintain a diet low in sodium and saturated fats, increase potassium intake, increase exercise and physical activity, avoid smoking and tobacco use, get enough folic acid, manage stress, lose excess weight, avoid beta-blockers and illicit drug use, maintain proper lipid levels, maintain proper glucose levels, and maintain proper albumin excretion and creatinine levels.

Treatment and prevention of third-degree atrioventricular block

Lifestyle modifications, pharmacologic management, and pacemaker implantation are the key treatment approaches for third-degree atrioventricular block. New-onset third-degree atrioventricular block is a medical emergency and treatment is dependent on the extent and degree of the block.

Patients undergoing treatment with pharmacologic agents that target the atrioventricular node should stop or titrate down the medication to help resolve the complete atrioventricular block.

Complete heart block associated with repeated abnormal pulse, inadequate escape rhythm or block below the atrioventricular node should be treated immediately with a pacemaker or pacing agents. Patients with third-degree atrioventricular block and bradycardia, other arrhythmias, and neuromuscular diseases should receive a permanent pacemaker. Individuals who undergo catheter ablation or with documented periods of asystole greater than or equal to 3 seconds should be considered for a pacemaker.

Individuals diagnosed with third-degree atrioventricular block should be on bed rest to avoid further complications. Sympathomimetic agents such as atropine and isoproterenol hydrochloride can be used to treat third-degree atrioventricular block, but pacemaker placement is standard of care in most cases.

Typically, third-degree atrioventricular blocks are not preventable unless induced by pharmacologic drugs and then the drug can be stopped or titrated down. Furthermore, family members and/or caregivers should learn cardiopulmonary resuscitation (CPR) and how to contact emergency medical services (EMS) in the event of cardiac arrest. Pacemaker education is necessary to make sure that patients do not have a problem with the battery or the device.

Patients should also maintain a diet low in sodium and saturated fats, increase potassium intake, increase exercise and physical activity, avoid smoking and tobacco use, get enough folic acid, manage stress, lose excess weight, avoid beta-blockers and illicit drug use, maintain proper lipid levels, maintain proper glucose levels, and maintain proper albumin excretion and creatinine levels.

Goals of treating of cardiogenic shock

Treatment of cardiogenic shock requires emergency and prompt attention to restore blood flow to various end organ systems. The goal of treatment is to initially treat the shock and then to treat the underlying cause of cardiogenic shock. Emergency life support treatment is required for cardiogenic shock, which aims to restore blood flow to brain, kidney, and other end organ systems. Patients experiencing cardiogenic shock will be given oxygen as well as fluids including blood products. The goal of pharmacologic treatment is to reduce mortality and morbidity as well as prevent further complications.

Pharmacologic and surgical interventions used for cardiogenic shock

Pharmacologic agents used to treat cardiogenic shock include vasopressors such as dopamine and dobutamine, phosphodiesterase enzyme inhibitors such as milrinone and inamrinone, vasodilators such as nitroglycerin, analgesics such as morphine sulfate, diuretics such as furosemide, and natriuretic peptides such as nesiritide.

More invasive surgical approaches used to treat cardiogenic shock include intra-aortic balloon pump and angioplasty. Other surgical approaches used to treat the underlying cause of cardiogenic shock include coronary artery bypass surgery, surgery to repair damaged cardiac valves, surgery to repair the wall between heart chambers, left ventricular assist device implantation, and heart transplant.

Prevention of cardiogenic shock

Although little can be done to prevent the onset of cardiogenic shock, patient education and increased awareness in individuals with a history of the condition or that have other comorbid cardiovascular or respiratory risk factors is important for prompt diagnosis and treatment. Prevention of cardiac disease and/or myocardial infarction is the best way to prevent the onset of cardiogenic shock. Prompt treatment of myocardial infarction and/or heart disease may prevent the onset of cardiogenic shock.

Patients should also maintain a diet low in sodium and saturated fats, increase potassium intake, increase exercise and physical activity, avoid smoking and tobacco use, get enough folic acid, manage stress, lose excess weight, avoid beta-blockers and illicit drug use, maintain proper lipid levels, maintain proper sugar levels, and maintain proper albumin excretion and creatinine levels.

Adrenergic group of drugs

The classes of agents included in the adrenergic group of drugs include sympathomimetics such as dobutamine, isoproterenol, dopamine, metaraminol, epinephrine, and norepinephrine; alpha-1 selective adrenergic agonists such as methoxamine, phenylephrine, and midodrine; alpha-2 selective adrenergic agonists such as clonidine, guanfacine, guanabenz, and methyldopa; alpha adrenergic antagonists such as doxazosin, prazosin, phenoxybenzamine, terazosin, phentolamine, and tolazoline; and beta-adrenergic antagonists such as acebutolol, atenolol, betaxolol, bisoprolol, carteolol, carvedilol, esmolol, labetalol, metoprolol, nadolol, penbutolol, pindolol, propranolol, sotalol, and timolol.

Sympathomimetic agents

Sympathomimetic agents stimulate both alpha and beta-adrenogenic receptors. Stimulation of alpha-adrenergic receptors induces vasoconstriction and stimulation of beta-adrenergic receptors increase cardiac contraction and heart rate. Sympathomimetic agents also target dopamine receptors, which also increases cardiac contraction and dilates renal blood vessels. Therapeutic uses of sympathomimetic agents include treatment of hypotension and cardiogenic shock associated with myocardial infarction.

Adverse events associated with sympathomimetic agents include gastrointestinal side effects such as nausea and vomiting, cardiovascular events such as tachycardia, dysrhythmia, hypertension, palpitations, and angina and central nervous system events such as throbbing headache and cerebral hemorrhage. Contraindications to sympathomimetic agents include tachydysrhythmia, ventricular fibrillation, and pheochromocytoma.

Alpha-1 selective adrenergic agents

The alpha-1 selective adrenergic agents stimulate vascular smooth muscle by targeting alpha-adrenergic receptors. Stimulation of alpha-adrenergic receptors increases peripheral vascular resistance and increase blood pressure through vasoconstriction. Therapeutic uses of alpha-1 selective adrenergic agents include the treatment of persistent hypotension, neurally mediated hypotension or orthostatic hypotension.

Adverse events associated with alpha-1 selective adrenergic agents include over stimulation that leads to high levels of blood pressure and profuse sweating. Contraindications of alpha-1 selective adrenergic agents include hypertension, tachycardia, vasospasm, and lactation.

These agents should not be stopped immediately, as sudden withdrawal could lead to reverse complications and sudden death. These agents should be tapered over a few days.

Alpha-2 selective adrenergic agents

The alpha-2 selective adrenergic agents stimulate the cardiovascular control centers of the central nervous system, activating alpha-2 receptors. Stimulation of alpha-2 receptors decreases blood pressure and heart rate. Therapeutically, alpha-2 selective adrenergic agents are used in the treatment of systemic hypertension.

Adverse events associated with alpha-2 selective adrenergic agents include central nervous system events such as depression, nightmares, sedation, drowsiness, fatigue, and headache, and cardiovascular events such as hypotension, congestive heart failure, and bradycardia. Other adverse events include dry mouth, sexual dysfunction, and decreased urinary output. Contraindications of alpha-2 selective adrenergic agents include severe coronary artery disease, vascular disease, and chronic renal failure. Sudden discontinuation of these agents could lead to withdrawal reactions, so practicing clinicians should titrate down dosages upon discontinuation.

Alpha-adrenergic antagonists

Alpha-adrenergic antagonists target both alpha-1 adrenergic and alpha-2 adrenergic receptors and block receptor action. Alpha-1 adrenergic receptors produce the effects of the sympathetic nervous system, while alpha-2 adrenergic receptors stimulate norepinephrine release. Drugs within this class of agents have different affinity for these receptors. Prazosin, terazosin, and doxazosin have more affinity for blocking alpha-1 receptors, while phenoxybenzamine and phentolamine have similar affinity for both alpha-1 and alpha-2 receptors.

Alpha-adrenergic antagonists decrease vascular tone, increase vasodilation and decrease blood pressure. Therapeutic uses of alpha-adrenergic antagonists include hypertension, pheochromocytoma, and extravasation of tissue-toxic agents.

Adverse events associated with alpha-adrenergic antagonists include cardiovascular events such as postural hypotension, dysrhythmia, edema, congestive heart failure, and angina; and central nervous system events such as dizziness, weakness, fatigue, drowsiness, and depression. Other adverse events include fainting and syncope up to 90 minutes post administration. Therefore, practicing clinicians should monitor patients starting treatment with these agents to assess side effects and titrate dose to get the desired effect with minimal adverse effects. Caution should be used when administrating these agents in patients with congestive heart failure, pregnancy, and renal failure.

Beta-adrenergic antagonists

Beta-receptor antagonists block beta-adrenergic receptor signaling. Beta-1 adrenergic receptors stimulate myocardial contraction and increase heart rate. Beta-2 receptors are found in vascular smooth muscle of lungs, blood vessels, and uterus and stimulate dilation and relaxation. Drugs within this class of agents have different affinity for these receptors, with most agents targeting both beta-1 and beta-2 receptors equally.

Beta-adrenergic antagonists decrease heart rate and blood pressure. Therapeutic uses include treatment of hypertension, ventricular dysrhythmia, chronic angina, prevention of reinfarction after myocardial infarction, congestive heart failure, supraventricular tachycardia, dysrhythmias, idiopathic hypertrophic subaortic stenosis, and pheochromocytoma.

Adverse events associated with beta-adrenergic antagonists include cardiovascular events such as bradycardia, heart block, congestive heart failure, hypotension and peripheral vascular insufficiency; pulmonary events such as shortness of breath, coughing, and bronchospasm; and central nervous system events such as fatigue, dizziness, depression, paresthesia, sleep disturbances, memory loss, and disorientation. Other adverse events include nausea, vomiting, diarrhea, colitis, decreased libido, sexual dysfunction, vomiting, slowed recovery from hypoglycemia, and decreased exercise dysfunction.

Contraindications include cardiovascular conditions such as bradycardia or heart block, pulmonary conditions such as bronchospasm, chronic obstructive pulmonary disease, or acute asthma. These agents should be used with caution in patients with heart failure and/or diabetes. Sudden discontinuation of these agents could lead to withdrawal reactions, so practicing clinicians should titrate down dosages over a 2-week period.

Ionotropic group of drugs

The classes of agents included in the ionotropic group of drugs include cardiac glycosides such as digitalis, digitoxin, and digoxin; phosphodiesterase inhibitors such as amrinone and milrinone; and sympathomimetics such as dopamine, dobutamine, isoproterenol, metaraminol, epinephrine and norepinephrine.

Sympathomimetic agents stimulate vasoconstriction and increase cardiac contraction. Sympathomimetic agents also target dopamine receptors, which also increases cardiac contraction and dilates renal blood vessels. Therapeutic uses of sympathomimetic agents include treatment of hypotension and cardiogenic shock associated with myocardial infarction.

Cardiac glycosides

Cardiac glycosides target the sodium/potassium pump, which maintains resting membrane potential of nerve and muscle cells of the heart. Cardiac glycosides allow for influx of calcium into myocardial cells during depolarization, which increases contraction of cardiac muscle, increases cardiac output, increases renal profusion, decreased heart rate, and decreased conduction velocity through the atrioventricular node. Therapeutically, cardiac glycosides are used to treat congestive heart failure, atrial flutter, atrial fibrillation, and paroxysmal atrial tachycardia.

Adverse events associated with cardiac glycosides include cardiovascular events such as premature ventricular contractions, dysrhythmia, and bradycardia; gastrointestinal events such as vomiting, anorexia, nausea and vomiting; central nervous system events such as changes to visual field, headaches, fatigue, confusion and depression.

Factors that can influence toxicity in patients undergoing treatment with cardiac glycosides include electrolyte imbalances such as decreased potassium levels as well as renal and hepatic insufficiency. Specifically, digitalis-related toxicities require treatment that includes decontamination, monitoring of plasma potassium levels, administration of anti-dysrhythmic agents, and digitalis antibodies.

Some drugs may decrease or increase the action of cardiac glycosides. Some specific examples include drugs that decrease effect of digoxin such as antacids, cholestyramine, neomycin, and sulfasalazine and drugs that increase effect of digoxin, such as albuterol, amiodarone, captopril, cyclosporine, diltiazem, erythromycin, nifedipine, omeprazole, tetracycline, and thyroxine.

Contraindications include ventricular tachycardia, ventricular fibrillation, atrioventricular block, idiopathic hypertrophic subaortic stenosis, myocardial infarction, and Wolff-Parkinson-White syndrome. Caution needs to be taken when administering cardiac glycosides, as their effective therapeutic dose is very close to their toxic dose.

Phosphodiesterase inhibitors

Phosphodiesterase inhibitors increase calcium levels within myocardial cells. These agents increase cardiac muscle contractions and cardiac output. However, these inhibitors have little impact on heart rate and blood pressure.

Phosphodiesterase inhibitors are typically prescribed over short periods due to a high degree of toxicity associated with these agents. They are used to treat decompensated congestive heart failure in patients who fail first line treatment approaches. Adverse events associated with phosphodiesterase inhibitors include cardiovascular events such as dysrhythmia and gastrointestinal events such as nausea, vomiting, and liver enzyme changes. Other adverse events include thrombocytopenia and bone marrow toxicity. Contraindications include aortic or pulmonary valvular disease, myocardial infarction, and ventricular dysrhythmia.

Anti-dysrhythmic group of drugs

The anti-dysrhythmic group of drugs includes 6 classes of agents and 2 additional agents. The 6 classes of agents include class IA, IB, IC, II, III and IV. Examples of class IA agents include quinidine, procainamide, moricizine, and disopyramide. Examples of class IB agents include lidocaine, tocainamide, mexiletine, and phenytoin. Examples of class IC agents include flecainide and propafenone. Examples of class II agents include propranolol, acebutolol and esmolol. Examples of class III agents include bretylium, amiodarone, ibutilide, dofetilide, and sotalol. Examples of class IV agents include verapamil and diltiazem. Other agents not categorized include digoxin and adenosine.

Adverse events associated with anti-dysrhythmic agents include cardiovascular events such as new dysrhythmia, heart block, hypotension, vasodilation, and cardiac arrest. Noncardiac events include nausea, vomiting, hypersensitivity, hemolytic anemia, tinnitus, headache, blurred vision, arthralgia, arthritis, dizziness, euphoria, perioral numbness, agitation, disorientation, paraesthesia, tremor, lightheadedness, slurred speech, seizures, bone marrow suppression, bronchospasm, photosensitivity, pulmonary fibrosis, liver enzyme dysfunction, thyroid dysfunction, constipation, lassitude, nervousness, peripheral edema, shortness of breath, flushing, and paresthesia. Specific agents within each class are more prone to certain adverse events than others, but all have potential for the above adverse events.

Contraindications include allergy, bradycardia, sick sinus syndrome, atrioventricular block, shock, hypotension, and respiratory depression. Caution should be used when administering these agents in patients with congestive heart failure.

Anti-dysrhythmic agents

Class I anti-dysrhythmic agents inhibit sodium channels. Class II drugs include beta-adrenergic receptor antagonists, which slow heart rate and increase cardiac muscle contraction. Class III drugs inhibit potassium efflux during repolarization. Class IV agents include calcium channel blocker. Unclassified agents such as digoxin decrease conduction velocity and adenosine activates adenosine receptors that play a role in potassium conductance.

Therapeutic uses of anti-dysrhythmic agents include atrial dysrhythmia, ventricular tachycardia, life-threatening ventricular dysrhythmias, ventricular dysrhythmias, sinus tachycardia, atrioventricular reentry, Wolff-Parkinson White syndrome, premature ventricular contractions, atrial fibrillation, atrial flutter, and atrial tachycardia.

Nitrates/nitrites

Nitrates and/or nitrates act directly on vascular smooth muscle and increase vasodilation. This class of agents increases blood flow and increases oxygen supply to myocardial cells. This class of agents has been shown to be ineffective in patients with coronary artery disease. Nitrates and/or nitrates are used to treat acute and chronic angina.

Adverse events associated with nitrates and/or nitrites include cardiovascular events such as hypotension, rebound tachycardia, bradycardia, flushing, and sweating and central nervous system events such as headache and dizziness. Other adverse events include nausea, vomiting, incontinence, and contact dermatitis. Contraindications include head trauma, cerebral hemorrhage, pregnancy, and lactation. Sublingual administration of nitrates/nitrates is the most preferred method of administration due to low bioavailability of these agents. Patients may develop resistance to these agents over time and may require higher doses to get the same effect.

Phosphodiesterase inhibitors

Phosphodiesterase inhibitors increase calcium levels within myocardial cells. These agents increase cardiac muscle contractions and cardiac output. However, these inhibitors have little impact on heart rate and blood pressure.

Phosphodiesterase inhibitors are typically prescribed over short periods due to a high degree of toxicity associated with these agents. They are used to treat decompensated congestive heart failure in patients who fail first line treatment approaches. Adverse events associated with phosphodiesterase inhibitors include cardiovascular events such as dysrhythmia and gastrointestinal events such as nausea, vomiting, and liver enzyme changes. Other adverse events include thrombocytopenia and bone marrow toxicity. Contraindications include aortic or pulmonary valvular disease, myocardial infarction, and ventricular dysrhythmia.

Vasodilator group of drugs

Classes of agents include in the vasodilator group include beta-blockers such as acebutolol, atenolol, betaxolol, bisoprolol, carteolol, carvedilol, esmolol, labetalol, metoprolol, nadolol, penbutolol, pindolol, propranolol, sotalol, and timolol; nitrates/nitrites, also known as anti-anginal vasodilators, such as amyl nitrate, isosorbide dinitrate, isosorbide mononitrate, and nitroglycerin; anti-hypertensive vasodilators such as diazoxide, minoxidil, fenoldopam, nitroprusside, hydralazine, and tolazoline; and calcium channel blockers such as amlodipine, bepridil, diltiazem, felodipine, isradipine, nicardipine, nifedipine, nimodipine, nisoldipine, and verapamil.

Beta-adrenergic inhibitors can also be classified as adrenergic agents. Beta-adrenergic inhibitors and calcium channel blockers indirectly act as vasodilators, whereas anti-anginal vasodilators and anti-hypertensive vasodilators directly act on vasodilator mechanisms.

Calcium channel blockers

Calcium channel blockers act by antagonizing L-type calcium channels in vascular smooth muscle, which leads to reduced cardiac muscle contractility, decreased SA pacemaker rate, and decreased atrioventricular conduction velocity in cardiac tissue.

Therapeutic uses include angina, hypertension, congestive heart failure, bradycardia associated with angina, Raynaud's phenomenon, atrial tachycardia, atrial flutter, and subarachnoid hemorrhage. Adverse events associated with calcium channel blockers include headache, dysrhythmias, edema, bleeding gums, agranulocytosis, dizziness, nausea, fatigue, severe gastrointestinal upset, constipation, tachycardia, flushing, diarrhea, hypotension, and myocardial depression.

Patients on concomitant calcium channel blocker and beta-blocker and/or nitrate should have their blood pressure monitored by a practicing clinician due to increased risk of hypotensive episodes. Degree of vasodilation should be monitored due to increased risk of edema.

Anti-hypertensive vasodilators

Anti-hypertensive vasodilators act directly on vascular smooth muscle and increase vasodilation. These agents decrease arteriolar resistance and decrease arterial blood pressure. Therapeutic uses include treatment of hypertension, hypertensive crisis, and pulmonary hypertension in newborns.

Adverse events associated with anti-hypertensive vasodilators include cardiovascular events such as sweating, flushing, edema, dizziness, hypotension, reflex tachycardia and central nervous system events such as headache. Other adverse events include systemic lupus like syndrome and hypertrichosis. Contraindications include pregnancy and lactation. Caution should be used when administering these agents in patients with peripheral vascular disease, coronary artery disease, congestive heart failure, and/or tachycardia. Practicing clinicians should take caution when administering nitroprusside in patients with renal failure.

Anticoagulant, anti-thrombotic, and thrombolytic group of drugs

The classes of agents within this group include anticoagulants, anti-thrombotic or anti-platelet agents, and thrombolytic or fibrinolytic agents. Anti-coagulants include anti-thrombin III, heparin, lepirudin, warfarin, danaparoid, and low molecular weight heparins such as ardeparin, dalteparin, enoxaparin and tinzaparin, argatroban and bivalirudin. Anti-thrombotic or anti-platelet agents include abciximab, aspirin, ibuprofen, sulfinpyrazone, clopidogrel, dipyridamole, eptifibatide, ticlopidine, and tirofiban. Thrombolytic or fibrinolytic agents include alteplase, streptokinase, anistreplase, urokinase, reteplase, and TNK t-PA.

This group of agents, which include anticoagulants, anti-thrombotic or anti-platelet agents and thrombolytic or fibrinolytic agents, prevent inhibition of platelet aggregation and clot formation.

Anticoagulants

Anti-coagulants prevent clot formation but each of the agents included in this class have various mechanisms of action. These agents prevent clot formation by depleting clotting factors, inhibiting their activity, and/or prolonging clotting times.

Antithrombin III prevents clotting, while heparin is a protein that inhibits the conversion of prothrombin to thrombin, which prevents fibrinogen being converted to fibrin. Lepirudin directly inhibits thrombin formation, while low molecular weight heparins block factors Xa and IIa, which inhibit thrombus and clot formation. Warfarin prevents clot formation by interfering with formation of vitamin K dependent clotting factors in the liver.

Practicing clinicians should not use warfarin during acute situations, as the onset of action is about 3 days and lasts for about 5 days. Heparin or low molecular weight heparins should be used during acute situations, but warfarin can be used over the long term due to the drug's long-lasting effects. Warfarin should be administered with caution, as the drug is contraindicated with a variety of drugs to treat a number of different conditions. Practicing clinicians should keep antidotes on hand in case of overdose including protamine sulfate for heparin overdose and vitamin K for warfarin overdose.

Therapeutic uses of anticoagulants include hereditary antithrombin III deficiency with potential for thromboembolism, acute deep venous thrombosis, prevention of deep venous thrombosis, acute pulmonary embolism, prevention of pulmonary embolism, atrial fibrillation with embolism, prevention of clotting in blood samples, dialysis, venous tubing, diagnosis and treatment of disseminated intravascular coagulation, myocardial infarction, stroke, heparin-induced thrombocytopenia, artificial heart valves, and valvular damage.

Adverse effects associated with anticoagulants include bleeding complications, hemorrhage, nausea, gastrointestinal upset, thrombocytopenia, and hepatic dysfunction. Contraindications include hemorrhagic disorders, recent trauma, spinal puncture, gastrointestinal ulcers, recent surgery, intrauterine device placement, tuberculosis, indwelling catheters and threatened abortion. More specifically, warfarin is contraindicated during pregnancy. Caution should be taken if anticoagulants are prescribed in patients with congestive heart failure, thyrotoxicosis, diarrhea, and fever.

Antithrombotic agents

Therapeutic uses of anti-thrombotic, or anti-platelet agents, include ischemia, percutaneous coronary intervention, risk reduction of recurrent TIAs in men, risk reduction of myocardial infarction or death in patients with history of cardiovascular disease, reduction of embolization in rheumatic valve disease, atrial fibrillation, peripheral arterial disease, stroke, prevention of thromboembolism, acute coronary syndrome, and prevention of cardiac ischemic complications.

Caution should be taken when prescribing anti-thrombotic or anti-platelet agents in patients who underwent recent surgery, or who are at risk of excessive blood loss or closed head injuries. Patients undergoing treatment with anti-thrombotic or anti-platelet agents should avoid cutting themselves and contact sports.

Anti-thrombotic or anti-platelet agents inhibit platelet aggregation. Specifically, abciximab, tirofiban, and eptifibatide are glycoprotein IIb/IIIa inhibitors that block platelet aggregation. Aspirin, ibuprofen, and sulfinpyrazone are cyclooxygenase inhibitors that inhibit the formation of thromboxanes, thereby blocking platelet aggregation. Clopidogrel and ticlopidine interfere with the ADP receptor blockade and prevent ADP from binding to platelets, thus inhibiting platelet aggregation. Dipyridamole is a phosphodiesterase inhibitor that increases cAMP, activating prostacyclin, and inhibiting platelet aggregation.

Adverse events associated with anti-thrombotic or anti-platelet agents include bleeding, hemorrhage, gastrointestinal ulcerations, angina, dizziness, headache, syncope, rash, thrombocytopenia, neutropenia, nausea, and diarrhea.

Thrombolytic or fibrinolytic agents

Thrombolytic or fibrinolytic agents open blood vessels and restore blood flow to dependent organ systems. These agents induce the production of plasmin through the digestion of fibrin, thereby degrading fibrin clots within blood vessels.

Specifically, streptokinase, urokinase, and anistreplase inhibit the formation of fibrin by disrupting the conversion of plasminogen to plasmin. Alteplase, tenecteplase, and reteplase activate the conversion of fibrin-bound plasminogen to plasmin.

Therapeutic uses of thrombolytic and fibrinolytic agents include lysis of thrombi in coronary arteries after myocardial infarction, stroke, pulmonary embolism, deep venous thrombosis, occluded cannulas in dialysis patients and peripheral artery thrombosis.

Adverse effects associated with thrombolytic or fibrinolytic agents include bleeding, bruising, anaphylaxis, and hematoma. Contraindications associated with use of thrombolytic or fibrinolytic agents include any condition that could be compromised by dissolution of clots such as recurrent surgery, hemorrhage, recent cerebrovascular accident, aneurysm, obstetric delivery, organ biopsy, serious gastrointestinal bleeding, major trauma, or hypertension.

Aminocaproic acid inhibits fibrin formation and is typically administered to antagonize the action of thrombotic or fibrinolytic agents.

Patients should be monitored for blood loss. Also, practicing clinicians should initiate treatment with thrombolytic or fibrinolytic within 3 hours of experiencing an acute myocardial infarction to prevent further cardiovascular complications if percutaneous coronary intervention is not available.

Angiotensin-converting enzyme inhibitors

Angiotensin-converting enzyme inhibitors inhibit the converting enzyme that hydrolyzes angiotensin I to angiotensin II, which increases bradykinin that is a potent vasodilator. By inhibiting the renin-angiotensin system, angiotensin-converting enzyme inhibitors prevent vasoconstriction by blocking angiotensin II formation, decreasing sodium and water reabsorption in the kidneys, and indirectly inducing bradykinin.

The pharmacologic effect of angiotensin-converting enzyme inhibitors is to decrease blood pressure through vasodilation and inhibiting salt reuptake through aldosterone. Therapeutic uses of angiotensin-converting enzyme inhibitors include hypertension treatment, diabetic nephropathy, congestive heart failure after myocardial infarction, and preservation of left ventricular function after myocardial infarction.

The classes of drugs that influence the renin-angiotensin system include angiotensin-converting enzyme inhibitors and angiotensin II antagonists. Angiotensin-converting enzyme inhibitors, also known as ACE inhibitors, include benazepril, moexipril, captopril, perindopril, enalapril, quinapril, fosinopril, ramipril, lisinopril, and trandolapril. Angiotensin II antagonists include candesartan, losartan, eprosartan, telmisartan, irbesartan, and valsartan.

Both angiotensin-converting enzyme inhibitors and angiotensin II antagonists induce vasodilation. However, angiotensin II antagonists are more specific in their mechanism of action than angiotensin-converting enzyme inhibitors. These drugs are mainly used for the treatment of hypertension, but have other cardiovascular effects.

Adverse events associated with angiotensin-converting enzyme inhibitors include hypotension, glomerular damage, acute renal failure, hyperkalemia, dry cough, wheezing, angioedema, agranulocytosis, gastrointestinal upset, skin rash and/or other hypersensitivities.

Contraindications of angiotensin-converting enzyme inhibitors include women during their second and third trimester of pregnancy due to risk of fetal hypotension, anuria, renal failure, fetal malformations, and/or death.

Patients with renal insufficiency should not be prescribed angiotensin-converting enzyme inhibitors due to elimination through the kidneys. However, fosinopril and moexipril are not eliminated through the kidneys and therefore can be administered in this patient population. Hypotension, potassium levels, and renal function should be monitored in patients undergoing treatment with angiotensin-converting enzyme inhibitors.

Angiotensin II antagonists

Angiotensin II antagonists are more specific in action than angiotensin-converting enzyme inhibitors. Angiotensin II antagonists block angiotensin II receptors by inhibiting a subtype of the angiotensin II receptor known as AT_1. Angiotensin II antagonists do not interfere with bradykinin metabolism. The pharmacologic effect of angiotensin II antagonists is decreased blood pressure caused by a decrease in both peripheral resistance and blood volume. Inhibition of the AT_1 receptors leads to inhibition of the pressor and aldosterone-releasing effects of angiotensin II, which causes the decrease in blood pressure.

Angiotensin II antagonists are mainly used to treat hypertension but have effects on other cardiovascular conditions.

Adverse events associated with angiotensin II antagonists include gastrointestinal upset, dry mouth, tooth pain, headache, dizziness, minor cough, dry skin and alopecia. Since angiotensin II antagonists do not impact bradykinin metabolism, angiotensin II antagonists present with limited cough and fewer side effects as compared to angiotensin-converting enzyme inhibitors. Angiotensin II antagonists provide a more specific approach to the treatment of hypertension as compared to angiotensin-converting enzyme inhibitors.

Contraindications associated with angiotensin II antagonists include pregnant women during their second and third trimesters due to risk of fetal malformations and death. Hypotension, potassium levels, and renal function should be monitored in patients undergoing treatment with angiotensin II antagonists.

Classes of agents included in the diuretic group of pharmacologic drugs

The classes of agents included in the diuretic group of pharmacologic agents include thiazide diuretics such as bendroflumethiazide, benzthiazide, chlorothiazide, chlorthalidone, hydrochlorothiazide, hydroflumethiazide, indapamide, methyclothiazide, metolazone, polythiazide, quinethazone and trichlormethiazide; loop diuretics such as bumetanide, ethacrynic acid, furosemide and torsemide; potassium-sparing diuretics such as amiloride, spironolactone, and triamterene; and osmotic diuretics such as glycerin and mannitol.

Diuretics prevent reabsorption of sodium in the kidneys, with each class of diuretic working on a slightly different site within the nephron of the kidney. Each of these classes of diuretics has a slightly different mechanism of action.

Thiazide diuretics

Therapeutic uses for thiazide diuretics include treatment of congestive heart failure, hypertension, and edema. The most common adverse effects associated with thiazide diuretics include electrolyte imbalance, fluid imbalance, hypotension, oliguria, anuria, dizziness, hypokalemia, hyponatremia, hypocalcemia, hyperglycemia, hyperuricemia, and gastrointestinal upset.

Contraindications of thiazide diuretics include patients with renal disease, hypokalemia, dysrhythmia, glucose intolerance, and gout. Thiazide diuretics should not be used prior to bedtime due to increase urine output. Caution should be used when using diuretics in combination with other antihypertensive agents. Practicing clinicians need to monitor electrolyte and renal function to prevent complications. Additionally, patients should monitor potassium intake due to potential for electrolyte imbalance and supplement accordingly.

Thiazide diuretics prevent the reabsorption of sodium within the nephron of the kidneys, which allow for sodium and other ions to be excreted in the urine and not reabsorbed in the blood stream. Specifically, thiazide diuretics inhibit sodium and chloride reabsorption in the nephron, resulting in excretion of potassium, chloride, and sodium in the urine. The excretion of sodium in the urine decreases the glomerular filtration rate and has been associated with moderate potassium loss, which needs to be monitored. Thiazide diuretic net effect is to decrease blood pressure, decrease cardiac stroke volume, and cardiac output.

Loop diuretics

Loop diuretics prevent the reabsorption of sodium and chloride within the nephron of the kidneys, which allow for sodium, chloride, and potassium to be excreted in the urine and not reabsorbed in the blood stream. Loop diuretics are more powerful than thiazide diuretics and are associated with increased potassium loss. Loop diuretic net effect is to decrease blood pressure, cardiac stroke volume, and cardiac output.

Therapeutic uses of loop diuretics include treatment of congestive heart failure, pulmonary edema, hypertension, and edema associated with congestive heart failure, renal disease, or liver disease.

The most common adverse effects associated with loop diuretics include electrolyte imbalance, fluid imbalance, hypotension, oliguria, anuria, dizziness, hypokalemia, hyponatremia, hypocalcemia, hyperglycemia, hyperuricemia, ototoxicity resulting from hearing loss, and gastrointestinal upset.

Contraindications of loop diuretics include patients with renal disease, hypokalemia, dysrhythmia, glucose intolerance, and gout. Loop diuretics should not be used prior to bedtime due to increased urine output. Caution should be used when using diuretics in combination with other antihypertensive agents. Practicing clinicians need to monitor electrolyte and renal function to prevent complications. Additionally, patients should monitor potassium intake due to potential for electrolyte imbalance and supplement accordingly.

Potassium-sparing diuretics

Potassium-sparing diuretics increase sodium excretion and decrease potassium secretion in the nephron of the kidneys, which allow for sodium and other ions to be excreted in the urine and not reabsorbed in the blood stream. However, potassium-sparing diuretics are associated with decreased potassium excretion compared to thiazide and loop diuretics, making potassium-sparing diuretics an attractive option. Potassium-sparing diuretics' net effect is to decrease blood pressure, decrease cardiac stroke volume, and cardiac output.

Therapeutic uses of potassium-sparing diuretics include hypertension and edema from congestive heart failure, renal disease, or liver disease. In patients undergoing treatment with thiazide or loop diuretics who develop hypokalemia, potassium-sparing diuretics are another option.

The most common adverse effects associated with potassium-sparing diuretics include electrolyte imbalance, fluid imbalance, hypotension, oliguria, anuria, dizziness, hyperkalemia, some hyponatremia, glucose intolerance in diabetic patients, gynecomastia, and gastrointestinal upset.

Potassium-sparing diuretics should not be used prior to bedtime due to increased urine output. Caution should be used when using diuretics in combination with other antihypertensive agents. Practicing clinicians need to monitor electrolyte and renal function to prevent complications. Additionally, patients should monitor potassium intake due to potential for electrolyte imbalance and supplement accordingly, even though potassium levels are not impacted to the same degree as with thiazide or loop diuretics.

Osmotic diuretics

Osmotic diuretics prevent the reabsorption water within the permeable regions of the nephron because these nonabsorbable agents create an osmotic gradient favoring increased urine volume. Osmotic diuretic net effect is to decrease blood pressure, decrease cardiac stroke volume, and cardiac output.

Therapeutic uses of osmotic diuretics include treatment of intracranial pressure and brain edema. The most common adverse effects associated with osmotic diuretics include electrolyte imbalance, fluid imbalance, hypotension, oliguria, anuria, and dizziness.

Osmotic diuretics should not be used prior to bedtime due to increased urine output. Caution should be used when using diuretics in combination with other antihypertensive agents. Practicing clinicians need to monitor electrolyte and renal function to prevent complications. Additionally, patients should monitor potassium intake due to potential for electrolyte imbalance and supplement accordingly.

Classes of agents included in the antihyperlipidemic group of pharmacologic drugs

The classes of agents included in the antihyperlipidemic group of pharmacologic drugs include resins, niacin, statins, also known as HMG-coenzyme A reductase inhibitors, and fibric acid derivatives. Drugs within the resin class of agents include cholestyramine, colestipol, and colesevelam. Drugs within the statins, or HMG-coenzyme A reductase inhibitors, include atorvastatin, pravastatin, fluvastatin, simvastatin and lovastatin. Drugs within the fibric acid derivatives include clofibrate, fenofibrate, and gemfibrozil.

Antihyperlipidemic classes of agents directly or indirectly affect lipid and cholesterol levels by lowering low-density lipid levels, increasing high-density lipid levels and decreasing triglyceride levels.

Resins

The pharmacologic effects of resins include decrease in low-density lipid levels, increase in high-density lipid levels and decrease in triglyceride levels. The mechanism of action of these agents is to act as bile acid sequestrants, which increase liver low-density lipoprotein receptors, removing low-density lipids from circulation and oxidizing the cholesterol from low-density lipids to form bile acids.

Therapeutic uses for resins include treatment of hypercholesterolemia and hyperlipidemia. Resins are recommended only when a patient fails first line therapy with diet modifications and exercise and their low-density lipid levels are above 160 mg/dL or above 130 mg/dL with more than 2 cardiovascular risk factors such as obesity, smoking or high-density lipid levels below 40 mg/dL. The goal of treatment when prescribing resins in patients with coronary heart disease or at high risk for coronary heart disease is low-density lipid levels below 100 mg/dL. Resins may also be used in children between the ages of 11 and 20.

Adverse effects associated with resins include gastrointestinal upset, bloating, constipation, and malabsorption of vitamins A, D, and K. Contraindications associated with resins include hypertriglyceridemia, biliary obstruction, abnormal intestinal function, pregnancy, and lactation.

Practicing clinicians should inform patients that these agents should not be taken in dry powder form, but mixed with fluids to be efficacious. Additionally, if prescribed resins in tablet form, the tablets should not be cut, chewed, or crushed, as they will become ineffective if that is done. Resins are designed to be broken down in the gastrointestinal tract and, if broken down sooner, the drugs will become ineffective.

Niacin

The pharmacologic effects of niacin include a decrease in low-density lipid levels, increase in high-density lipid levels and decrease in triglyceride levels. The mechanism of action of niacin is inhibition of lipolysis of triglycerides in fatty tissue, which decreases synthesis of triglycerides in the liver. In turn, decreased triglyceride synthesis decreases low-density lipid synthesis, decreasing low-density lipid levels. Niacin is the most effective agent for increasing high-density lipid levels, but also has effects on lowering low-density lipid levels and triglyceride levels.

Therapeutic uses include hypertriglyceridemia, hypercholesterolemia, and hyperlipidemia. Niacin is recommended only when a patient fails first line therapy with diet modifications and exercise and their low-density lipid levels are above 160 mg/dL or above 130 mg/dL with more than 2 cardiovascular risk factors such as obesity, smoking or high-density lipid levels below 40 mg/dL. The goal of treatment when prescribing niacin in patients with coronary heart disease or at high risk for coronary heart disease is low-density lipid levels below 100 mg/dL.

Adverse events associated with niacin include flushing, pruritus, abnormal glucose tolerance, and hyperuricemia. The most common adverse events associated with niacin include flushing and dyspepsia. These common adverse events decrease patient compliance and effectiveness of niacin treatment. However, flushing tends to decrease with treatment duration. Patients may also take aspirin 30 minutes prior to taking niacin to reduce flushing. They may also reduce hot beverage or alcohol intake to reduce extent and degree of flushing.

Contraindications associated with niacin treatment include pregnancy and gout. Patients should not take oral nicotinamide as treatment for hypertriglyceridemia, hypercholesterolemia, and hyperlipidemia because this source of niacin does not have any impact on lipid levels. The effective dose for antihypertensive treatment ranges between 1 and 2 grams per day or more.

HMG coenzyme A reductase inhibitors or statins

Statins compete for inhibition of HMG coenzyme A reductase, which impacts cholesterol biosynthesis. Statins are well tolerated and effective agents for the treatment of hyperlipidemia and hypercholesterolemia. The pharmacologic effects of statins include decrease in low-density lipid levels, increase in high-density lipid levels and decrease in triglyceride levels. Higher doses of more potent statins such as atorvastatin and simvastatin are more effective in reducing triglyceride levels.

Therapeutic uses of statins include hypertriglyceridemia, hypercholesterolemia, and hyperlipidemia. Statins are recommended only when a patient fails first line therapy with diet modifications and exercise and their low-density lipid levels are above 160 mg/dL or above 130 mg/dL with more than 2 cardiovascular risk factors such as obesity, smoking or high-density lipid levels below 40 mg/dL. The goal of treatment when prescribing statins in patients with coronary heart disease or at high risk for coronary heart disease is low-density lipid levels below 100 mg/dL.

Adverse events associated with HMG coenzyme A reductase inhibitors or statins include liver dysfunction, increase liver transaminases, myopathy, rhabdomyolysis associated with myalgia and fatigue, hypersensitivity, and renal failure. Due to risk of liver dysfunction and liver transaminases, practicing clinicians should monitor patients' alanine aminotransferase (ALT) levels. Measurements should be taken upon initiation of treatment and should be repeated every 3 months. Practicing clinicians should also monitor patients for cataract development, especially in elderly patients.

Additionally, due to increased risk for myopathy and rhabdomyolysis, practicing clinicians should inform patients to tell them if they experience any muscle or joint pain, as that may be early indication for rhabdomyolysis, which is a serious complication.

Contraindications associated with statins include liver disease and pregnancy. Statins should be administered prior to bedtime since the highest rates of cholesterol synthesis occur between the hours of midnight and 5 AM.

Fibric acid derivatives

The pharmacologic effects of fibric acid derivatives include decrease in low-density lipid levels, increase in high-density lipid, and decrease in triglyceride levels. However, the exact mechanism of action of fibric acid derivatives is unknown.

Therapeutic uses of fibric acid derivatives include treatment of hypertriglyceridemia primarily, with minimal effect on hypercholesterolemia and hyperlipidemia. Fibric acid derivatives are recommended only when a patient fails first-line therapy with diet modifications and exercise and their triglyceride levels still remain very elevated.

Adverse events associated with fibric acid derivatives include gastrointestinal upset, rash, alopecia, fatigue, headache, impotence, and anemia and myositis flu-like syndrome.

Contraindications associated with fibric acid derivatives include renal failure and liver failure. Caution needs to be taken when prescribing fibric acid derivatives with other agents, as fibric acid derivatives also have anti-platelet effects. Gemfibrozil should not be administered with statins due to increased risk of rhabdomyolysis. However, if gemfibrozil is administered with a statin, practicing clinicians need to monitor patients very closely for the any indication of rhabdomyolysis. Therefore, due to increased risk for myopathy and rhabdomyolysis, practicing clinicians should inform patients to tell them if they experience any muscle or joint pain, as that may be early indication for rhabdomyolysis.

Role of hormone replacement therapy

Hypertension:
Recent data has demonstrated that the use of antihypertensive agents reduces cardiovascular complications such as risk for stroke, myocardial infarction, and congestive heart failure. In women, undergoing treatment with hormone replacement therapy, these agents have been shown to have no effect on blood pressure or risk of stroke but estrogen may improve compliance of large blood vessels. However, hormone replacement therapy with estrogen is contraindicated in postmenopausal women with a history of cardiovascular complications such as thromboembolic disorders.

Therefore, use of hormone replacement therapy for the treatment of hypertension and other cardiovascular complications remains controversial.

Coronary heart disease:
The use of hormone replacement therapy to prevent acute myocardial infarction or recurrent myocardial infarction remains controversial. Initial observational studies have demonstrated the benefit of hormone replacement therapy in the prevention of acute myocardial infarction or recurrent myocardial infarction. However, the Women's Health Initiative (WHI) showed that although estrogen replacement has a beneficial effect on lipids, it may increase the risk of cardiovascular complications and, additionally, breast cancer.

Estrogen antagonists and selective estrogen receptor modulators may have similar impact, not reducing coronary heart disease as compared with estrogen or estrogen-progesterone combination. Currently, no evidence exists that demonstrates that estrogen antagonists and/or selective estrogen receptor modulators have any effect on coronary artery disease.

Percutaneous transluminal coronary angioplasty (PTCA) procedure

The goal of percutaneous transluminal coronary angioplasty is to increase blood flow to the coronary arteries by reducing plaque build-up. The procedure involves the use of a catheter introduced through the femoral, brachial, or radial artery into the diseased coronary artery. The catheter has a balloon at the end of the device to be used to tamponade plaque in the diseased vessel. Once the catheter is inserted, balloon pressure is applied to the area of plaque formation to decrease plaque size and/or stretch the vessel wall. The balloon is threaded over a wire after the wire is placed properly in the diseased vessel through angiography. A stent is often placed after ballooning opens the vessel.

Percutaneous transluminal coronary angioplasty is indicated for patients with refractory angina, unstable angina, evidence of cardiac ischemia, acute myocardial infarction, angina post coronary bypass surgery, unsuitable coronary anatomy for coronary bypass surgery, and restenosis after successful percutaneous transluminal coronary angioplasty or stent placement.

Prior to percutaneous transluminal coronary angioplasty, practicing clinicians should take the patient's medical history, perform a physical examination, and evaluate the patient's overall health. Patients should be screened for drug-drug interactions, allergies, vital signs such as heart rate and blood pressure and cardiovascular blood indicators such as potassium levels, prothrombin time, and hematocrit and creatinine levels. Patients should also undergo electrocardiogram and echocardiogram prior to procedure.

During the procedure, patients should only receive medications via intravenous access, except for aspirin, which is given orally prior to procedure. Pharmacologic agents used during the procedure include heparin, nitroglycerin, and/or glycoprotein IIb/IIIa receptor inhibitor such as abciximab.

Post percutaneous transluminal coronary angioplasty, practicing clinicians should perform electrocardiogram, echocardiogram, perform physical assessment, monitor peripheral blood flow and look for swelling and evaluate cardiac pain. Hospital protocols for aftercare should be followed. Prior to patient release, practicing clinicians should perform additional physical assessment and laboratory tests such as hematocrit, potassium levels, creatinine levels, and cardiac enzymes. Cardiac stress testing should be completed 2 to 6 months post-procedure.

Stent

A stent is defined as a small mesh tube that is inserted into diseased cardiac vessel that is narrowed or weakened to increase blood flow and restore cardiac function. Stents are typically implanted during an angioplasty procedure. Stents can be made of metal such as stainless steel, tantalum, cobalt alloy, platinum or nitinol, fabric, and/or also drug coated to prevent restenosis.

A stent procedure is very similar to a percutaneous transluminal coronary angioplasty. There are several types of stent procedures including balloon expandable stent procedures and self-expanding stents. With balloon expanding stents, the stent is placed over the balloon and is placed once the balloon is expanded at the plaque site within the diseased coronary vessel. Self-expanding stents are covered by a sheath that allows the stent to expand when removed.

Stent procedures are indicated for patients with refractory angina, unstable angina, evidence of cardiac ischemia, acute myocardial infarction, angina post coronary bypass surgery, unsuitable coronary anatomy for coronary bypass surgery, focal de novo lesions, stenosis of previously placed saphenous vein grafts and restenosis after successful percutaneous transluminal coronary angioplasty or stent placement.

Contraindications for a stent procedure include high-risk coronary anatomy, severe coronary artery disease, bleeding disorder and/or multiple episodes of percutaneous transluminal coronary angioplasty restenosis. If glycoprotein IIb/IIIa inhibitors are used, other contraindications include gastrointestinal bleeding, inability to take antiplatelet agents, intracranial hemorrhage, recent surgery, or trauma.

Complications associated with stent procedures include abrupt closure of diseased coronary artery, periprocedural myocardial infarction, coronary restenosis, bleeding, or hematoma at catheter introduction site, arterial embolism, pseudoaneurysm, retroperitoneal bleeding, and sudden death.

Prior to a stent procedure, practicing clinicians should take a patient's medical history, perform a physical examination, and evaluate the patient's overall health. Patients should be screened for drug-drug interactions, allergies, vital signs such as heart rate and blood pressure and cardiovascular blood indicators such as potassium levels, prothrombin time, hematocrit, and creatinine levels. Patients should also undergo electrocardiogram and echocardiogram prior to procedure.

During the procedure, patients should only receive medications via an intravenous route, except for aspirin, which is given orally prior to the procedure. Pharmacologic agents used during the procedure include heparin, nitroglycerin, and/or glycoprotein IIb/IIIa receptor inhibitor such as abciximab.

Post stent procedure, practicing clinicians should perform electrocardiogram, echocardiogram, perform physical assessment, monitor peripheral blood flow and look for swelling and evaluate cardiac pain. Hospital protocols for aftercare should be followed. Prior to patient release, practicing clinicians should perform additional physical assessment and laboratory tests such as hematocrit, potassium levels, creatinine levels, and cardiac enzymes. Cardiac stress testing should be completed 2 to 6 months post-procedure.

Coronary atherectomy

There are 3 currently available atherectomy procedures that include directional coronary atherectomy, rotational atherectomy, and transluminal extraction atherectomy.

Directional coronary atherectomy is a procedure that involves the use of a catheter with a balloon and cutting tool at the end of the catheter. During the procedure, the catheter is inserted into the diseased tissue, the balloon is inflated to remove or disrupt the plaque, and the cutting tool is used to remove the rest of the plaque.

Rotational atherectomy is a procedure that is also a catheter-based procedure that uses a metal cutting tool coated with diamonds, which breaks up the plaque into tiny particles to be removed.

Transluminal extraction atherectomy is a procedure involves the use of a hollow tube with a cutting tool at the end of the device. The hollow tube also has suction bottles that collect removable plaque build-up.

An atherectomy procedure, also known as a rotablator procedure, is a technique that involves a catheter with a grinding/cutting tool at the end of the device that is used to clear plaque build-up within diseased coronary arteries. An Atherectomy procedure can be done in combination with percutaneous transluminal catheter angioplasty and/or stent procedure.

The procedure involves the use of catheter introduced through the femoral, brachial, or radial artery into the diseased coronary artery. The catheter has a grinding/cutting tool at the end of the device to be used to reduce plaque build-up in the diseased vessel.

Directional coronary atherectomy is indicated for bifurcation lesions, ostial lesions and eccentric lesions. Rotational atherectomy is indicated for calcified lesions, ostial lesions, 15- to 25-mm-length lesions, and in-stent restenosis. Transluminal extraction atherectomy is indicated for lesions that require removal of thrombus or debris such as patients with unstable angina, acute myocardial infarction, and failed thrombolytic therapy.

Contraindications for coronary atherectomy include high-risk coronary anatomy, severe coronary artery disease, bleeding disorder, and/or multiple episodes of percutaneous transluminal coronary angioplasty restenosis.

Complications associated with coronary atherectomy include abrupt closure of the diseased coronary artery, periprocedural myocardial infarction, coronary restenosis, bleeding, or hematoma at catheter introduction site, arterial embolism, pseudoaneurysm, retroperitoneal bleeding, vascular spasm, distal embolization, vessel perforation, and sudden death.

Prior to a coronary atherectomy procedure, practicing clinicians should take patient's medical history, perform a physical examination, and evaluate the patient's overall health. Patients should be screened for drug-drug interactions, allergies, vital signs such as heart rate and blood pressure and cardiovascular blood indicators such as potassium levels, prothrombin time, and hematocrit and creatinine levels. Patients should also undergo an electrocardiogram and echocardiogram prior to the procedure.

During the procedure, patients should only receive medications via an intravenous route, except for aspirin, which is given orally prior to the procedure. Pharmacologic agents used during the procedure include heparin, nitroglycerin, and/or glycoprotein IIb/IIIa receptor inhibitor such as abciximab.

Post coronary atherectomy procedure, practicing clinicians should perform an electrocardiogram, echocardiogram, perform a physical assessment, monitor peripheral blood flow and look for swelling and evaluate cardiac pain. Hospital protocols for aftercare should be followed. Prior to patient release, practicing clinicians should perform additional physical assessments and laboratory tests such as hematocrit, potassium levels, creatinine levels, and cardiac enzymes. Cardiac stress testing should be completed 2 to 6 months post-procedure.

Percutaneous transluminal angioplasty

The lower extremity:
The types of percutaneous transluminal angioplasty of the lower extremity include iliac percutaneous transluminal angioplasty and stenting, femoropopliteal percutaneous transluminal angioplasty, and tibioperoneal percutaneous transluminal angioplasty.

Iliac percutaneous transluminal angioplasty is a procedure that involves access through a retrograde approach or an iliac crossover approach. Access can also be gained from the axillary or brachial arteries. The catheter has a balloon at the end of the device to be used to reduce plaque build-up in the diseased vessel. Once the catheter is inserted, balloon pressure is applied to the area of plaque formation to cause plaque rupture, endothelial disruption, and/or stretching of the vessel wall.

Femoropopliteal percutaneous transluminal angioplasty is a procedure that involves access through an antegrade femoral approach or femoral crossover approach. The role of stents in this approach is currently being investigated.

Percutaneous transluminal angioplasty of the lower extremity is a procedure used for the treatment of peripheral arterial disease. The procedure involves balloon angioplasty of the diseased peripheral vessel to improve blood flow to extremities. The procedure is similar to percutaneous transluminal coronary angioplasty. The catheter has a balloon at the end of the device to be used to reduce the plaque in the diseased vessel. Once the catheter is inserted, balloon pressure is applied to the area of plaque formation to decrease plaque size and/or stretch the vessel wall. The procedure can be done with stents, thrombolytic agents and with arthrectomy approaches.

Percutaneous transluminal angioplasty of the lower extremity is indicated for symptoms of severe claudication and critical limb ischemia. Percutaneous transluminal angioplasty of the lower extremity can be done in combination with surgical bypass surgery.

Percutaneous transluminal angioplasty of the lower extremity is contraindicated in patients who are medically unstable, have long arterial occlusions, have poor distal runoff, or who have diabetes.

Complications associated with percutaneous transluminal angioplasty of the lower extremity include vasospasm, thrombus formation, arterial dissection, vessel perforation, compartment syndrome, arterial dissection, restenosis, and sudden death. Other complications may occur due to the patient's overall health, allergies, and other comorbid conditions. Therefore, practicing clinicians need to take careful medical history and perform physical examination prior to the procedure.

Prior to a percutaneous transluminal angioplasty of lower extremity, practicing clinicians should take the patient's medical history, perform a physical examination, and evaluate the patient's overall health. Patients should be screened for drug-drug interactions, allergies, vital signs such as heart rate and blood pressure and cardiovascular blood indicators such as potassium levels, prothrombin time, and hematocrit and creatinine levels. Patients should also undergo an electrocardiogram and echocardiogram prior to the procedure.

During the procedure, patients should only receive medications via an intravenous route, except for aspirin, which is given orally prior to the procedure. Pharmacologic agents used during the procedure include heparin, nitroglycerin, and/or glycoprotein IIb/IIIa receptor inhibitor such as abciximab. Post percutaneous transluminal angioplasty of the lower extremity, practicing clinicians should perform an electrocardiogram, echocardiogram, perform physical assessments, monitor peripheral blood flow and look for swelling and evaluate ischemic pain. Hospital protocols for aftercare should be followed. Prior to patient release, practicing clinicians should perform additional physical assessments and laboratory tests such as hematocrit, potassium levels, creatinine levels, and cardiac enzymes.

<u>The carotid artery</u>:

Percutaneous transluminal angioplasty of the carotid artery is indicated for stenosis of the internal carotid artery, stenosis associated with transient ischemic attacks, bilateral stenosis, contralateral carotid artery occlusion, previous neck irradiation, radial neck dissection, increased operative risk such as severe coronary artery disease, and systemic restenosis.

Percutaneous transluminal angioplasty of the carotid artery is contraindicated in patients with major thrombus formation and thick circular or semicircular stenosis. Complications associated with percutaneous transluminal angioplasty of the carotid artery include transient ischemic attacks, stroke, cerebral hemorrhage, amaurosis fugax, stent restenosis, cranial nerve injury, and sudden death.

Percutaneous transluminal angioplasty of the carotid artery is a procedure that involves increasing blood flow by reducing plaque build-up within the brain. The procedure can be done alone or in combination with stenting. Vascular approaches include the femoral artery to access the internal carotid artery, but access through the axillary and brachial arteries can be done. During the procedure, a wire is guided from the vascular access to the site within the carotid artery and a stent is put into place. Balloon angioplasty may be done prior to wire access to dilate the blood vessel and reduce plaque build-up.

Prior to percutaneous transluminal angioplasty of the carotid artery, practicing clinicians should take the patient's medical history, perform a physical examination, and evaluate the patient's overall health. Patients should be screened for drug-drug interactions, neurological status, allergies, vital signs such as heart rate and blood pressure and cardiovascular blood indicators such as potassium levels, prothrombin time, hematocrit, and creatinine levels. Patients should also undergo an electrocardiogram and echocardiogram prior to the procedure. Also, patients are premedicated with heparin, atropine, and nifedipine.

During the procedure, patients should only receive medications via an intravenous route, except for aspirin, which is given orally prior to procedure. Pharmacologic agents used during the procedure include heparin, nitroglycerin, and/or glycoprotein IIb/IIIa receptor inhibitor such as abciximab.

Post percutaneous transluminal angioplasty of the carotid artery, practicing clinicians should perform an electrocardiogram, echocardiogram, perform physical assessments, monitor peripheral blood flow and look for swelling and evaluate cardiac pain. Hospital protocols for aftercare should be followed. Prior to patient release, practicing clinicians should perform additional physical assessments and laboratory tests such as hematocrit, potassium levels, creatinine levels, and cardiac enzymes. Follow-up examination 1-week post procedure is completed to check neurological status. Additionally, Doppler ultrasound is performed every 3 to 6 months and then every year. Magnetic resonance imaging will be performed 3-months postprocedure as well.

<u>The renal artery</u>:

Percutaneous transluminal angioplasty of the renal artery is indicated for renovascular hypertension caused atherosclerotic disease, renal transplant artery stenosis, renal artery or vein bypass graft stenosis and renal insufficiency with more than 50% renal artery stenosis.

Percutaneous transluminal angioplasty of the renal artery is contraindicated for borderline lesions, long section of occlusion, aortic plaque extending to renal artery and other unstable comorbid medical conditions.

Complications of percutaneous transluminal angioplasty include vascular access complications, worsening of renal failure, thrombus, nonocclusive dissection, embolism to peripheral artery, rupture of artery, and sudden death.

Percutaneous transluminal angioplasty of the renal artery is a procedure that involves increasing blood flow to the kidney, decreasing associated secondary hypertension, and improving renal function. Percutaneous transluminal angioplasty of the renal artery is typically done for fibromuscular dysplasia, but stenting can be used as an adjunctive approach for atherosclerotic plaque formation.

The procedure involves the use of a catheter introduced through the femoral or brachial arteries into the renal artery. The catheter has a balloon at the end of the device to be used to reduce plaque build-up in the diseased vessel. Once the catheter is inserted, balloon pressure is applied to the area of plaque to decrease size and/or stretch the vessel wall.

Prior to percutaneous transluminal angioplasty of the renal artery, practicing clinicians should take the patient's medical history, perform a physical examination, and evaluate the patient's overall health. Patients should be screened for drug-drug interactions, urine output, allergies, vital signs such as heart rate and blood pressure and cardiovascular blood indicators such as potassium levels, prothrombin time, hematocrit, and creatinine levels. Patients should also undergo electrocardiogram and echocardiogram prior to procedure.

During the procedure, patients should only receive medications via an intravenous route, except for aspirin, which is given orally prior to the procedure. Patients undergoing the procedure with stent placement may receive clopidogrel post procedure.

Postpercutaneous transluminal angioplasty of the renal artery, practicing clinicians should perform an electrocardiogram, echocardiogram, physical assessment, monitor peripheral blood flow and look for swelling and evaluate cardiac pain. Hospital protocols for aftercare should be followed. Prior to patient release, practicing clinicians should perform additional physical assessment and laboratory tests such as hematocrit, potassium levels, creatinine levels, and cardiac enzymes. Cardiac stress testing should be completed 2 to 6 months postprocedure.

Percutaneous balloon valvuloplasty

Percutaneous balloon valvuloplasty is a procedure that involves restoring blood flow and cardiac function by opening a constricted heart valve. Two types of percutaneous balloon valvuloplasty include percutaneous balloon mitral valvuloplasty and percutaneous balloon aortic valvuloplasty.

The percutaneous balloon mitral valvuloplasty procedure involves the use of a catheter introduced through the femoral, brachial, or radial artery into the diseased valve. Transeptal catheterization is performed and a large balloon catheter is placed over the mitral valve. Once the catheter is inserted, balloon pressure is applied to the area of the mitral valve. Please note that 2 balloon catheters can be used for this procedure as well.

The percutaneous balloon aortic valvuloplasty involves the use of a catheter introduced through the femoral, brachial, or radial artery into the diseased valve. Transeptal catheterization is performed and a large balloon catheter is placed over the aortic valve. Once the catheter is inserted, balloon pressure is applied to the area of aortic valve.

Percutaneous balloon mitral valvuloplasty is indicated for symptomatic mitral valve stenosis with or without valvular disease with a small degree of mitral valve regurgitation and nonsurgical candidates with severely calcified or fused mitral valves.

Percutaneous balloon aortic valvuloplasty is indicated for short-term relief of valve surgery candidates, left ventricular dysfunction, and symptomatic patients subject to undergo noncardiac surgery.

Contraindications associated with percutaneous balloon valvuloplasty include atrial thrombus, severely fused or calcified leaflets, severe coronary artery disease, and severe aortic regurgitation.

Complications associated with percutaneous balloon valvuloplasty include periprocedural myocardial infarction, emergency coronary artery bypass surgery, coronary restenosis, bleeding, or hematoma at catheter introduction site, arterial embolism, pseudoaneurysm, retroperitoneal bleeding, hemopericardium or tamponade, mitral regurgitation, atrial septal defects and sudden death.

Prior to percutaneous balloon valvuloplasty, practicing clinicians should take the patient's medical history, perform a physical examination, and evaluate the patient's overall health. Patients should be screened for drug-drug interactions, allergy, vital signs such as heart rate and blood pressure and cardiovascular blood indicators such as potassium levels, prothrombin time, hematocrit, and creatinine levels. Patients should also undergo electrocardiogram and echocardiogram prior to procedure.

During the procedure, patients should only receive medications via an intravenous route, except for aspirin, which is given orally prior to the procedure. Pharmacologic agents used during the procedure include heparin, nitroglycerin, and/or glycoprotein IIb/IIIa receptor inhibitor such as abciximab. After percutaneous balloon valvuloplasty, practicing clinicians should perform an electrocardiogram, echocardiogram, physical assessment, monitor peripheral blood flow and look for swelling and evaluate cardiac pain. Hospital protocols for aftercare should be followed. Prior to patient release, practicing clinicians should perform additional physical assessments such as the patient's heart sounds and laboratory tests such as hematocrit, potassium levels, creatinine levels and cardiac enzymes. Patients should follow-up with their practicing clinician 1 week post procedure and should undergo an echocardiogram 3 to 6 months postprocedure.

Artificial pacemakers

Artificial pacemakers provide electrical stimulation to the cardiac muscle when the heart is not able to keep up with the demands of the body. This occurs when the intrinsic heart rate is not able to provide enough cardiac output. The artificial pacemaker is made up of a pulse generator, unipolar or bipolar lead and is implanted in the right atrium or ventricle in contact with the cardiac walls.

The types of pacemakers include permanent pacemakers and temporary pacemakers. Temporary pace makers include transvenous pacing, transcutaneous pacing, epicardial pacing, and transthoracic pacing. Other types of pacing include single chamber pacing, dual chamber pacing, rate modulating pacing, atrial overdrive pacing, and anti-tachycardia pacing.

<u>Indications of permanent and temporary pacemakers</u>
Permanent pacing is indicated for third-degree atrioventricular block, second-degree atrioventricular block with symptomatic bradycardia, intermittent third-degree atrioventricular

block, type II second-degree atrioventricular block, sinus node dysfunction with symptomatic bradycardia or third-degree heart block, symptomatic chronotropic incompetence, persistent second-degree atrioventricular block with bilateral bundle branch, or third-degree atrioventricular block, transient advanced second or third-degree infranodal atrioventricular block and associated bundle block, ventricular tachycardia, recurrent syncope caused by carotid sinus stimulation, and symptomatic recurrent supraventricular tachycardia.

Temporary pacing is indicated for symptomatic bradycardia after acute myocardial infarction or associated hyperkalemia and/or drug toxicity, prior to permanent pacing, bradycardia nonresponsive to atropine or isoproterenol, bifascicular bundle block, alternating bundle branch block associated with acute myocardial infarction, transient right bundle block, and post-cardiovascular surgery to address bradycardia.

In transvenous pacing, vascular access is gained by percutaneous puncture of the internal jugular, subclavian, antecubital or femoral vein. Access can also be gained by venous cutdown in an antecubital vein. A bipolar, transvenous pacing lead is usually placed and maintained.

Transcutaneous pacing requires a nonsurgical approach where electrodes are attached to the anterior and posterior chest walls and connected to an external generator. This approach is typically used during emergency situations.

In epicardial pacing, surgery is done to attach leads to the atria and/or ventricle. The other end of the lead is connected externally to a generator.

In transthoracic pacing, a long needle is used to thread a lead to the right ventricle, which is then connected to an external generator. This approach is reserved for emergency situations.

Contraindications and complications of permanent and temporary pacemakers
Contraindications for implantation of pacemakers include first-degree atrioventricular block, asymptomatic second-degree atrioventricular block, transient atrioventricular block, atrioventricular block due to interior wall myocardial infarction, asymptomatic sinus node dysfunction, and suppression of ventricular tachycardia.

Complications associated with pacemaker implantation can vary depending on whether permanent or temporary pacing is being used. Complications associated with permanent pacing include pneumothorax, hemothorax, inadvertent entry into an artery, perforation of cardiac tissue or vein, damage to cardiac valve, inadequate or improper connection to leads, pain or infection in pacemaker pocket, migration of pacemaker, intravascular thrombus, bradycardia, tachycardia, endocarditis, and manual disruption of pacing.

Complications associated with temporary pacing include malfunction of the pacing system, ventricular tachycardia, thromboembolism, endocarditis, infection, phlebitis, failure to capture or sense properly, pneumothorax, hemothorax, perforation of atria, ventricle, or cardiac tissue/vessels and cardiac tamponade.

Single chamber pacing, rate modulated pacing, atrial overdrive pacing and anti-tachycardia pacing
Single chamber pacing involves either the atrium or ventricle being paced, but not both chambers in combination. However, dual chamber pacing involves both the atria and ventricles to be paced together.

Rate modulated pacing involves the pacing of the atria and ventricles based on physiological stress with increased heart rate. This type of pacing uses sensors to modulate pacing. Upon muscle or body movement, the sensor responds and modulates pacing.

Atrial overdrive pacing is a technique used to treat atrial flutter and tachycardia by providing atrial pacing rates of 200 to 500 impulses per minute.

Anti-tachycardia pacing is a technique that sends impulses to the heart to disrupt tachycardia. This approach can be used with implantable cardioverter defibrillators.

Generic pacemaker code

Pacemakers are classified using a 5-position code, which describes the different types of pacemakers and their function. Position one (I) indicates the chamber or chambers being paced. Position two (II) indicates the chamber or chambers being sensed. Position three (III) indicates the device's response to sensing. Position four (IV) indicates the programmability and rate of modulation function. Position five (V) is only used for tachycardia functions.

Each position, I through V, has addition subsets to describe the function taking place. For example, for position III, response to sensing, O=none, T=triggered, I=Inhibited and D=dual (triggered and inhibited). In positions I and II, there will be an A (atrial), V (ventricle), or D (dual) for the chamber(s) paced and sensed.

Operating settings for pacemakers

Operational settings for pacemakers are described based on rate, output, and sensitivity. Rate is defined as the number of times per minute that the pacemaker will fire when the patient's rate goes below that of the set rate. Output is described as the intensity of the electrical stimulus used to depolarize the cardiac tissue. Sensitivity is defined as the ability of a pacemaker to sense the patient's intrinsic heart rate. The sensitivity of the pacemaker increases as the number decreases.

The operational settings vary based on the type of pacemaker and whether it is for permanent pacing or temporary pacing.

Follow-up required post-permanent and temporary pacemaker placement

Patients should be instructed to follow-up with their practicing clinician 1 week post permanent pacemaker placement and then follow-up every 3 to 6 months to check programming and settings of the device. Elderly patients should be checked on a regular basis for risk of infection, heart sounds, and cardiac risk factors. Patients at risk for other cardiovascular complications should be monitored on a regular basis.

Some patients may be followed via telephone for pacemaker battery status with trans-telephonic monitoring. This method of monitoring sends a telephone transmission of a rhythm strip that allows the pacemaker battery status to be measured.

Role of practicing clinician pre-, during, and post-temporary pacemaker implantation

Practicing clinicians need to understand how the pacemaker works in terms of operational settings as well as programming to be able to intervene if a problem arises.

Prior to temporary pacemaker placement, a sterile environment needs to be established. A clean insertion site needs to be established to prevent infection. Guidelines for care of central venous catheters and dressing should be followed for this procedure.

Post-temporary pacemaker placement and daily iodine cleaning of areas where leads exit the body needs to be performed. Electrical safety is necessary in the care of these patients. Practicing clinicians should always wear gloves when handling pacing and/or wiring, insulate exposed metal ends of pacing leads, keep dressing dry, and make sure all other electrical equipment in the room is grounded.

<u>Role of the practicing clinician pre-, during, and post-permanent pacemaker implantation</u>
Practicing clinicians need to understand how the pacemaker works in terms of operational settings as well as programming to be able to intervene if a problem arises.

Prior to permanent pacemaker implantation, practicing clinicians should take patient's medical history, perform a physical examination, and evaluate a patient's overall health. Patients should be screened for drug-drug interactions, allergies, vital signs such as heart rate and blood pressure and cardiovascular blood indicators such as potassium levels, prothrombin time, hematocrit, and creatinine levels. Patients should also undergo electrocardiogram and echocardiogram prior to procedure. Additionally, they should take prophylactic antibiotic therapy.

Post permanent pacemaker implantation, practicing clinicians should perform an electrocardiogram, echocardiogram, perform a physical assessment, monitor peripheral blood flow and look for swelling and evaluate cardiac pain. Hospital protocols for aftercare should be followed. Prior to patient release, practicing clinicians should perform additional physical assessment such as assess patient's heart sounds and laboratory tests such as hematocrit, potassium levels, creatinine levels, and cardiac enzymes. Chest X-ray should also be performed pre and post pacemaker placement.

Implantable cardioverter defibrillator

Implantable cardiac defibrillators are used to treat life-threatening irregular heartbeat. They are small devices implanted in the chest or abdomen to control heart rate and cardiovascular function. The device consists of a pulse generator and lead system, which is available for pacing, sensing and shocking.

The implantation of cardiac defibrillator is very similar to that of permanent pacemakers. The transvenous lead system is inserted into the right ventricle and then connected to pulse generator. Also, a patch is connected from the ventricle to the pulse generator. However, some systems may have more than 1 lead and more than 1 patch.

Implantable cardiac defibrillators are capable of defibrillation, cardioversion, anti-tachycardia pacing, and anti-bradycardia pacing.

Implantable cardiac defibrillators are indicated for cardiac arrest due to ventricular fibrillation or ventricular tachycardia, sustained ventricular tachycardia, undetermined syncope or fainting, nonsustained and inducible ventricular tachycardia due to coronary heart disease, left ventricular dysfunction or previous myocardial infarction, hypertrophic cardiomyopathy with high risk for sudden death, and prolonged QT syndrome.

Contraindications associated with implantable cardiac defibrillators include myocardial ischemia, electrolyte abnormalities, terminal illness with short life expectancy, and ventricular tachycardia or ventricular fibrillation due to dysrhythmia.

Patients should be instructed to follow-up with their practicing clinician 1 week post implantable defibrillator placement and then follow-up every 3 to 6 months to check programming and settings of the device. Practicing clinicians should assess stored data and provide any treated episodes of dysrhythmia. Elderly patients should be checked on a regular basis for risk of infection, heart sounds, and cardiac risk factors. Other patients at risk for cardiovascular complications should be monitored on a regular basis.

Chest x-rays should be should be done annually to evaluate the implantable cardioverter. If the implantable defibrillator discharges, the patient should notify the provider. Emergency services should be contacted if the device discharges multiple times and/or the patient feels ill.

Practicing clinicians need to understand how the implantable defibrillator works in terms of operational settings as well as programming to be able to intervene if a problem arises.

Prior to implantable defibrillator placement, practicing clinicians should take the patient's medical history, perform a physical examination, and evaluate the patient's overall health. Patients should be screened for drug-drug interactions, allergies, vital signs such as heart rate and blood pressure and cardiovascular blood indicators such as potassium levels, prothrombin time, hematocrit, and creatinine levels. Patients should also undergo electrocardiogram and echocardiogram prior to procedure. Additionally, they should take prophylactic antibiotic therapy.

Post implantable defibrillator placement, practicing clinicians should perform an electrocardiogram, echocardiogram, perform a physical assessment, monitor peripheral blood flow and look for swelling and evaluate cardiac pain. Hospital protocols for aftercare should be followed. Prior to patient release, practicing clinicians should perform additional physical assessment such as assess the patient's heart sounds and laboratory tests such as hematocrit, potassium levels, creatinine levels, and cardiac enzymes. Chest X-ray should also be performed pre and post implantable defibrillator placement to assess for pneumothorax.

Coronary artery bypass graft surgery

Coronary artery bypass graft surgery is a procedure that uses a vessel graft to treat ischemic areas of cardiac tissue. Surgical revascularization uses vessel grafts including internal mammary artery, saphenous vein graft, gastroepiploic artery, and radial artery.

The procedure is performed under general anesthesia and requires opening of the sternum and putting the patient on cardiopulmonary bypass while the procedure is being completed. During the procedure, the cardiac muscle is arrested using a pharmacologic agent and hypothermia.

The procedure can also be performed minimally invasively as well as without the assistance of cardiopulmonary bypass.

Coronary artery bypass graft is indicated for angina refractory to drugs and other surgical interventions, significant left cardiac main disease, triple vessel coronary artery disease, acute myocardial infarction, and left ventricular failure due to cardiogenic shock or congestive heart failure.

Contraindications associated with coronary artery bypass graft include lack of adequate graft, small coronary arteries, severe aortic stenosis and severe left ventricular failure and coexisting peripheral vascular, renal, and pulmonary disease.

Complications associated with coronary artery bypass graft procedures include postoperative bleeding such as heparin induced thrombocytopenia, disseminated intravascular coagulopathy and diluted anemia, myocardial depression, cardiac tamponade, perioperative myocardial infarction, dysrhythmia including atrial tachycardia or atrial fibrillation, pulmonary edema, pulmonary atelectasis, pneumothorax, renal impairment, abdominal distention, cerebral ischemia, postcardiotomy delirium, peripheral neurological deficits, postpericardiotomy syndrome, wound infection and sudden death.

Prior to coronary artery bypass graft procedure, practicing clinicians should take patient's medical history, perform a physical examination, and evaluate the patient's overall health. Patients should be screened for drug-drug interactions, allergies, vital signs such as heart rate and blood pressure and cardiovascular blood indicators such as potassium levels, prothrombin time, hematocrit, and creatinine levels. Patients should also undergo electrocardiogram and echocardiogram prior to procedure. Additionally, they should take prophylactic antibiotic therapy and undergo chest x-ray. Overall, a full cardiovascular work-up should be conducted prior to the procedure.

During the procedure, patients should only receive medications via intravenous route, except for aspirin, which is given orally prior to procedure.

Post coronary artery bypass graft, practicing clinicians should perform an electrocardiogram, echocardiogram, perform a physical assessment, monitor peripheral blood flow and look for swelling and evaluate cardiac pain. Hospital protocols for aftercare should be followed. Prior to patient release, practicing clinicians should perform additional physical assessments such as assess patient's heart sounds and laboratory tests such as hematocrit, potassium levels, creatinine levels and cardiac enzymes. Overall, a full cardiovascular work-up should be conducted prior to releasing the patient.

Valvular replacement

Valvular replacement is a procedure that is used when repair will not be effective for fixing a dysfunctional valve. Two types of valvular replacements are currently available including mechanical valve replacements such as bileaflet, tilting-disk and caged ball valves and biologic valve replacements such as xenografts, homografts or allografts.

The procedure can be performed as standard cardiovascular procedure with sternum access, minimally invasive approaches or through port access. However, cardiac arrest is required to perform the procedure; therefore, patients need to undergo general anesthesia and cardiopulmonary bypass. Valvular replacement may be performed for aortic stenosis and aortic insufficiency.

Two types of valvular replacements are currently available including mechanical valve replacements such as bileaflet, tilting-disk, and caged ball valves and biologic valve replacements such as xenografts, homografts, or allografts. Mechanical valve replacements require life-long anticoagulation therapy due to risk of thrombosis.

Mechanical valves last longer and are typically used for patients under 65 or patients over 65 that have a long life expectancy. Biologic valves deteriorate at a rate inversely proportional to the patient's age (wear out faster in younger patients). Thus, biological valves are typically great for elderly patients in whom the expected lifespan is less than the life of the valve (15-20 years). Women that would like to become pregnant should also have biologic valves placed to avoid long-term teratogenic anticoagulants.

Valvular repair

Valvular repair is a procedure that involves repair of calcified or nonfunctioning cardiac valve. Several types of valve repair procedures may be performed including commissurotomy, annuloplasty, and chordoplasty. Commissurotomy is a procedure that separates fused leaflets of a cardiac valve. Annuloplasty is a procedure that repairs the junction between the cardiac valve leaflet and cardiac muscle. Two different approaches can be used to perform annuloplasty including the use of ring prosthesis and/or sutures. Chordoplasty is a procedure that involves the repair of an elongated or ruptured chordae tendinea.

The procedure can be performed open or through minimally invasive approaches or through port access. However, cardiac arrest is required to perform the procedure; therefore, patients need to undergo general anesthesia and cardiopulmonary bypass. Valvular repair may be performed for mitral valve stenosis and mitral insufficiency.

Indications, contraindications, and complications of valvular repair and valvular replacement

Valvular repair or valvular replacements are indicated for aortic or mitral valve disease. Contraindications for valve repair and/or replacement include presence of other cardiovascular comorbidities or poor health status as well as those patients at high surgical risk.

Complications of valvular repair and/or valvular replacements include postoperative bleeding such as heparin induced thrombocytopenia, disseminated intravascular coagulopathy and diluted anemia, myocardial depression, cardiac tamponade, perioperative myocardial infarction, dysrhythmia including atrial tachycardia or atrial fibrillation, pulmonary edema, pulmonary atelectasis, pneumothorax, renal impairment, abdominal distention, cerebral ischemia, postcardiotomy delirium, peripheral neurological deficits, postpericardiotomy syndrome, wound infection, and sudden death.

Role of practicing clinician pre, during, and post valvular repair or valvular replacement

Prior to valvular repair or replacement, practicing clinicians should take a patient's medical history, perform a physical examination, and evaluate a patient's overall health. Patients should be screened for drug-drug interactions, allergies, vital signs such as heart rate and blood pressure and cardiovascular blood indicators such as potassium levels, prothrombin time, and hematocrit and creatinine levels. Patients should also undergo an electrocardiogram and echocardiogram prior to procedure. Additionally, they should take prophylactic antibiotic therapy and undergo a chest x-ray. Overall, a full cardiovascular work-up should be conducted prior to the procedure.

During the procedure, patients should only receive medications via an intravenous route, except for aspirin, which is given orally prior to procedure.

Post-valvular repair or replacement, practicing clinicians should perform an electrocardiogram, echocardiogram, perform a physical assessment, monitor peripheral blood flow, look for swelling, and evaluate cardiac pain. Hospital protocols for aftercare should be followed. Prior to patient release, practicing clinicians should perform additional physical assessments such as assess the patient's heart sounds and laboratory tests such as hematocrit, potassium levels, creatinine levels, and cardiac enzymes. Overall, a full cardiovascular work-up should be conducted prior to releasing the patient.

Arterial bypass surgery

In cases of severe ischemia or occlusion of cardiac blood vessels, bypass grafts may be used to reroute blood flow and improve cardiac function. Bypass vessels that can be used to reroute cardiac blood flow include femoral artery bypass grafting or axillofemoral reconstruction. Bypass grafts can be made from the patient's own tissue or of synthetic nature. Synthetic graft materials include expanded polytetrafluoroethylene and woven or knitted Dacron.

Various approaches may be used to perform arterial bypass surgery including aortobifemoral bypass, aortoiliac endarterectomy, or femoral to popliteal graft. Other approaches may be used dependent on the extent and degree of the patient's disease and/or presence of other comorbid conditions.

Arterial bypass surgery is indicated for severe unilateral or bilateral aortoiliac disease, distal aortic occlusion, and critical limb ischemia with diffuse disease and severe occlusion.

Contraindications for arterial bypass surgery include patients who are medically unstable and have poor distal runoff. Complications of arterial bypass surgery include thrombosis, embolization, bleeding, arterial dissection, infection, restenosis, compartment syndrome, mesenteric ischemic, mesenteric infarction, and/or sudden death. Other complications may arise due to the presence of other comorbid conditions such as diabetes and various cardiovascular conditions as well as due to patient's overall health.

Prior to arterial bypass surgery, practicing clinicians should take the patient's medical history, perform a physical examination, and evaluate the patient's overall health. Patients should be screened for drug-drug interactions, allergies, vital signs such as heart rate and blood pressure and cardiovascular blood indicators such as potassium levels, prothrombin time, and hematocrit and creatinine levels. Patients should also undergo an electrocardiogram and echocardiogram prior to the procedure. Additionally, they should take prophylactic antibiotic therapy and undergo a chest x-ray. Overall, a full cardiovascular work-up should be conducted prior to the procedure.

During the procedure, patients should only receive medications via an intravenous route, except for aspirin, which is given orally prior to the procedure. Post arterial bypass surgery, practicing clinicians should perform an electrocardiogram, echocardiogram, perform a physical assessment, monitor peripheral blood flow and look for swelling and evaluate cardiac pain. Extremity swelling of legs and feet is typical after arterial bypass surgery and should be monitored and treated if it becomes severe. Additionally, patients should be evaluated for compartment syndrome and/or infection.

Pharmacologic management post-surgery may include anticoagulants, antiplatelet agents, aspirin, and/or board spectrum antibiotics.

Hospital protocols for aftercare should be followed. Hemodynamic blood flow should be monitored and patients should be assessed for hemorrhagic shock. Doppler evaluation of vessels may also be completed. Prior to patient release, practicing clinicians should perform additional physical assessments such as assess patient's heart sounds and laboratory tests such as hematocrit, potassium levels, creatinine levels, and cardiac enzymes. Overall, a full cardiovascular work-up should be conducted prior to releasing the patient.

Aneurysm repair

Aneurysm repair involves aneurysm resection and bypass grafting. Aneurysms can be categorized as abdominal, thoracic, aortic, subclavian, femoral, or popliteal. Aneurysm repair procedures may be done on an emergency basis or as a routine procedure to prevent other cardiovascular complications such as stroke, myocardial infarction, or congestive heart failure.

The procedure requires removal of the aneurysm by accessing the location of the aneurysm, clamping above and below the site as well as opening the aneurysm and inserting a graft. Types of aneurysm repair procedures include endovascular grafting, abdominal aortic aneurysm grafting and ascending thoracic aneurysm grafting.

Aneurysm repair is indicated for abdominal aortic aneurysms and thoracic aneurysms. Contraindications for aneurysm repair include patients who are medically unstable. However, in the case of dissection, emergency surgery may be performed.

Complications associated with aneurysm repair procedures include post-operative bleeding, cardiac tamponade, myocardial infarction, pulmonary complications such as pulmonary edema or embolism, renal impairment, gastrointestinal upset such as abdominal distension, ileus, hepatic dysfunction or mesenteric ischemia, hematoma, infection, endocarditis, ischemia, embolism, spinal cord ischemia and/or sudden death. Other complications may arise due to the presence of other comorbid conditions such as diabetes and various cardiovascular conditions as well as due to the patient's overall health.

Prior to aneurysm repair, practicing clinicians should take the patient's medical history, perform a physical examination, and evaluate the patient's overall health. Patients should be screened for drug-drug interactions, allergy, vital signs such as heart rate and blood pressure and cardiovascular blood indicators such as potassium levels, prothrombin time, hematocrit and creatinine levels. Patients should also undergo an electrocardiogram and echocardiogram prior to the procedure. Additionally, they should take prophylactic antibiotic therapy and undergo a chest x-ray. Overall, a full cardiovascular work-up should be conducted prior to the procedure.

Practicing clinicians should also assess the patient for signs of impending aneurysm rupture. Symptoms associated with abdominal aneurysm that can lead to rupture include back or abdominal pain. Symptoms associated with thoracic aneurysm include severe chest, back, shoulder, or abdominal pain. Other associated symptoms include hypotension, congestive heart failure, and/or falling hematocrit.

During the procedure, patients should only receive medications via an intravenous route, except for aspirin, which is given orally prior to procedure. Post-aneurysm repair, practicing clinicians should perform an electrocardiogram, echocardiogram, perform a physical assessment, monitor peripheral blood flow, look for swelling, and evaluate cardiac pain.

Hospital protocols for aftercare should be followed. Hemodynamic blood flow should be monitored and patients should be assessed for hemorrhagic shock. Doppler evaluation of vessels may also be completed. Prior to patient release, practicing clinicians should perform additional physical assessment such as assessing a patient's heart sounds and laboratory tests such as hematocrit, potassium levels, creatinine levels, and cardiac enzymes. Overall, a full cardiovascular work-up should be conducted postsurgery and prior to releasing the patient, including cardiac status, respiratory status, neurological status, peripheral vascular status, gastrointestinal status, pain status, psychosocial status, and potential high-risk complications associated with aneurysm repair.

Carotid endocardiectomy

Carotid endocardiectomy is a common procedure that removes plaque build-up within the carotid artery that serves cerebral blood flow. The procedure involves clamping of the carotid artery and then removal of the plaque build-up to restore blood flow. In an effort to monitor blood flow to the brain, Doppler and electroencephalogram may be used during the procedure.

Carotid endarterectomy is indicated for patients with severe asymptomatic or symptomatic carotid stenosis, ulcerated or intermediate degrees of stenosis that are not effectively treated with anticoagulation therapy and severe stenosis with contralateral internal carotid occlusion.

Carotid endocardiectomy is contraindicated in patients with thick circular calcification, completely blocked arteries, and other cardiovascular comorbid conditions that may be better treated with percutaneous transluminal angioplasty or stent procedure.

Complications associated with carotid endocardiectomy include thrombus formation, embolism, transient ischemic attack, stroke, cranial nerve injury, infection, hematoma, intracranial hemorrhage, restenosis, and/or sudden death. Other complications may arise due to the presence of other cardiovascular comorbid conditions such as diabetes, congestive heart failure, hypertension, or hyperlipidemia as well as due to patient's overall health status. Elderly or severely ill patients with cardiovascular comorbid conditions should be monitored closely pre- and post-carotid endocardiectomy.

Prior to carotid endocardiectomy, practicing clinicians should take a patient's medical history, perform a physical examination, and evaluate a patient's overall health. Patients should be screened for drug-drug interactions, allergies, vital signs such as heart rate and blood pressure and cardiovascular blood indicators such as potassium levels, prothrombin time, and hematocrit and creatinine levels. Patients should also undergo an electrocardiogram and echocardiogram prior to procedure. Additionally, they should take prophylactic antibiotic therapy and undergo a chest x-ray. Overall, a full cardiovascular work-up should be conducted prior to the procedure. Additionally, patient's neurological status should be assessed as well.

During carotid endocardiectomy, patients should only receive medications via an intravenous route, except for aspirin, which is given orally prior to the procedure. Post-procedure, practicing clinicians should perform an electrocardiogram, echocardiogram, perform a physical assessment, monitor peripheral blood flow and look for swelling and evaluate cardiac pain. Neurological assessment including level of consciousness, vocal cord functioning, reflexes, motor strength, level of sensation, pupil size, and reaction to light should be made every 1 to 2 hours post-surgery.

Hospital protocols for aftercare should be followed. Hemodynamic blood flow should be monitored and patients should be assessed for hemorrhagic shock. Doppler evaluation of vessels may also be completed. Prior to patient release, practicing clinicians should perform additional physical assessments such as assess patient's heart sounds and laboratory tests such as hematocrit, potassium levels, creatinine levels, and cardiac enzymes. Overall, a full cardiovascular work-up should be conducted post-surgically and prior to releasing the patient.

Patients should be instructed to follow-up with their practicing clinician 1 week post procedure and then follow-up after 3 months should be done. At 3 months, Doppler evaluation should be performed to assess artery patency. At 6 months and then yearly, Doppler evaluation should be performed to assess for restenosis. Elderly patients should be checked on a regular basis for risk of infection, heart sounds, and cardiac risk factors. Patients at risk for other cardiovascular complications should be monitored on a regular basis. Patients should also be assessed for other cardiovascular risk factors and managed for these risks.

Peripheral thromboembolectomy

Peripheral thromboembolectomy is a procedure that uses a balloon catheter to remove an arterial embolism and restore blood flow through the peripheral circulation. For aortic or iliac occlusions, bilateral ventricle groin incisions followed by embolectomy balloon catheter approach is typically performed. The procedure can be performed on both legs once the initial clot is removed from the occlusion.

For femoral and popliteal occlusions, incisions in the distal common femoral artery followed by embolectomy balloon catheter approach are typically performed. If thromboembolectomy fails, then adjuvant balloon dilatation and/or atherectomy may also be performed. However, anticoagulation therapy may be initiated prior to peripheral thromboembolectomy.

Peripheral thromboembolectomy is indicated for patients with acute symptomatic arterial occlusion as well as patients with gangrene to achieve lower level amputation.

Contraindications of peripheral thromboembolectomy include advanced ischemia up to 2 days. Patients with advanced ischemia after 48 days have a higher risk of amputation. Complications associated with peripheral thromboembolectomy include thrombus formation, vessel vasospasm, hemorrhage, bleeding, hematoma formation, artery dissection, compartment syndrome, venous thrombosis, edema, hyperkalemia, cardiac arrhythmia, renal failure, and rhabdomyolysis. Complications may arise due to the presence of other cardiovascular comorbid conditions such as diabetes, congestive heart failure, hypertension, or hyperlipidemia as well as due to the patient's overall health status.

Prior to peripheral thromboembolectomy, practicing clinicians should take a patient's medical history, perform physical examination, and evaluate the patient's overall health. Patients should be screened for drug-drug interactions, allergies, vital signs such as heart rate and blood pressure and cardiovascular blood indicators such as potassium levels, prothrombin time, hematocrit, and creatinine levels. Patients should also undergo electrocardiogram and echocardiogram prior to procedure. Additionally, they should take prophylactic antibiotic therapy and undergo a chest x-ray. Overall, a full cardiovascular work-up should be conducted prior to the procedure. Additionally, patients should be administered heparin prior to the procedure.

During peripheral thromboembolectomy, patients should only receive medications via an intravenous route, except for aspirin, which is given orally prior to the procedure.

Post-procedure, practicing clinicians should perform an electrocardiogram, echocardiogram, perform a physical assessment, perform pedal pulse assessment with Doppler and/or ankle brachial indices, monitor peripheral blood flow, look for swelling, and evaluate cardiac pain.

Hospital protocols for aftercare should be followed. Hemodynamic blood flow should be monitored and patients should be assessed for hemorrhagic shock. Doppler evaluation of vessels may also be completed. Prior to patient release, practicing clinicians should perform additional physical assessments such as assess patient's heart sounds and laboratory tests such as hematocrit, potassium levels, creatinine levels, and cardiac enzymes. Overall, a full cardiovascular work-up should be conducted postsurgically and prior to releasing the patient.

Patients should be instructed to follow-up with their practicing clinician 1 week postprocedure and then follow-up with Doppler and/or duplex ultrasound evaluation should be performed. Elderly patients should be examined on a regular basis for risk for infection, heart sounds, and cardiac risk factors. Other patients at risk for other cardiovascular complications should be monitored on a regular basis. Patient should also be assessed for other cardiovascular risk factors and managed for these risks. Patients should also be referred to a podiatrist or foot surgeon to address any additional limb and/or foot complications.

Cardiac transplantation

Cardiac transplantation involves the replacement of a patient's own heart with a donor heart. The procedure is performed in patients with progressive end stage cardiovascular disease. Cardiac transplantation is indicated for patients with class III or IV end stage cardiovascular disease, with life expectancy of less than 1 year, under 65 years of age, medically stable, and with no underlying comorbid conditions such as systemic infection, irreversible renal insufficiency, irreversible pulmonary insufficiency, irreversible hepatic insufficiency, active peptic ulcer, or recent pulmonary embolism.

Practicing clinicians and nurses need to work as a team to prepare a patient for cardiac transplantation. Pre-operative care focuses on immunosuppression, acute renal failure, bradycardia, and right ventricular dysfunction.

Long-term complications associated with cardiac transplantation include rejection, infection, transplant coronary artery disease, nephrotoxicity, hypertension, hyperlipidemia, transplant lymphoproliferative disease, and malignancy. Long-term pharmacologic management to prevent these complications includes use of immunosuppressive agents, antibiotics, antihypertensive agents, diuretics, and lipid-lowering agents.

Postpericardiotomy syndrome (PPS)

Postpericardiotomy syndrome is an inflammatory response most often occurring when a patient has undergone a surgical procedure involving the pericardium. Symptoms can develop 1–6 weeks after surgery. The key symptom is high fever (even if the patient has no other complaints of illness). Other symptoms might include malaise, chest or lung pain, trouble breathing, joint pain, irritability and lack of appetite. Physical examination and testing will often exhibit friction rubs, pleural effusions, lung inflammation and cardiac tamponade. Laboratory testing results show negative cultures, but high erythrocyte sedimentation rate (ESR), C-reactive protein (CRP) and anti-heart antibodies. Treatment involves pericardial draining and anti-inflammatory medications.

Evaluation

Complications and prognosis

Raynaud's phenomenon

Raynaud's phenomenon is typically not severe, but can lead to digit deformity due to lack of proper oxygenation and blood flow to digits. Other complications include skin ulcers, infection, and gangrene. Patients with Raynaud's phenomenon should address any cuts or scrapes in the affected areas to prevent infection. A clinical practitioner should address any cuts or scrapes that do not heal properly or in a timely manner. In severe cases of Raynaud's phenomenon, patients may have to undergo surgery and/or have digits amputated.

In terms of prognosis, primary Raynaud's phenomenon is rarely life threatening and more often annoying and a cause of discomfort. Over time, with proper management and care, the phenomenon typically improves. However, secondary Raynaud's phenomenon may be a sign of a rheumatic condition and should be monitored closely by a specialist.

Buerger's disease

Buerger's disease is a rare disorder involving inflammation and subsequent blockage of the veins and arteries. It mainly affects men younger than 40 of Middle Eastern or Far Eastern descent. It causes patchy numbness, cold, burning or tingling of one or more limbs and eventually causes necrosis in the tissues surrounding blocked areas. The principal cause is always tobacco use, therefore of primary concern to the healthcare provider is facilitating smoking and tobacco (of any kind) cessation in order to halt the disease process. Other areas of concern might be pain control, stress management and lifestyle changes that encourage tobacco abstinence. Other less effective treatment options include medications and compression devices to increase blood circulation. If circulation cannot be maintained and infection occurs, amputation of the affected limb may be needed.

Cardiomyopathy

The prognosis of cardiomyopathy varies by the type and extent of disease. Current treatments reduce symptoms and complications of disease. However, in some patients the disease can progress rapidly and result in serious complications such as heart attack and death.

The complications of cardiomyopathy include congestive heart failure, arrhythmias, heart murmur, endocarditis, cardiac arrest, and sudden death. Blood clots may also occur, which can lead to heart attacks and strokes. Patients need to be aware of these complications and manage these risks effectively with self-care, proper pharmacologic regimens, and clinical follow-up on a regular basis.

Congestive heart failure

Complications of congestive heart failure include end organ system dysfunction such as renal failure, pulmonary edema, liver dysfunction due to fluid buildup, and insufficient absorption of nutrients and pharmacologic agents by the small intestines.

Congestive heart failure is typically a progressive disease. The prognosis of the disease varies by the degree and extent of progression. Current treatments reduce symptoms and complications of disease. However, in some patients the disease can progress rapidly, while in others the disease can become chronically maintained.

Factors that determine prognosis include underlying comorbid conditions, symptoms, response to pharmacologic management, and degree and severity of the end organ system involvement

Cor pulmonale

The prognosis of cor pulmonale depends on the underlying cause of disease. The more severe the underlying cause, the greater the risk for complications, and the lower the chance of survival. The administration of supplemental oxygen is typically effective in increasing survival and improving quality of life.

Complications of cor pulmonale include severe fluid retention, life-threatening shortness of breath, shock, and/or death. Other complications include syncope, hypoxia, pedal edema, and/or hepatic congestion. Additionally, complications associated with underlying disease leading to cor pulmonale may arise.

Type I and type II diabetes

Acute complications associated with type I and type II diabetes include diabetic ketoacidosis (type I), nonketotic hyperosmolar coma (type II), hyperglycemia and hypoglycemia. Acute complications need to be addressed immediately; otherwise, individuals are at risk for seizures and/or coma.

Other long-term complications include vascular disease, coronary artery disease, stroke, peripheral vascular disease, diabetic myonecrosis, diabetic retinopathy, diabetic neuropathy, osteoporosis, Alzheimer disease, infections, foot ulcers, and diabetic nephropathy. In an effort to avoid these complications, patients need to comply with blood sugar management and control other environmental risk factors.

In an effort to prevent long-term complications, diabetic patients should undergo yearly physicals and eye examinations, get necessary immunizations, maintain teeth and feet, avoid stress, maintain proper cholesterol and blood pressure levels, and avoid smoking and/or tobacco use.

The prognosis of diabetes depends on the individual patient and the presence of other comorbid conditions. It also depends on an individual's compliance to lifestyle modifications and pharmacologic management.

Metabolic syndrome

The main complication of metabolic syndrome is cardiovascular disease such as coronary artery disease, congestive heart failure, heart attack, stroke, and sudden death. Another complication in patients diagnosed with metabolic syndrome who have not already been diagnosed with diabetes, is the development of type II diabetes. Most patients diagnosed with metabolic syndrome have abdominal obesity, which puts them at a high predisposition for developing type II diabetes. Patients diagnosed with metabolic syndrome who have comorbid type II diabetes are at a much higher risk for the development of cardiovascular disease.

Patients diagnosed with metabolic syndrome are also at an increased risk for blood clotting abnormalities and peripheral vascular disease.

Patients diagnosed with metabolic syndrome should have their 10-year risk of developing cardiovascular disease calculated by a specialist.

The National Cholesterol Education Program (NCEP) provides a risk calculator of developing cardiovascular disease within the next 10 years.

Individuals with a 10-year risk score more than 20% are considered high risk for developing cardiovascular disease.

Individuals with a 10-year risk score between 10% and 20% are considered moderately high risk for developing cardiovascular disease.

Individuals with a 10-year risk score less than 10% are considered at moderate risk for developing cardiovascular disease.

Individuals with 10-year risk score of zero or 1 percent are considered at low risk for developing cardiovascular disease.

Hypertension

Persistent hypertension is a risk factor for developing complications such as stroke, heart attack, congestive heart failure, aneurysm, aortic dissection, arteriosclerosis, vision loss, and chronic renal failure. Other complications include intracerebral hemorrhage, lacunar infarcts, congestive heart failure, angina, encephalopathy, myocardial infarction, cardiomyopathy, retinopathy, and nephropathy.

The prognosis of hypertension is associated with the blood pressure level and the presence of other comorbid conditions and complications. Untreated hypertension increases the risk of cardiovascular complications, end organ system failure, and mortality. Untreated mild to moderate hypertension, after 8 to 10 years post onset, has been shown to be associated with atherosclerotic disease in 30% of individuals and end organ system damage in 50% of individuals.

Myocardial infarction

Complications associated with myocardial infarction can be acute or develop post acute attack. Complications include recurrent myocardial infarction, congestive heart failure, valve problems, myocardial rupture, myocardial damage, life-threatening arrhythmia, pericarditis, and cardiogenic shock.

The prognosis of individual who experience a myocardial infarction depends on the degree and extent of the attack. It also depends on the presence of underlying comorbid conditions. Prognosis further depends on patient compliance with lifestyle modifications and pharmacologic management post acute attack. Increased prognosis is associated with early reperfusion, preserved left ventricular function, and compliance with short-term and long-term pharmacologic agents.

Stroke

Complications associated with stroke depend on the extent and degree of damage to brain and associated tissues. It also depends on the location of the brain affected by the stroke. Complications include numbness and weakness on 1 side of the body, confusion, slurred speech, difficulty speaking, vision loss, double vision, difficulty walking, dizziness, loss of balance and coordination, pain, memory loss, problems with spatial orientation and swallowing, loss of bladder or bowel function, and perception loss.

Complications of stroke may be improved with physical therapy and/or rehabilitation. Practitioners involved in rehabilitation include psychiatrists, physical therapists, occupational therapists, recreational therapists, and/or speech therapists. Family or loved ones should keep in close touch with a patient who has had a stroke. They should also keep conversations at an adult level using a normal tone of voice and speaking at a comfortable pace.

Approximately 75% of individuals who experienced a stroke are unable to maintain employment. Also, 30% to 50% of individuals who experience a stroke suffer depression.

Peripheral arterial disease
The main complications of peripheral arterial disease include limb ischemia, limb loss, pain, wound infection, poor wound healing, and decreased limb function.

Individuals diagnosed with peripheral arterial disease are at a greater risk of cardiovascular disease, heart attack, stroke, and/or transient ischemic attack than the general population.

Patients with diabetes and peripheral arterial disease are at a higher risk for developing critical limb ischemia, sometimes requiring amputation of affected limbs.

Inflammation
Examples of acute inflammation include acute appendicitis, acute dermatitis, acute infective meningitis, and acute tonsillitis.

Complications of chronic inflammation can lead to prolonged activation of the inflammatory cascade and inflammatory disorders caused by presence of viral or bacterial infections or signaling malfunctions. Chronic inflammation can lead to development of inflammatory disorders such as asthma; autoimmune disease such as lupus, psoriasis and rheumatoid arthritis; bursitis; gout; prolonged inflammation; chronic prostatitis; glomerulonephritis; hypersensitivities such as allergies; myopathies; leukocyte defects; inflammatory bowel disease such as Crohn disease and ulcerative colitis; pelvic inflammatory disease; reperfusion injury; transplant rejection; obesity; and vasculitis.

Pericarditis
The complications of pericarditis include pericardial effusion, arrhythmias, constrictive pericarditis, and cardiac tamponade. Early diagnosis of pericarditis can reduce the risk of developing these complications.

Constrictive pericarditis is permanent thickening of the pericardium, which hinders proper function of the heart muscle. Complications of constrictive pericarditis include swelling of the abdomen and legs as well as shortness of breath.

Cardiac tamponade is accumulation of fluid in the pericardium leading to improper functioning of the heart. The excess fluid does not allow the heart to pump blood effectively and can lead to sudden death if not properly treated.

Pericarditis can range from mild to very severe cases and prognosis depends on the extent and degree of disease. Most cases resolve within 2 weeks to 3 months.

Vasculitis

Complications of vasculitis are dependent on the degree and extent of disease as well as the blood vessels systems and end organ systems involved. Most cases of vasculitis are minor and resolve on their own without medical intervention. However, some cases are severe and involve major end organ systems and result in serious complications. Serious complications include end organ system damage, cardiovascular disease, heart attack, stroke, and death.

Other complications include renal insufficiency, digital gangrene, pulmonary hemorrhage, central nervous system infarction, arterial or venous thrombosis, and subglottic stenosis.

The prognosis of individuals diagnosed with vasculitis depends on the type, extent, and degree of vasculitis as well as end organ involvement.

Endocarditis

Complications associated with endocarditis are dependent on the extent and degree of disease. In more severe cases, where debris and bacteria reside in the endocardium, individuals may experience heart attack, stroke, other end organ system damage, and sudden death. Other complications include arrhythmias, blood clots, brain abscess, brain or nervous system damage, congestive heart failure, glomerulonephritis, jaundice, cardiac valvular insufficiency, aneurysm, cardiac abscesses and severe heart failure.

Untreated endocarditis can be very serious and permanently damage inner lining of heart cambers and valves, leading to congestive heart failure due to an inability of the heart to pump effectively.

The prognosis in individuals who receive early intervention is better for those who receive delayed treatment. However, complications such as heart attack and stroke can lead to sudden death.

Renal artery occlusion

Complications associated with renal artery occlusion include hypertension, chronic renal failure and malignant hypertension. Hypertension associated with renal artery occlusion may be difficult to control and require intervention with multiple pharmacologic approaches including angiotensin-converting enzyme inhibitors such as captopril and enalapril and angiotensin II receptor antagonists such as losartan.

Untreated renal artery occlusion can result in chronic renal failure and potentially death. Although balloon angioplasty and stenting may improve blood flow from arteries of kidneys, blockage may reoccur. Early diagnosis and careful monitoring can prevent progression of the disease and improve outcomes.

Renal vein thrombosis

Renal vein thrombosis typically improves overtime, with limited permanent damage to kidneys and other end organ systems. However, complications that can arise from renal vein thrombosis include acute renal failure if occurring due to dehydration in an infant or adolescent, embolization of blood clot to lungs, heart, brain or other organ systems, and formation of new blood clots.

The prognosis of renal vein thrombosis depends on the degree and extent of the condition and the impact on other organ systems such as the lungs and/or brain. It also depends largely on the extent of renal system damage. The effects on kidney function depend on whether 1 or both kidneys are affected, whether blood flow can be restored and health of the kidney prior to the presence of renal vein thrombosis. Death is typically rare but can occur due to an underlying comorbid condition.

Atheroembolic renal disease

The complications of atheroembolic renal disease are similar to that of atherosclerotic disease. Complications associated with atheroembolic disease include acute renal failure, chronic renal failure, high blood pressure, embolization of blood clots, and formation of blood clots in other organ systems such as heart, intestines, lungs, and legs.

Complications associated with atherosclerosis include risk of blood clotting, in which a plaque increases in size to reduce blood flow and risk of rupture, which can lead to heart attack and/or stroke. If blood flow is reduced to the peripheral vasculature then patients may have walking and dexterity complications, erectile dysfunction and abdominal aortic aneurysms.

Atherosclerosis leads to altered vascular function including coronary heart disease, myocardial ischemia and myocardial infarction, cerebrovascular insufficiency, stroke, aortic aneurysm and vasculitis. The prognosis of atheroembolic renal disease depends on the degree and extent of disease as well as presence of other comorbid conditions. The disease typically progresses overtime and outcomes are generally poor.

Lifestyle modifications may slow the progression of the disease but progression typically occurs.

Marfan syndrome

Complications of Marfan syndrome include aortic dissection due to weakening of the aorta, heart value disease that can lead to enlargement of the heart, mitral valve prolapse, mitral valve regurgitation, endocarditis, optical complications, lung complications such as breathing difficulties, abnormal heart sounds, as well as aortic aneurysm. Aortic aneurysm accounts for the most deaths associated with Marfan syndrome.

Vision complications associated with Marfan syndrome include shifting or dislocation, extreme nearsightedness, glaucoma, cataract and/or detachment or tear in the retina. Skeletal complications include scoliosis, spondylolisthesis, and foot pain. Other complications include stretch marks and dural ectasia.

Pregnant women with Marfan syndrome are at greater risk for aortic dissection or rupture due to increased stress to the aortic walls.

Atrial septal defect

The prognosis for patients with small atrial septal defect is very good, with most living a normal life span without symptoms. However, patients with larger defects may have complications later in life including disabilities due to shunting of blood between atria and increased blood flow in pulmonary circulation.

Complications associated with atrial septal defects include pulmonary hypertension, arrhythmias such as atrial fibrillation, Eisenmenger syndrome, right-sided heart failure, shortened life expectancy, stroke, and heart failure. Patients with larger defects have a higher risk of high blood pressure leading to lung problems and congestive heart failure. If surgery is not performed, patients with these comorbid conditions are at a higher risk for death. Eisenmenger syndrome occurs when pulmonary resistance increases because of prolonged high blood flow from the shunt. Eventually, the shunt reverses and causes cyanosis.

Surgical mortality rate is less than 0.1%. In younger adolescents, surgical closure is effective in preventing complications, with excellent prognosis.

Pulmonary embolism

Complications associated with pulmonary embolism depend on the extent and degree of disease. The most common complications associated with the condition include pulmonary hypertension, cor pulmonale, heart failure, heart attack, and stroke.

Pulmonary embolism can lead to death if left untreated. Approximately 33% of undiagnosed or untreated individuals die of the condition due to complications. Also, reoccurrence of the condition increases with initial diagnosis of the disease. Early treatment of pulmonary embolism decreases the risk of serious side effects and proactive continued monitoring of the condition prevents the reoccurrence of pulmonary embolism.

Patients who develop pulmonary embolism from a deep venous thrombosis may develop permanent leg swelling, discomfort, discoloration, chronic nonhealing ulcerations, and atrophic skin changes.

Deep venous thrombosis

The complications of deep venous thrombosis include pulmonary embolism and postphlebitic syndrome. Blood clots in the thigh have a higher rate of leading to pulmonary embolism than deep venous thrombosis of the lower leg.

The prognosis of deep venous thrombosis is good with early intervention. However, untreated deep venous thrombosis can lead to serious complications such as pulmonary embolism, stroke, heart attack, and sudden death. Also, maintaining regular check-ups, being compliant with pharmacologic agents, using graduated compression stockings, and increasing physical activity, all decrease complications of deep venous thrombosis.

Venous insufficiency

Complications of venous insufficiency include chronic pain, dermatitis, chronic nonhealing ulcers, hemorrhage, recurrent cellulitis, deep and superficial thrombophlebitis, pulmonary embolism, heart attack, stroke and even sudden death. Complications associated with nontreatment of venous insufficiency include recruitment of veins, deep venous thrombosis, pulmonary embolism, venous ulceration, and secondary lymphedema.

Potential complications associated with surgical ablation include infection, peripheral nerve damage, and arterial injury. Adverse events associated with radiofrequency ablation and endovenous laser therapy include skin burns, injury to adjacent tissues, and injury to deep veins. Additionally, side effects associated with sclerotherapy include allergic reaction, cutaneous necrosis, and loss of limb.

The prognosis of venous insufficiency depends on the extent and degree of the condition, presence of other comorbid conditions, and patient's age and overall general health.

Valvular disease

Most patients diagnosed with valvular disease can live their normal lifespan without any interruption of quality of life or become impacted by symptoms. However, in some patients diagnosed with the condition, the disease progresses over time leading to complications such as congestive heart failure, stroke, blood clot formation, myocardial infarction, and sudden death.

The prognosis of individuals diagnosed with valvular disease depends on the extent and degree of the condition, age of the patient and presence of other comorbid conditions. Pharmacologic management and lifestyle changes may improve a patient's prognosis and prevent the onset of more serious complications such as congestive heart failure, stroke, blood clot formation, myocardial infarction, and sudden death.

Cardiac vasospasm
Complications associated with cardiac vasospasm include myocardial infarction, arrhythmias, tachycardia, ventricular fibrillation, heart failure, stroke, and sudden death. Complications depend on the degree and extent of cardiac vasospasm, age of patient and presence of other comorbid conditions.

General preventive measures that individuals can take to reduce the risk of cardiac vasospasm and disease complications include avoiding the triggers of vasospasm such as cocaine or stress. Decreasing risk factors for heart disease in general is also beneficial.

Angina pectoris
In most cases, angina pectoris is typically a symptom and dissipates as the underlying condition is treated. It is not a typically a serious condition and most patients will not experience any complications such as myocardial infarction, heart failure, or stroke due to angina pectoris.

Treating underlying causes of angina pectoris decreases the risk of developing complications or other comorbid conditions. However, in more severe cases in individuals with comorbid cardiovascular conditions, patients may experience myocardial infarction and/or arrhythmias. Elderly patients who are in poor health with other comorbid conditions are more likely to experience more-serious complications compared to younger patients who are in good health.

Angina pectoris, especially unstable angina and cases not responding to nitrates, should always be taken seriously.

Atrial fibrillation
Chronic atrial fibrillation leads to complications that include clot formation, thromboembolism, heart failure, and potential for heart attack and stroke. Acute atrial fibrillation can lead to more-serious complications, as the body is unable to handle the severity of the condition.

Nearly half of patients experiencing atrial fibrillation treated with pharmacologic agents including dysrhythmia agents do not experience a reoccurrence at 12 months. However, individuals with underlying comorbid conditions should have those conditions addressed to prevent reoccurrence of atrial fibrillation as well as other comorbid cardiovascular complications. Severe complications, including myocardial infarction, thromboembolism, and stroke occur more often in undiagnosed individuals and those who are noncompliant with treatment.

Arrhythmias
Complications of arrhythmias include stroke, congestive heart failure, and thromboembolism. Severe complications including myocardial infarction, thromboembolism, and stroke occur more often in undiagnosed individuals and those noncompliant with treatment.

Treating the underlying causes of arrhythmias and the arrhythmia itself decreases the risk of developing complications. However, in more severe cases, especially in individuals with comorbid cardiovascular conditions, patients may experience myocardial infarction and/or arrhythmias. Elderly patients who are in poor health with other comorbid conditions are more likely to experience more-serious complications compared to younger patients who are in good health.

Atrial flutter

Typically, atrial flutter is not considered as life threatening as atrial fibrillation. However, complications associated with atrial flutter include stroke, embolization, rate related complications, clot formation, sudden cardiac death, congestive heart failure, severe bradycardia and myocardial rate-related ischemia.

The risk of developing stroke with atrial fibrillation and atrial flutter is approximately 4%. In more severe cases of atrial flutter, especially those with comorbid cardiovascular conditions, patients may experience myocardial infarction or stroke. Elderly patients who are in poor health with other comorbid conditions are more likely to experience more serious complications compared to younger patients who are in good health.

Wolff-Parkinson-White syndrome

Complications of Wolff-Parkinson-White syndrome include hypotension, congestive heart failure, and other comorbid cardiovascular conditions.

The prognosis of patients diagnosed with Wolff-Parkinson-White syndrome varies depending on the degree and extent of disease. However, most patients respond well to lifestyle modifications and pharmacologic management. Also, more invasive approaches such as radiofrequency catheter ablation cure the condition by ablating the extra pathway, which has demonstrated good outcomes. Elderly patients who are in poor health with other comorbid conditions are more likely to experience more-serious complications compared to younger patients who are in good health.

Ventricular fibrillation

Ventricular fibrillation is a very serious condition with severe complications including congestive heart failure and sudden cardiac death. The degree and extent of complications depends on when a patient receives treatment for the condition or if the patient recognizes the symptoms and seeks treatment.

Other complications in patients who survive an acute ventricular fibrillation episode include coma, reduced mental perception, neurological problems, congestive heart failure, central nervous system (CNS) ischemic injury, myocardial injury, post defibrillation arrhythmias, aspiration pneumonia, defibrillation injury, injuries from cardiopulmonary resuscitation, skin burns, stroke, and other cardiovascular conditions.

The prognosis for patients who experience an acute ventricular fibrillation episode depends on the length the patient was in fibrillation. However, for those patients who survive an acute ventricular fibrillation episode, the survival rate averages between 2% to 25% post hospital stay. Patients who seek treatment sooner than later tend to have better outcomes over the longer term. Elderly patients who are in poor health with other comorbid conditions are more likely to experience more serious complications compared to younger patients who are in good health.

Ventricular tachycardia

Complications associated with ventricular tachycardia can be benign or very serious including congestive heart failure and cardiac sudden death. The prognosis of patients with ventricular tachycardia depends on the degree and extent of the condition. Patients who seek treatment sooner than later tend to have better outcomes over the longer term. Elderly patients who are in poor health with other comorbid conditions are more likely to experience more-serious complications compared to younger patients who are in good health.

The mortality rate of ventricular tachycardia in patients with cardiomyopathy and nonsustained disease averages 30% in 2 years. In patients with idiopathic disease, prognosis is excellent. However, patients with long QT syndrome, right ventricular dysplasia, and hypertropic cardiomyopathy are at an increased risk of sudden cardiac death.

Intermittent claudication

The prognosis of individuals diagnosed with intermittent claudication is good because the condition typically stabilizes or improves over time. The condition tends to improve over a few months, when new smaller blood vessels form to make up for the blockage or lack of blood flow to larger blood vessels in the legs.

Typically, approximately 1/3 of patients with intermittent claudication tend to improve over time, while 1/3 remains stable and another 1/3 deteriorate, mainly due to continued smoking. Graduated increased physical activity can improve the condition over time, as regular walks have demonstrated improvement in the condition.

Early intervention with physical activity provides better outcomes and improvements in the condition. Patients who seek treatment sooner than later tend to have better outcomes over the longer term. Elderly patients who are in poor health with other comorbid conditions are more likely to experience more serious complications as compared to younger patients who are in good health.

Hypotension

Complications associated with hypotension or low blood pressure include dizziness, fainting, confusion and in more serious cases, severe heart, endocrine, and/or neurological disorders. Shock is a complication of very severe hypotension, where the brain and other organ systems are deprived of oxygen and vital nutrients.

Most healthy individuals with hypotension can maintain their condition with lifestyle modifications. However, in more severe cases, practicing clinicians will prescribe pharmacologic agents and treat the underlying cause of the condition. Individuals with hypotension including neurally mediated hypotension or orthostatic hypotension need to be careful to avoid fainting and dizziness, which can be dangerous. In very severe cases of hypotension, shock is a life-threatening condition that is fatal if not treated immediately.

Compartment syndrome

Prompt diagnosis and treatment of compartment syndrome results in good outcomes, with recovery of affected nerves and blood vessels of the muscle. However, the prognosis of compartment syndrome is determined by the underlying injury leading to the condition. Delayed diagnosis and treatment can result in permanent nerve damage and loss of muscle function. Other complications include impaired function due to muscle damage, infection, cosmetic deformity, and death and limb amputation.

Increased education in patients at high risk for compartment syndrome improves prognosis and prevents serious complications due to early diagnosis and treatment.

Pulmonary edema

Complications associated with pulmonary edema include leg swelling, abdominal swelling and pleural effusion. If treated promptly, individuals diagnosed with pulmonary edema have a good prognosis. However, individuals who are not promptly diagnosed or treated may have more-serious complications or death.

Early intervention provides better outcomes and improvements in the condition. Patients who seek treatment sooner than later tend to have better outcomes over the longer term. Elderly patients who are in poor health with other comorbid conditions are more likely to experience more serious complications as compared to younger patients who are in good health.

First-degree atrioventricular block

Complications associated with first-degree atrioventricular block include progression of condition to a higher degree of atrioventricular block, reduction in left ventricular stroke volume and cardiac output leading to left ventricular systolic dysfunction, and pacemaker syndrome. Patients who progress usually progress to Mobitz type I, second-degree atrioventricular block but sometimes progress to complete atrioventricular block.

The prognosis associated with first-degree atrioventricular block is excellent, especially in patients with asymptomatic disease. First-degree atrioventricular block does not present with increased mortality or morbidity. However, patients that present with comorbid intranodal blocks have an increased risk of developing complete atrioventricular block, which comes with a high risk of serious complications including death.

Second-degree atrioventricular block type I

Second-degree atrioventricular block type I is typically a benign condition that does not require immediate treatment. The complications associated with more mild forms of the condition are minimal, except in patients with poor health or other cardiovascular comorbid conditions.

Patients undergoing treatment with agents that have the potential to induce second-degree atrioventricular block type I should be monitored closely and doses should be adjusted if the condition is induced by the medication.

The prognosis of second-degree atrioventricular block type I depends on the extent and degree of the block. Atrioventricular nodal blocks, which make up most of the type I blocks carry a better prognosis than intra or infra bundle blocks. Intra- and/or infra- bundle blocks can progress to higher degrees of atrioventricular block including complete atrioventricular block.

Second-degree atrioventricular block type II

The prognosis for patients with second-degree atrioventricular block type II is not as good as the prognosis for patients with second-degree atrioventricular block type I. Typically, second-degree atrioventricular block type II progresses to complete heart block and carries risk of syncope, stroke, myocardial infarction, and congestive heart failure. In particular, intra- and/or infra- bundle blocks can progress to higher degrees of atrioventricular block including complete atrioventricular block.

Patients undergoing treatment with agents that have the potential to induce second-degree atrioventricular block type II should be monitored closely and doses should be adjusted if the condition is induced by the medication.

Third-degree atrioventricular block

The prognosis of third-degree atrioventricular block is excellent for patients who receive treatment with permanent pacing. However, patients who are untreated or seek treatment too late are at higher risk for serious complications. Patients with other comorbid cardiovascular health conditions and/or are in poor health have a poorer prognosis. Patients diagnosed with third-degree atrioventricular block are at a high risk for stroke, congestive heart failure, and myocardial infarction.

Patients undergoing treatment with agents that have the potential to induce third-degree atrioventricular block should be monitored closely and doses should be adjusted if the condition is induced by the medication.

Cardiogenic shock

Complications associated with cardiogenic shock include cardiopulmonary arrest, dysrhythmia, renal failure, multisystem organ failure, ventricular aneurysm, thromboembolic disease, stroke, congestive heart failure, and death.

The prognosis for patients diagnosed with cardiogenic shock is very poor. Approximately 50% of patients who experience cardiogenic shock do not survive. The reason that patients diagnosed with cardiogenic shock are able to survive is prompt treatment with pharmacologic agents and/or surgical intervention. The ability to restore blood flow to vital organ systems improves outcomes and prognosis. Patients who undergo treatment promptly with pharmacologic intervention or surgical intervention have an improved prognosis. Evidence of right ventricular dilation on echocardiogram may indicate worse prognosis than other underlying causes of the condition.

Percutaneous transluminal coronary angioplasty (PTCA)

Contraindications for a percutaneous transluminal coronary angioplasty procedure include high-risk coronary anatomy, severe coronary artery disease, bleeding disorder, and/or multiple episodes of percutaneous transluminal coronary angioplasty restenosis.

Complications associated with percutaneous transluminal coronary angioplasty include abrupt closure of diseased coronary artery, periprocedural myocardial infarction, coronary restenosis, bleeding, or hematoma at catheter introduction site, arterial embolism, pseudoaneurysm, retroperitoneal bleeding, and sudden death. Bleeding from the site of catheter insertion (usually the femoral artery) and anaphylaxis to the dye used are also major risk factors.

Other complications may occur due to the patient's overall health, allergies, and other comorbid conditions. Therefore, practicing clinicians need to take a careful medical history and perform a physical examination prior to the procedure.

Coronary artery bypass graft (CABG)

Potential risk factors:
- Death
- Pain: incisional or related to new-onset myocardial infarction
- Bleeding: surgical trauma, thrombocytopenia, anemia or disseminated intravascular coagulopathy (DIC)
- Myocardial depression: cardiac dysfunction
- Cardiac tamponade: increased pericardial fluid
- Myocardial infarction: additional injury occurring after surgery

- Dysrhythmia: most commonly atrial fibrillation
- Pulmonary complications: pulmonary edema, atelectasis, pneumothorax
- Renal impairment: mild to acute renal failure
- Neuropsychological problems: cerebral ischemia, infarction, emboli, postcardiotomy delirium (ranging from elation and denial to hallucinations and neurological symptoms), brachial plexus or ulnar nerve injury
- Postpericardiotomy syndrome: autoimmune response to surgical injury
- Infection: wound, sepsis
- Gastrointestinal problems: distention, ileus, hepatic dysfunction, mesenteric ischemia

Cardiac tamponade

Swift identification and treatment of cardiac tamponade (a buildup of fluid in the pericardial space) is a critical factor in patient mortality. Key symptoms include the classic Beck triad: increased jugular vein pressure with visual vein distention (Kussmaul sign), decreased blood pressure (pulsus paradoxus) and diminished heart sounds. Other signs and symptoms might include increased heart rate, cold and clammy hands and/or feet, cough, dyspnea, decreased consciousness or fainting and anxiety. In advanced cases, Ewart (Pins) sign may also be present: an area of breath sound dullness or bronchophony (very audible and high-pitched voice sounds in the lung) is evident below the left scapula.

Abdominal aortic aneurysms

Most aortic aneurysms are asymptomatic, making early detection more difficult. If the patient presents with symptoms the most common will be pain that is dull and deep within the abdominal cavity and radiating into the back. The pain may be alleviated or eased by change of position. The other noticeable symptom that might be detected by the patient or medical personnel is a palpable, abnormal pulsation within the abdominal cavity. Identification of the aneurysm is made with ultrasound or CT scan. Surgical repair is the primary route of treatment. When the aneurysm is small enough that it doesn't require surgery, then treatment will focus on preventing growth or rupture through smoking cessation, controlling blood pressure, and cholesterol levels while monitoring the aneurysm size every 6–12 months.

Differences between a coronary artery bypass graft (CABG) and minimally invasive direct coronary artery bypass (MIDCAB)

Traditional CABG surgery involves restoring cardiac blood flow by grafting in a new vein or artery to direct blood around a blockage in the coronary artery. This procedure requires a large incision, stopping the heart and use of a heart-lung machine.

MIDCAB uses a smaller incision and can be performed on a still-beating, but slowed, heart. Prime candidates for this operation are those patients with proximal left anterior descending lesion. This requires less time and therefore, shorter exposure to anesthesia with earlier extubation. Initial pain during recovery may be greater than with CABG, but it is relieved more quickly. There are fewer risks associated with the procedure and expenses are reduced. Patients receiving MIDCAB report better physical activity and sleeping conditions than those undergoing CABG.

Medications that can cause variations in the effectiveness of digoxin

Antacids, amiloride, cholestyramine, neomycin and sulfasalazine reduce the effect of digoxin. Herbal remedies such as plantain and St. John's wort may also decrease effectiveness.

Albuterol, amiodarone, captopril, cyclosporine, diltiazem, erythromycin, nifedipine, omeprazole, quinidine, tetracycline, thyroxin and verapamil can cause higher blood levels of digoxin and risk toxicity. Herbal remedies of gossypol, horsetail, licorice, oleander, Siberian ginseng and squill (scilla) also carry a greater risk for digoxin toxicity.

Betel pal, fumitory, goldenseal, hawthorn, lily of the valley, motherwort, rue and shepherd's purse should be avoided completely.

Therapeutic digoxin blood levels are between 0.8–2 ng/ml. Monitor lab results and pulse prior to each administration of digoxin.

Medications and foods that may alter the effectiveness of warfarin sodium (Coumadin)

Multiple medications will react with Coumadin and vary the effectiveness. Monitor PT and INR levels closely to maintain therapeutic levels. Review all medications and supplements carefully. Pay special attention to pain relievers, hormones (oral contraceptives, testosterone, estrogen and thyroid), steroids, hypolipidemics, antidiabetics, antibiotics and tricyclic antidepressants. Most common herbal remedies, including garlic, ginger, ginkgo, ginseng, licorice and angelica, should not be combined with warfarin use. Alcohol use should be minimized, and any source of vitamin K (green leafy vegetables, vitamin supplements and green tea) should be kept at a constant level.

Medications and foods that may alter the effectiveness of Lipitor

Antacids, colestipol and isradipine may decrease the effectiveness of Lipitor. Erythromycin, fluconazole, itraconazole, ketoconazole and voriconazole may increase Lipitor blood levels. Lipitor also interacts unfavorably with digoxin and contraceptives, changing the effectiveness of these medications. Lipitor in combination with antifungal, cyclosporine, erythromycin, fibric acid and niacin can increase the risk of developing muscle weakness. Herbal supplements including eucalyptus, kava and red yeast rice can cause adverse reactions. Grapefruit juice should not be ingested while taking Lipitor. Use cautiously in the patient with a known history of heavy alcohol use, liver and/or renal disease.

Risks associated with vascular repair

Vascular repair procedures include aortic aneurysm repair, bypass grafting, vena cava filter insertion and embolism removal. Postoperatively, monitor for
- Bleeding: external at incision site or internal, causing low blood pressure, increased heart rate, diminished respirations, restlessness, confusion, abdominal pain, increased girth or rigidity.
- Occlusion: diminished or absent peripheral pulses, abnormal sensation and/or pain, reduced oxygen saturation and cyanosis.
- Infection: fever; redness; warmth; drainage; pain; abnormal heart rate, respiration, or blood pressure; or cough and congestion.
- Renal impairment: swelling, weight gain, low urinary output and increased blood urea nitrogen (BUN) and creatinine levels.

Arrhythmias as seen on ECG

<u>Sinus node</u>
The sinus node is the primary pacemaker for the heart, setting a normal rate and rhythm of 60–100.
- Sinus arrhythmia: ECG rate falls within normal limits, but there is a slight change in rhythm correlating to breathing (increased pulse with inspiration, slowing with expiration).
- Sinus bradycardia: Rhythm is normal, all parts of the ECG appear normal, with a rate below 60 beats per minute.
- Sinus tachycardia: Rhythm is normal, ECG is normal, but rate is greater than 100 beats per minute.
- Sinus arrest: Rate is normal, but rhythm is interrupted by occasional missing PQRST complexes. This is referred to as a sinus pause if only one or two beats are dropped; sinus arrest refers to 3 or more missing complexes.
- Sick sinus syndrome: Irregular rhythm in which the waves and complexes vary instead of forming a predictable pattern.

<u>Junctional</u>
Premature junctional contraction (PJC): Rate and rhythm are fundamentally regular with occasional early, inverted P wave and following QRS complex.

Junctional escape rhythm: Regular rate and rhythm appears to be normal sinus rhythm except for inverted P waves.

Accelerated junctional rhythm: Regular rhythm of 60–100 beats per minute. P wave may be absent or appear inverted before or after the QRS complex. Everything else appears normal.

Junctional tachycardia: Regular rhythm with a rate of 100–200 beats per minute. P wave is inverted and occurs after the QRS complex.

<u>Ventricular</u>
Premature ventricular contraction (PVC): Underlying regular rate and rhythm, with occasional early, wide and bizarre-looking QRS complex.

Ventricular tachycardia: No P wave, wide and bizarre QRS complex with rapid rate of 100–200 beats per minute.

Ventricular fibrillation: No identifiable rhythm, no identifiable wave forms. ECG shows only a fine or coarse chaotic wavy line. Patient is unresponsive and pulseless.

Idioventricular rhythms: Ventricular rate of 20–40 beats per minute, independent or no P wave (PR interval unmeasurable) with bizarre-looking QRS complex longer than 0.12 seconds.

Asystole: No electrical conduction, displayed as an almost flat line only disturbed by medical interventions such as CPR. Patient is unconscious and pulseless.

Types of heart block as seen on ECG

First-degree AV block: Rhythm is regular and appears very similar to a normal sinus rhythm. The only difference is a PR interval longer than 0.20 seconds.

Type I second-degree AV block: Regular atrial rhythm with a repeating pattern of progressively longer PR intervals until a QRS complex no longer appears behind the P wave.

Type II second-degree AV block: Atrial rhythm is regular, ventricular rhythm maybe either regular or irregular. Look for missing QRS complexes.

Third-degree AV block: Atrial and ventricular rates are regular, but independent of each other. PR interval will vary.

Left bundle-branch block: QRS complex is wider than 0.12 seconds, R wave may not be detected or may be "slurred."

Right bundle-branch block: QRS complex is wider than 0.12 seconds and has an unusual appearance (may look like rabbit ears or the letter M). T wave is inverted.

Ventricular assist devices (VAD)

A ventricular assist device is a 1–2 pound pump, usually placed internally by the left ventricle. It is electrically controlled from outside the body. It re-routes the blood flow from the ineffective or damaged ventricle through a series of tubes that will pump the blood more efficiently than the body is able to do on its own. This treatment is not without significant risk, but the patient with chronic heart failure that can no longer be controlled with medication or pacemaker may be assessed for eligibility. The most likely candidate is a younger, healthy patient who is awaiting transplant.

Enhanced external counterpulsation (EECP)

Enhanced external counterpulsation (EECP) is a pain control method that may be effective for patients with recurring stable angina. Treatment involves sequential compression of the patient's entire leg length to promote blood flow and increase cardiac output. The patients who might receive the most benefit from this type of treatment are those who refuse invasive treatment measures, have not responded to medication and revascularization efforts or are not candidates for such treatments. EECP should be used cautiously in the patient with preexisting decreased left ventricular ejection fraction or heart failure.

Outcome evaluation

Outcome evaluation is a necessary step taken by practicing clinicians to assess a patient's recovery from cardiovascular procedures. The process is used to evaluate the patient's status, evaluate effectiveness of interventions, and identify areas of improvement.

Commonly used patient outcomes include morbidity, mortality, hemodynamic parameters, laboratory values such as blood sugar, lipid levels, and prothrombin time, symptoms such as nausea, vomiting, pain, fatigue, angina, anxiety and depression, and functional status. Commonly used practicing clinician parameters include change in knowledge or skill level and compliance with patient standards. Commonly used system outcomes include service utilization, length of hospital stay, and cost of care or services. Outcome evaluation is often used to identify factors associated with complications post cardiovascular intervention.

Stages of Prochaska's transtheoretical model of motivation and change

Prochaska states there are five stages a person must go through in order to accept the value of change and take action accordingly:

- Precontemplation: The patient is resistant to change. This stage can last up to 6 months after a need for change has been initially identified.
- Contemplation: For the next 6 months to a year, the patient begins to visualize what changing would actually be like.
- Preparation: The patient begins taking tentative steps, such as option exploration, toward change. This stage's timeframe can vary greatly.
- Action: For approximately the next 6 months the patient begins taking active steps toward change; relapse and setbacks may occur, but overall the patient remains resolved toward change.
- Maintenance: For at least 6 months following completion of the change goal, the patient works to maintain the changes achieved. Setbacks may still occur but become less frequent.

The nurse must meet the patient at whatever stage he/she is currently in and promote progress toward the next stage.

Benefits of cardiac rehabilitation

Endorsed by both the American Heart Association (AHA) and American College of Cardiology, cardiac rehabilitation is an individualized program designed for the patient with cardiac disease, including those recovering from myocardial infarction and treatment surgeries. Cardiac rehabilitation focuses on education, including diet and lifestyle changes, and developing an individualized exercise program that will return the cardiac patient to his/her highest functioning capacity and reduce the risk of further cardiac injury.

For the first 3–6 months, care is focused on gradual exercise progression and probable consults with cardiologists, health educators, dietitians, physical and occupational therapists and psychologists/psychiatrists.

Exercise options might include both endurance and strength training. Lifestyle education and counseling focuses on disease management, risky behavior reduction, diet and mental health.

Attending cardiac rehabilitation increases the cardiac patient's chances of survival and effective healing.

Subacute care facilities

General: Patients discharged to this level of care are stable and healing well, but still require skilled care for such things as long-term intravenous treatments.

Chronic: Chronic care facilities are for terminal and end-of-life patients who cannot be cared for in an at-home setting because of choice or complexity of care such as ventilator dependency.

Transitional: At this level the patient still needs complex medical and nursing care, such as deep wound management.

Long-term transitional: Identifies a need for continued complex medical care that is expected to have an extended treatment time.

End-of-life care related to heart failure

If treatments fail to control the patient's heart failure, it is possible for the disease to progress to a point where even heart transplant is no longer an option. At this point, it is time to educate the patient and family regarding his/her end-of-life care options. Many patients choose the support of hospice. This option allows for care at home surrounded by family and friends. Those involved in the care might include nurses, nursing aides, social workers and even trained volunteers to help ease the passage from life to death by giving support to all facets of a person's life: health, social, mental, emotional and spiritual. Other options might be continued care within the hospital or transfer to a chronic care facility. Discussions must be held regarding end-of-life care parameters and wishes and these decisions documented and expressed to family and friends.

Education and Health Promotion

Qualities of an excellent nurse-teacher

Confidence: An excellent teacher provides a comfortable and appropriate learning environment and is prepared ahead of time regarding what and how to teach the individual or group according to their needs.

Competence: Prioritize learning goals and material, focusing on the most critical first. Care should be taken to ensure patient safety and confidentiality during teaching exercises.

Communication: Speak clearly and concisely on a level that is comfortable for the patient. Provide for an interpreter or any available resources in the patient's native language. Materials should be presented in a variety of ways to accommodate different learning styles.

Caring: The most effective teacher is able to show empathy toward the patient and his/her emotions and concerns. He/she is unhurried and willing to address any questions the patient might have while encouraging and providing positive feedback in the patient's efforts to learn.

Standards established by JCAHO for evaluating the effectiveness of education efforts

- Did the effort promote open and honest communication between the nurse and the participants?
- Was patient understanding of the concept improved after the experience?
- Was the patient actively involved in the learning and decision-making processes?
- Was the information provided pertinent to the patient's individual needs, values, abilities and concerns at the time of the teaching event?
- Can the patient easily demonstrate the needed skills being taught?
- Is the patient aware of his/her responsibility related to any treatments and goals that will be employed toward a healthy lifestyle?
- Does the knowledge gained improve the patient's ability to cope with circumstances and to participate in his/her care?
- Will the patient be able to follow and accomplish any care goals that have been set?

Kleinman model

The Kleinman model relies on a series of questions to help a nurse prepare to teach a patient from an unfamiliar cultural background. These questions allow the patient to define his/her own healthcare beliefs and problems. The questions include:
- The patient's name for a problem or condition.
- The patient's perception of the problem's cause and initiating events, as well as their timing.
- How the problem is affecting the patient—what problems result from the illness or variance in health.
- The patient's beliefs regarding the severity of the problem and its anticipated progression.
- The patient's confidence in various treatments.
- What the patient hopes intervention will accomplish for him/her.
- What fears the patient possesses regarding the illness and the proposed treatments.

Adult learning

Adult learning is defined as a consistent change in behavior due to life experiences. The characteristics of adult learning include motivation to know more information, self-direction, life experiences that positively or negatively impact the learning process and ability to enhance an already established knowledge base. Adult learning is most effective when an individual can relate to an immediate need, problem, or deficit. These individuals are self-directed by a need to know more information based on their current situation. They will take a proactive approach to gain more insight due to a current situation or based on a need to build on past experience.

Three conditions for adult learning
The 3 conditions necessary for adult learning include motivation to learn, ability to learn and the learning environment. Motivation is a condition that is defined as the effect of internal and external factors that drive an individual's need to learn, change, and maintain behavior. It is a willingness of an individual to want to acquire knowledge or insight. Motivation can be driven by different factors including reinforced or rewarded behavior, need for survival, ability to recognize a previous behavior that caused a negative outcome, personality, perceived ability to achieve a specific goal, and coping style.

Three domains of adult learning
The domains of adult learning include cognitive learning, affective learning, and psychomotor learning. Each type of learning impacts how an individual addresses adult learning and affects the knowledge the individual can acquire. Cognitive learning is defined as the ability to acquire knowledge or intellectual information through acquisition of facts, data, making decisions or drawing conclusions. Affective learning is defined as the ability of an individual to change their attitude, feeling, emotions, or interests toward a particular event or idea. Psychomotor learning is defined as an individual's ability to master physical or motor skills and/or activities.

Impact of environment on adult learning
External factors and the environment may affect an individual's ability to learn. Many external factors may need to be addressed in order for an individual to have the ability to learn, as these external factors may pose barriers to learning. Understanding how individuals learn most effectively is key to addressing environmental factors. Some individuals learn better on a one-on-one basis, while others learn more effectively in small groups, where others learn better in large groups. Understanding the environmental factors that impact learning can positively or negatively influence an individual's learning process. Providing a comfortable learning environment that includes a moderate temperature, sufficient lighting, minimal noise, adequate ventilation, and comfortable furniture will facilitate the learning process.

Learning ability
Learning ability plays an important role in the learning process, as the ability to learn is dependent on an individual's developmental level, physical wellness, and intellectual thought process. The developmental level of learning depends on the individual's stage in life.

Literacy level involves reading, comprehension, problem solving, and mathematics. Health literacy is defined as an individual's level of literacy required to function in a health environment and independent of educational literacy. Language can also influence an individual's ability to learn, especially if English is a second language. Physical wellness is defined as the level of strength, coordination, and sensory acuity to learn.

Reduced visual acuity

Individuals that present with reduced visual acuity can effectively learn if certain teaching approaches are taken. Practicing clinicians should make sure that an individual with reduced visual acuity has clean glasses and adequate light, and is wearing contacts or using magnifying glasses. In reading documents, make sure the letters used are in large font and of a contrasting color. Black ink on a white paper is the best for individuals with vision problems. The use of auditory tapes or CDs may also be effective in getting information across to patients with reduced visual acuity.

Reduced hearing acuity

Individuals that present with reduced hearing acuity can effectively learn if certain teaching approaches are taken. A practicing clinician should speak slowly and clearly. He/she should get the individual's attention prior to speaking and use simple sentences. Facing the patient and standing in close proximity is most effective in teaching a patient with reduced hearing acuity. Requesting feedback from the individual will provide information if the patient understands the clinical practitioner and if he or she is getting information across effectively. Additionally, if the patient is still having problems hearing the clinical practitioner, make sure that the individual's hearing aid is working properly and check to see if the patient hears more effectively in 1 ear versus the other.

Strategies for effective teaching and learning

The role of the clinical practitioner is to facilitate learning, while the role of the patient is to learn. Structured learning environments are more effective than unstructured learning environments. The strategy most effective for teaching depends on the learning and what works best for that individual. Teaching strategies include lecturing, question and answer sessions, demonstrations, role playing, oral or written exams, simulation, illustrations, case studies, books, pamphlets, pictures, film, computer-assisted learning programs, and video tapes/DVDs. Clinical practitioners need to take into account the patient's learning level and adjust teaching strategies to that learning level. The practitioner should also make sure that the learning material is relevant, relatable, and organized.

Assessment

Assessment, in the patient education process, involves defining learning needs and developing a teaching plan to meet the needs of an individual. Assessment involves understanding an individual's need to learn, motivation to learn and readiness to learn. If individuals have an internal locus of control, then they will be more proactive in the approach to their health, while an individual with an external locus of control will not be as proactive in the approach to their health. Therefore, practicing clinicians need to take different approaches depending on the patient's ability to take control of their own health. Practicing clinicians also need to take into account any external factors that may affect an individual's readiness to learn including cultural or religious beliefs, perceived benefits of changing behaviors, and belief that individuals can effectively influence their own health. Other factors include physical well-being, comfort, sensory, and physical and intellectual maturity.

Strategies for patient education and counseling

The strategy used should be employed based on the patient's perception. Practicing clinicians should inform the patient the expected goals of these strategies and issue small goals rather than large unattainable goals. Setting out specific goals is much more effective than being vague. Patients are more apt to follow specific recommendations rather than just giving them ideas. New behaviors should be linked to old behaviors and it is typically easier to establish new behaviors rather than eliminate old habits. Follow-up with the patient and having them monitor their goals are essential for the individual to achieve the goals laid out for them. Multiple members of the healthcare staff should be involved in the process, including nurses, doctors, counselors, and nutritionists.

Strategies for effective evaluation and reteaching

Evaluation requires the practicing clinician to assess a patient's performance, health-related outcomes, and determine competence. Evaluation is used to assess whether a patient is effectively learning and changing their health related behaviors. If the approach is not effective, practicing clinicians can alter their approach to better suit the patient's needs. Direct and indirect measurements can be used for evaluation assessment. Direct measurement involves observing the patient and recording behaviors. Indirect measurement assumes that learning has occurred, as the patient has reached a predetermined learning level. Oral questioning and written examinations are examples of indirect learning measurements.

Three health self-management issues

Health self-management issues include health maintenance, disease prevention and health promotion. Health maintenance is defined as strategies that help maintain and/or improve health over time. Health maintenance is dependent on 3 factors, which include health perception, motivation for behavioral change, and compliance to set goals. Disease prevention is an effort to limit the development or progression of lifestyle related illness. Disease prevention can be categorized into primary, secondary, and tertiary prevention. Primary prevention measures are employed prior to disease onset and are used in health populations. Secondary prevention measures are used to screen, detect, and treat disease in earlier stages to prevent further progression or development of other complications. Tertiary prevention measures are used to prevent onset of other complications or comorbid conditions. Health promotion strategies include risk reduction strategies applied to general population.

Barriers that might interfere with the patient's ability to learn

Language: Is English the patient's primary language? Are interpreters available to help the patient hear and understand the information in his/her native tongue?

Hearing impairment: Is there a known, or suspected, hearing deficit? Is hearing equipment in use and functioning? Improve communication by facing the patient and using short sentences.

Sight impairment: Is there a known, or suspected, sight deficit? Are eyeglasses clean and in use? Accommodate for the use of a magnifying glass and provide high-contrast, large-print material as needed. Offer auditory rather than written teaching supplements when available.

Pain: Is the patient adequately medicated in order to pay attention and think clearly, but not drowsy?

Physical restriction: Is the patient physically able to perform the tasks you are teaching him/her about?

Intellectual development: Is the patient developmentally able to understand the concepts being presented?

Motivation: Is the patient ready to learn, or is anger, denial or other emotion impairing his/her readiness and receptiveness to new information?

Ways to recognize low health literacy

The patient may:
- Express frustration or inaccurate knowledge about how and where to find needed healthcare services.
- Express frustration or difficulty following through with treatments, including medications or testing.
- Be unable to provide an accurate personal health history or fill out detailed health surveys.
- Have little or no knowledge and regard for preventative measures and the consequences of risky behaviors and may express belief in healthcare misconceptions.
- Appear disinterested in provided materials, often expressing that someone else outside of themselves will meet their healthcare needs.

These concerns can be addressed by:
- Assuring that communication is provided in the patient's primary language and at a level appropriate to his/her developmental and learning level.
- Avoiding the use of medical jargon and complex explanations that can be misunderstood and frequently assessing the amount of learning.
- Prioritizing information according to its perceived value to the patient.
- Providing multiple learning methods and supplemental materials as needed to reinforce learning.

Self-efficacy theory of learning

Self-efficacy learning models are based on the core belief within the patient that change can be accomplished. This belief can be supported through educational efforts in four key ways.

Personal mastery is the most vital component. Personal mastery is directly based on the patient's belief that a new skill can be mastered or a solution to a problem found.

Vicarious experience allows the patient to observe and learn from demonstration by others, either patient or nurse. Role models with similar experiences as teaching agents are particularly helpful.

Verbal persuasion provides positive reinforcement in the patient's efforts toward change and expresses the third party's (including the teacher or care provider) belief that a skill can be mastered by the patient.

Physiologic feedback provides tangible evaluation methods (physical appearance of a bandage, lab results, resolution of nausea, etc) the patient can utilize to see if his/her work has succeeded or failed.

Conditions and motivations that encourage learning

There are three domains of learning that need to be addressed. Cognitive: actual knowledge of facts; affective: attitudes and feelings associated with the subject; and psychomotor: hands-on skills and actions.

Learning in these three areas is based on the patient's motivation and ability to learn as well as the environment in which he/she is expected to learn. A desire to learn and change must be present, and knowledge must be presented in a manner that enables and sparks the individual's ability to learn. Knowledge and learning opportunities must be presented in an atmosphere that is respectful, encouraging and comfortable for the patient.

Signals that a patient needs expanded teaching and discharge planning

- Patients older than 70
- Anyone living alone, in another state or country, or whose housing arrangements are in question
- Anyone suspected of being abused or neglected
- Patients with multiple admissions
- Patients transferring from other care centers
- Patients with new or multiple diagnoses
- Anyone with a terminal illness or diseases requiring long-term intensive treatments and other significant life changes
- Patients with known or potential financial burdens related to care or basic needs
- Patients with few visitors or family/support system problems
- Those with little or no English-speaking ability or with learning disabilities
- Substance abusers

Maslow's hierarchy of needs

Basic physiological and survival needs must always be met first. Learning cannot take place in an environment of personal emergency. Basic health needs that preserve life are addressed at this stage.

Patient concerns progress from there to include fears for safety and security including pain control.

When these areas are addressed the patient is then ready to begin taking an active role in his/her current health care.

The next step is a more active interest in promoting current and future health and wellness. Focus is still on problem solving and affirming positive health practices. Then, a desire to reach fulfilling life goals can be addressed.

Individual versus group teaching sessions

Lecture can be appropriate for teaching large groups, but when used in small groups it has better results when coupled with discussion and/or question and answer.

Discussion alone is appropriate for a one-on-one instruction setting. Question and answer time should only be used in a single-learner setting when prior knowledge has been given and absorbed by the learner, or as a method to assess how much learning may have taken place.

Demonstration and practice work best in small groups or individual settings. Practicing skills can include return demonstration or role playing in either setting.

Supportive teaching tools such as written material or audio-visual treatments are helpful in both group and individual learning environments and provide reinforcement of material in different methods to accommodate various learning styles.

Patient and family teaching

Invasive treatment procedures
Pre-operative: Provide information regarding the procedure, including who will be present in the room and his/her function, what sights and sounds are typical, sensations and amount of discomfort both during and after the procedure, and an estimate of the amount of time required for the procedure.

Review consents and other documentation including living will/advanced directives.

Post-operative: Review the procedure and its outcomes, provide visual documentation of the procedure including before and after images of the area(s) treated.

Assess pain and instruct patient and family about expected pain levels and locations during recovery. Review expected progression of activity levels.

Review what constitutes an emergency and how to contact help in the event of an emergency. Provide clear written instructions.

Review all medications with clear written instructions and follow-up care plans, as well as referrals to other institutes that promote further wellness interventions.

Cardiovascular disease and depression
Depression is a major risk factor for developing cardiovascular disease, particularly myocardial infarction. Depression affects the patient's decision-making ability, his/her interest in self-care and motivation toward healing and rehabilitation. If depression is caught and treated it can help prevent disease development and improve quality and length of life in those with active disease processes. The first line of treatment is stress management and counseling for anxiety. Medications are carefully considered after taking into account the patient's condition, other medications and treatments. Signs and symptoms of depression should be discussed with every cardiovascular patient before discharge from a healthcare setting. You should be particularly aware of symptoms of depression in postmenopausal women.

Recovering coronary artery bypass graft (CABG) patient
Notify doctor of signs and symptoms of infection at the incision sites (leg and chest) or postpericardiotomy syndrome (fever, muscle and joint pain, weakness and chest discomfort).

Seek medical care immediately if the patient experiences symptoms of heart failure or myocardial infarction.

Monitor weight and notify the doctor if there is a sudden gain.

Verbalize explanations and tips for following prescribed diet, activity, rest and exercise programs including cardiac rehabilitation.

Obtain written and verbal instructions regarding all medications including purpose, dose, frequency and common side effects.

Accept referrals and information for lifestyle modifications such as smoking cessation and other support organizations.

Percutaneous coronary intervention (PCI)

Preoperative: Information regarding the procedure, including who will be present in the room and his/her function, what sights and sounds are typical, sensations and amount of discomfort during and after the procedure, and an estimate of the amount of time required for the procedure.

Review consents and other documentation including advanced directives.

Postoperative: Review the procedure and its outcomes, provide visual documentation of the procedure including before and after images of the lesions.

Assess pain and instruct patient and family about expected pain levels and locations (chest, back, insertion site) during recovery.

Review what constitutes an emergency and how to contact help in the event of an emergency. Provide clear written instructions.

Review all medications (aspirin, antiplatelets, beta-blockers, antihypertensives, antilipids and nitrates) with clear written instructions.

Review diet and activity expectations and progression including referrals to consultations for diet or lifestyle modifications and cardiac rehabilitation.

Define follow-up care plans as well as referrals to other institutes that promote further wellness interventions.

Pacemaker placement

Preoperative: Information regarding the procedure, including who will be present in the room and his/her function, what sights and sounds are typical, sensations and amount of discomfort during and after the procedure, and an estimate of the amount of time required for the procedure.

Review consents and other documentation including advanced directives.

Postoperative: Expected and unexpected pain levels and locations (chest, insertion site) during recovery.

Review what constitutes an emergency and how to contact help in the event of an emergency. Provide clear written instructions.

Review all medications (including antibiotics) with clear written instructions and follow-up care plans, as well as referrals to other institutes that promote further wellness interventions.

Review activity expectations and progression including referrals to consultations for diet or lifestyle modifications and cardiac rehabilitation.

Review lifestyle modifications, including carrying a pacemaker identification card and informing all healthcare providers (including dentists) of the pacemaker. Include safety precautions: may safely operate microwaves and cell phones, but should avoid high-strength radiation fields such as MRI.

Carotid endarterectomy

Preoperative: Information regarding the procedure, including who will be present in the room and his/her function, what sights and sounds are typical, sensations and amount of discomfort during and after the procedure, and an estimate of the amount of time required for the procedure.

Review consents and other documentation including advanced directives.

Postoperative: Review the procedure and its outcomes, provide visual documentation of the procedure.

Assess pain and instruct patient and family about expected pain levels and locations (chest, back, insertion site) during recovery.

Review what constitutes an emergency (including neurological impairment) and how to contact help in the event of an emergency. Provide clear written instructions.

Review all medications (aspirin, clopidogrel) with clear written instructions and follow-up care plans, as well as referrals to other institutes that promote further wellness interventions.

Review diet and activity expectations and progression including referrals to consultations for diet and weight loss or lifestyle modifications for hypertension, cholesterol, diabetes management and smoking cessation.

Heart failure

Disease process: Heart failure causes and disease progression should be covered. This teaching should include signs and symptoms of worsening conditions and self-monitoring techniques such as daily weights.

Life expectancy: The patient should have a clear understanding of the length and quality of life he/she will experience as part of the disease process. End-of-life choices should be discussed and advanced directives should be reviewed.

Activity levels: Based on the current stage of the disease and diagnostic testing, parameters are set for all activities of daily life.

Diet: Detailed instruction on what constitutes a low-sodium diet is generally required; fluid restriction may also be needed.

Medications: Education regarding medications should include clear and written instructions regarding dosage, timing and frequency of each administration as well as what the expected treatment result will be, common side effects, interactions and negative reactions.

Therapeutic support: Every effort should be made to encourage compliance with treatment plans and acceptance of referrals to other health and education resources for top priority health needs such as smoking cessation and mental health.

Acute or chronic illnesses

Diagnosis: Establish a basic understanding of the disease process, including areas of body affected, causes, prognosis and whether or not it is contagious.

Complications: Clarify possible signs and symptoms, early warning signs and signals of disease progression and healing.

Management: Define what the patient can expect from his/her care and recovery, including treatments, diet, activity levels and medications.

Aggravating factors: Help the patient understand what behaviors or triggers may increase his/her symptoms and what can be done to avoid or control them.

Prognosis: Patients need both an immediate idea as well as a long-term picture of what to expect.

Prevention: Establish self-care habits that can help prevent recurrence of the problem.

Resources: Make sure the patient is informed of all available resources for help on his/her healthcare journey.

Crisis

A crisis is a change in well-being that has a definite beginning and end. It is marked by an inability to cope either because of exhaustion of normal coping mechanisms or sudden and dramatic change in circumstances. A nurse's role during times of crisis is to first ensure the safety of the individual, then improve coping strategies and assist the patient in returning to a stable level of functioning. This can be done by use of medication, therapies, controlling environmental influences, offering reassurance, suggestions for change and support in decisions and actions toward crisis resolution.

Benefits of a learning contract

A learning contract establishes a formal agreement that learning will take place. Learning contracts are a concrete indication of a learner's willingness to begin the learning and change process. It spells out expectations of both teacher and learner to maintain a positive and productive relationship. Goals are set and ways to evaluate progress are outlined so that both parties know what will be expected of them. Goals should be centered on patient needs and wishes and decided upon with his/her input. Learning contracts can be employed in a number of healthcare settings and provide measurable outcomes for intervention evaluation.

Professional Role

Legal regulation of nursing practice

Legal regulation of nursing practice protects the health, safety, and welfare of patients. All states require nurse licensing and most states require additional accreditation for advanced nursing practice. Nursing practice acts are state laws that grant the right to practice nursing to individuals who meet predetermined standards. Regulatory boards are responsible for determining eligibility for licensing and relicensing, approving and supervising educational programs, enforcing statutes, and writing rules and regulations. Licensing requirements, state statutes and monitoring, advisory boards, and guidelines effectively protect patients and aim to ensure optimum care by nurses.

Code of ethics for nurses as defined by the American Nurses Association

1. Practice with compassion and respect for each patient as a unique individual.
2. Maintain the patient as highest priority.
3. Support practices that promote patient safety.
4. Maintain a high level of individual accountability.
5. Utilize practices that will promote the health and well-being of the nurse as a practitioner and individual.
6. Establish and maintain environments of high quality care.
7. Actively participate in the advancement and improvement of the profession.
8. Coordinate care efforts with other healthcare and community resources.
9. Maintain integrity and set a public example of the values and excellence of the profession.

Patient rights as identified by the American Hospital Association

- Right to considerate and respectful care.
- Right to information about diagnosis, treatment and prognosis.
- Right to make decisions about the plan of care.
- Right to have advance directives.
- Right to privacy.
- Right to confidentiality.
- Right to review clinical records.
- Right to responsible care and services, including the right to transfer institutions, and payors that might influence care and treatment.
- Right to reasonable continuity of care.
- Right to be informed of hospital policies and procedures that regulate patient care, treatment and responsibilities; includes the right to grievance and dispute resolution.

(American Hospital Association, Patients' Bill of Rights, 1990)

Differences between licensure and certification

Licensure is the meeting of legal parameters established by government to identify that an individual has met a minimum standard of competence and safety in his/her profession. No one is allowed to practice in that profession without qualifying to do so under the laws of the state in which he/she is intending to practice.

Certification is a step above and beyond licensure that is pursued by the individual nurse or required by an institution for employment in specialty areas. Guidelines and testing for certification are established by the profession with the backing of independent agencies to ensure standards of quality. Certification implies a higher level of competency within a specialized area of care.

Negligence and malpractice

Negligence and malpractice are classified as unintentional torts (wrongful acts). Negligence refers to harm caused by carelessness or failure to act. Malpractice is a specific form of negligence that results from harm caused by not meeting reasonable standards of care set within the profession of nursing. Malpractice cases can be pursued if the wronged party is able to prove that the nurse in question was responsible for performing, or not performing, an intervention within his/her scope of practice. It must be reasonably proven that this action by the nurse was directly related to the harm and suffering of the patient.

Some of the most common areas of nursing malpractice include medication errors, inadequate assessment or monitoring of the patient (including allowing a patient to fall), performing activities for which the nurse has not been trained, and failure to communicate and document events or follow proper procedure.

Major tenets of the federal Health Insurance Portability and Accountability Act (HIPAA) legislation

HIPAA expands on a patient's basic right to know that his/her personal health information is held in confidence and only shared on a "need to know" basis that is clearly defined for the patient. If knowledge of the patient's information is required for those outside of the patient's direct care, it cannot be provided without his/her specific consent. It requires all persons and institutions with access to this information to practice high levels of protection for that information. Every healthcare institution is required by law to establish and enforce policy and procedure that enforces patient confidentiality.

Being a patient advocate

The American Nurses Association (ANA) regards patient advocacy as a basic cornerstone that helps define the profession of nursing. Advocacy denotes the nurse's commitment to promoting optimal health and safety for his/her patient (whether that is an individual, group or community). Nurses assume the responsibility of preserving a patient's basic rights for informed care that promotes the highest quality of life. This standard is maintained in communication and cooperation with all healthcare team members providing treatment, education, pain relief, comfort and safety while avoiding harm to the patient.

Consumerism, paternalism and patient advocacy approaches toward promoting change

Consumerism: This impersonal view presents the patient with the cost-effectiveness and anticipated outcomes of various treatments but does not take into account personal belief systems.

Paternalism: The care provider, or other influential person in the patient's life, assumes the role of parent and tries to dictate the patient's healthcare decisions for him/her.

Patient advocacy: The healthcare provider works directly with the patient, involving him/her in making decisions about what is best at any given time and respecting these wishes. Being an advocate involves creating a therapeutic relationship, presenting options and promoting understanding that allows the patient to make an informed decision and, as needed, defending the patient's decisions to other care providers or individuals in his/her life who might question or try to negate the power to be in control of his/her own health.

Ethical decision making

The most important aspect of ethical decision making is the fact that these decisions are not made by just one person. When an ethical dilemma exists, the problem is brought to the attention of a committee of which the nurse and the patient, or his/her representative if incapacitated, are members. Questions addressed would include an in-depth analysis of all the facts; then options are presented and prioritized. Paramount to any decision made should be consideration for the patient's wishes. Once a decision is reached the nurse must act as a patient advocate and facilitate actions related to that decision regardless of his/her personal feelings about the dilemma.

Leadership

Leadership is the personal characteristics or qualities that an individual uses to influence others to achieve set goals. Key characteristics and qualities associated with a leader include working well with others, facilitating communication, and motivating others. Leadership styles include autocratic, participative, laissez-faire, transactional, and transformational. Autocratic leadership uses power to influence members of a team. Participative leadership uses a democratic process for decisions among team members. Laissez-faire leadership involves minimal guidance from a leader and provides little feedback to team members. Transactional leadership focuses on daily activities and is comfortable with the status quo. Transformational leadership involves a vision and commitment to meet a team's goals.

The leader works well in a group/team setting and is able to coordinate patient care with multiple groups and areas of healthcare.

He/she promotes communication between all members of the group, streamlining and coordinating care (participative leader).

A leader appropriately motivates the team toward common goals, emphasizes and rewards productive work environments (transactional leader).

A leader appropriately motivates the team toward positive change as needed (transformational leader).

The leader provides respect, support and encouragement to all contributors and listens to all voices before making final decisions.

Of the generally recognized leadership styles, those possessing a participative or transformational style appear to have the best outcomes in healthcare and interdisciplinary settings. Unfavorable leadership methods tend to be autocratic (firm control with little group input) and laissez-faire (hands-off, unmotivated leadership).

Positive attributes of a mentor

A mentor is a role model and a guide to successful care and skill building experiences. He/she exhibits higher knowledge and experience than the individual he/she is guiding. The mentor is not in a leadership role over the student, but is seen as a more experienced equal. He/she does not take over and make decisions for the student; rather he/she provides options and information to help the student make positive decisions on his/her own. The mentor is honest and trustworthy, supportive, has effective communication and teaching skills and is respected by those he/she is leading to higher skill levels.

How to delegate appropriately

There are 5 basic responsibilities associated with delegating.
- Right Task: The task must be clearly defined and achievable.
- Right Circumstances: Can the task be completed in a timely manner? Are the needed tools easily accessible?
- Right Person: Is the person giving direction within his/her scope of practice to delegate the task, and is the person being asked to complete the task able to complete it within his/her own scope of practice?
- Right Communication: Is the task and the expected outcome clearly outlined so that both parties understand what needs to be done?
- Right Supervision: Appropriate monitoring, intervention and accountability needs to be maintained regardless of who is ultimately assigned the task.

Effective communication

Listening
Listening is often overlooked as an important communication skill because it seems natural to many. It is actually a learned skill that allows the communicator to overcome barriers such as stress, anger and distraction to truly process all aspects of the message being conveyed by the other party. It enables problem identification, sensitivity to emotions, relieves stress and facilitates problem solving. Active listening is a two-way process that allows both parties to express their thoughts and feelings with the knowledge that they will be heard and the other person truly wants to understand the message and work for resolution.

Assertiveness
Assertiveness should not be confused with aggression, a negative communication method used to manipulate and control interactions rather than collaborate and share respect. Assertiveness empowers the communicator to feel comfortable speaking freely and defending his/her own thoughts and feelings in a given situation using "I" statements. The assertive communicator also processes others' opinions and uses "you" statements in a positive manner. He/she is not passive or

silent when there is a need to speak out, but uses positive language that is appropriate to the situation and those who will be listening and trying to understand.

CARE method for dealing with conflict.

The CARE approach stands for Clarify, Articulate, Request and Encourage.

Clarify: Be specific in identifying the problem that needs to be addressed.

Articulate: Clearly define the reason(s) why a particular behavior or attitude is a problem.

Request: Define an acceptable means of change that will help resolve the problem.

Encourage: Offer support and respect toward others as you work together on creating change and resolving conflict.

Regardless of the other party's behavior, it is the nurse's personal responsibility to act with calm respect and dignity in the face of confrontation in order to facilitate positive change rather than contributing further to the problem.

Steps toward win-win conflict resolution

- Identify the need that is not being met rather than placing blame for dissatisfaction and frustration. Be specific in defining problem parameters.
- Acknowledge differences of opinion and attempt to see the problem from all perspectives.
- Involve all parties that are affected by the problem while searching for a solution.
- Remember that win-win solutions may not always be what one person considers the easiest or most obvious. Base the solution on what reaches the greatest compromise and satisfaction for all concerned.
- Agree on the action to be taken with all other involved parties.
- Plan for the success of the solution with goals and definitions of roles and expectations.
- Review the plan and solution's effectiveness after it has been carried out to identify areas of further improvement or recognize the need to re-address the problem.

Roles of a cardiac rehabilitation nurse

Clinician: Uses the nursing process to devise individualized care plans for his/her patients.

Collaborator: Works with other professionals to facilitate comprehensive care that meets the patient's needs.

Educator: Identifies the learning needs of the patient and facilitates positive health changes through providing knowledge and encouragement toward better wellness.

Manager: Identifies needs and coordinates care with other professions to provide comprehensive services and acts as an advocate for the patient's healthcare choices.

Researcher: Continually seeks creative and effective ways to improve the quality of care that can be provided to the patient.

Basic keys to providing competent and culturally sensitive nursing care

Care should always be specifically geared to the individual patient. Do not make assumptions about his/her needs or wishes based on personal views or previous interactions and circumstances.

Take time to identify the patient's unique cultural values and belief systems before establishing care goals.

Nursing interventions enable and include the patient and the primary decision maker about his/her own care, according to his/her cultural values and belief system.

Nurses and the care they provide should never reflect a personal judgment regarding the patient's culture or unique beliefs.

Key components of a helpful and therapeutic nurse-patient relationship

The nurse and patient should both be actively working together on a common goal regarding the patient's healthcare and recovery. The plan of action, means and evaluation of the intervention are completed jointly.

The patient should feel respected by the nurse and understand his/her privacy will be protected in order to encourage an involvement in his/her own care.

Emotional bonds may form but should be kept in proper context and boundaries. There will always be a beginning, middle and end to a nurse-patient relationship.

The nurse must be prepared on all levels—mental, physical and emotional—to be a positive, patient and helping influence in the relationship.

Collaboration and coordination among healthcare team members

Tools developed for this specific purpose in a healthcare setting include practice guidelines to help define each participant's role in care and clinical protocols or pathways to focus care and clarify procedures and strategies to be followed. The goal is to create a team where the members understand their own, and each other's, role within the group, understand the goals of the team, share responsibility, reach collective decisions and actively include the patient and his/her family in the care process. An effective collaboration effort includes all stages of care, from assessment of needs to action, communication and evaluation of goals upon completion. A primary key is streamlined communication and respect for each individual's unique contribution. The nurse often plays a primary role as mediator and advocate for the patient, making sure he/she understands the purposes and joint goal of the group and its members.

Coping

Coping is a mechanism that is used by an individual to deal with internal and external factors that arise. It involves continuously changing one's behavioral and cognitive actions to deal with challenging circumstances. Coping is an evolving process that involves an individual changing their actions based on internal and external factors. The functions of coping include reducing stress, maintaining equilibrium, facilitating independence, enhancing personal decision making, meeting external demands, managing stressors, avoiding negative self evaluation, and maintaining a stable psychosocial state. Coping varies from one individual to another but includes the above functions.

Positive coping mechanisms

Positive coping mechanisms utilize the patient's natural responses to crisis in order to facilitate his/her own independence and ability to make decisions and do not compromise the patient's self-worth perceptions, mental, social or physical stability. Positive techniques reduce tension and conflict while confronting and resolving the problem in a constructive manner. The patient who is coping positively will seek out knowledge and be involved in his/her own care. He/she will grieve appropriately and adjust to changes in health, social roles and relationships and maintain a sense of hope and confidence in his/her abilities and choices.

Coping styles

An individual's approach to coping may change based on internal and external factors. It may also change based on the situation the individual is presented with. A flexible coping style is much more effective than a rigid approach, as different situations will arise that require different modes of coping. Adaptive response to coping include lifestyle modification, enhancing knowledge and self care strategies, maintaining positive goals, adjusting to changes in relationships with family, loved ones, healthcare providers and/or co-workers, grieving over losses, dealing with role changes, adjusting to discomfort, maintaining a sense of control, maintaining hope and confronting impending death. Maladaptive responses to coping include anxiety, anger, depression, denial and dependence.

Maladaptive responses

Treatment of maladaptive responses to coping includes nonpharmacologic approaches and pharmacologic approaches. Nonpharmacologic strategies include cognitive behavioral therapy, psychotherapy, electroconvulsive therapy and/or light therapy. Pharmacologic approaches are used for cases where cognitive behavior therapy or psychotherapy is not completely effective. They are typically used in combination with these strategies. Pharmacologic approaches include selective serotonin reuptake inhibitors (SSRIs) such as fluoxetine, sertraline, paroxetine and fluoxetine; tricyclic antidepressants such as imipramine, nortriptyline, desipramine, amitriptyline and doxepin; benzodiazepines such as diazepam, lorazepam and oxazepam; monoamine oxidase inhibitors (MAOIs) such as phenelzine, tranylcypromine, L-deprenyl and moclobemide; and atypical antidepressants such as bupropion, mirtazapine, nefazodone, and trazodone.

Negative coping mechanisms

Negative responses do not allow the patient to adjust to the challenges he/she faces. While any of these responses may occur as part of the journey to positive action, they will not be sustained over a long period of time. If negative responses continue, they may require outside intervention and treatment to assist the patient in making positive coping and self-care decisions. Negative responses can include anxiety, depression, anger, denial, noncompliance with treatment or increased dependence on others for self-esteem and decision making abilities. Negative coping compromises the patient's sense of independence, mental, social or physical stability. They increase tension and conflict without confronting and resolving the problem. The patient who is coping negatively will not seek out knowledge and be involved in his/her own care, and cannot adjust to changes in health, social roles and relationships while maintaining a sense of hope and confidence.

Nursing interventions to enhance coping and adaptation

Nurses and clinical practitioners need to take a proactive approach to helping patients deal with coping and providing them with more adaptive coping strategies. Assessing and following a patient's response to illness and treatment is necessary to determine if any interventions are needed. Practicing clinicians need to make sure that there are no maladaptive responses such as anxiety, depression, or denial that need to be addressed with nonpharmacologic or pharmacologic approaches. It is necessary to provide the patient with educational material regarding their disease and treatment. Encouragement for patients to join support groups is a good approach for some patients who would like to discuss their condition with other patients. Nursing and practicing clinician interventions can be changed and revised as needed, depending on the patient's psychosocial state.

Stress

Physiologic responses to stress include the interaction between the sympathetic nervous system, anterior and posterior pituitary gland, and adrenal gland. Physiologic responses cause the release of hormones and cytokines such as norepinephrine, epinephrine, adrenocorticotropic hormone (ACTH), vasopressin, and antidiuretic hormone. These hormones and cytokines are released during the alarm stage also known as flight or fight. Psychologic responses to stress such as palpitations may result in the use of adaptive or maladaptive coping mechanism. Psychologic responses can be treated with nonpharmacologic management and/or pharmacologic agents. Coping mechanisms are best used adaptively to address psychologic responses.

General adaptation syndrome
General adaptation syndrome is defined as the stages associated with the body's response to a stressor. The 3 stages of general adaption syndrome include the alarm stage, stage of resistance or adaptation, and stage of exhaustion. The alarm stage is the initial response to a stressor, which is the fight or flight syndrome. The stage of resistance or adaptation is the process whereby the individual continues the fight or flight response. The stage of exhaustion is the point at which the stressor becomes dysfunctional and can lead to disease or illness.

Management techniques
Stress management techniques include autogenics, cognitive restructuring, imagery, progressive muscle relaxation, meditation, and aerobic exercise. Autogenics is a technique that involves the use of repetitive verbal phases and concentrating on sensations to lead to deep relaxation. Cognitive restructuring involves the use of the mind to alter the stress response. Imagery is another method for stress reduction. Additionally, progressive muscle relaxation reduces stress by interfering with the sympathetic nervous system. Meditation is a process that leads to deep relaxation through use of mantras and concentration. Aerobic exercise reduces anxiety and stress by increasing endorphins.

<u>Self-monitoring techniques</u>
Self-monitoring techniques include lifestyle modifications, reducing exposure to stressful situations, alteration of thinking, and modification to reactions. Patients should maintain a well-balanced diet, increase physical activity, get adequate sleep, apply stress management techniques and monitor blood pressure, cholesterol, and glucose levels. Reduce exposure to stressful situations by managing time and finances effectively and applying problem solving techniques to problems that arise. Patients should try to maintain a positive attitude and decrease negative thoughts. Modifying reactions to stressful situations can help reduce stress and anxiety. Applying self-monitoring techniques can help patients improve their quality of life and reduce maladaptive behaviors.

Factors that influence an individual's perception of his/her quality of life

The factors that influence an individual's perception of his/her quality of life include health, functional status, symptoms, and life satisfaction. The acute or chronic nature of an individual's condition influences an individual's perception of his/her quality of life. Health includes not only physical well-being, but also mental and social well-being. Functional status is defined as an individual's ability to perform activities of daily living. Symptoms are an individual's responses to his/her physical, emotional, or cognitive status. Life satisfaction is defined as an individual's contentment with their quality of life including family, health, sexuality, spirituality, friendships, job, education, housing, standard of living, and finances.

Practice Test

Practice Questions

1. A patient presents with pulmonary edema, tachypnea, tachycardia, hypertension, fever, and cough with frothy sanguineous sputum. What treatments are most commonly ordered initially with this clinical presentation?
    a. Oxygen, nitroglycerine, loop diuretics, and morphine
    b. Oxygen, thiazide diuretics, and angiotensin-converting enzyme inhibitors
    c. Oxygen and thiazide diuretics
    d. Oxygen, morphine, and calcium channel blockers

2. An 86-year old patient with end-stage cardiac disease has a do-not resuscitate (DNR) order as a result of an advance directive and has been explicit about her desire to avoid life-prolonging procedures; however, when she goes into cardiac arrest, her daughter demands that the nurses perform cardiopulmonary resuscitation (CPR). In this situation, the staff should do which of the following?
    a. Proceed with CPR as the patient can no longer make decisions.
    b. Proceed with CPR while calling the patient's physician to request verification of DNR order.
    c. Contact the ethics committee for guidance.
    d. Advise the daughter that a valid DNR order is in place and that CPR will be withheld in accordance with patient's wishes.

3. A patient with ventricular tachycardia at 200 bpm and multiple premature ventricular contractions loses consciousness. What treatment is most common in this situation?
    a. Antiarrhythmic medications
    b. Emergency defibrillation
    c. Digoxin
    d. Procainamide

4. The nurse notes that a patient who has just had cardiac surgery has decreased chest tube drainage, muffled heart sounds, tachycardia, and pulsus paradoxus. The most probable cause of these symptoms is:
    a. fluid overload.
    b. cardiac failure.
    c. cardiac tamponade.
    d. infection.

5. Ischemia is characterized on the electrocardiogram by:
    a. elevation of ST segments and elevated symmetrical T waves.
    b. inverted T waves.
    c. development of Q or QS waves.
    d. abnormal Q waves or decreased elevation of R waves without alteration of ST and T waves.

6. A patient complains of sharp pain in the substernal area or to the left of the sternum, which is referred to the neck, arms, and back. It occurs intermittently and suddenly and increases in intensity with inspiration, coughing, swallowing, or turning of the trunk. It is somewhat relieved by sitting upright. The most likely diagnosis is:
    a. angina.
    b. myocardial infarction.
    c. anxiety.
    d. pericarditis.

7. If a patient has an ankle systolic pressure of 90 and a brachial systolic pressure of 120, what is the ankle–brachial index?
    a. 0.75
    b. 1.33
    c. 0.13
    d. 7.5

8. Which heart sound indicates atrial gallop, which is often associated with left ventricular hypertrophy, hypertension, or aortic stenosis?
    a. S1
    b. S2
    c. S3
    d. S4

9. Anticoagulation therapy should be given before which of the following procedures?
    a. Emergency defibrillation
    b. Direct current cardioversion
    c. Direct current and chemical cardioversion
    d. Chemical cardioversion

10. Is a person who drinks heavily on one occasion in danger of cardiovascular impairment?
    a. No, only chronic drinking leads to cardiovascular impairment.
    b. Yes, but only if there is underlying cardiac disease.
    c. Yes, but only if alcohol use is combined with drugs, such as cocaine.
    d. Yes, drinking heavily on one occasion can cause cardiovascular impairment.

11. After cardiac surgery, urinary output should be monitored to ensure adequate renal perfusion. Urinary output should be:
    a. 20 mL/hr
    b. 25 mL/hr
    c. 50 mL/hr
    d. 75 mL/hr

12. Which of the following cardiac symptoms are typical of cocaine use?
    a. Hypertension and increased heart rate
    b. Hypertension and decreased heart rate
    c. Hypotension and increased heart rate
    d. Hypotension and decreased heart rate

13. Venous ulcers commonly have which of the following characteristics?
    a. They are deep and circular.
    b. They are superficial and irregularly shaped.
    c. They are often necrotic.
    d. They appear primarily on the toes and toe webs.

14. What preparation is necessary for a patient scheduled for a radionuclide ventriculogram?
    a. No special preparation is needed.
    b. Patients must fast for 4–6 hours.
    c. Cardiac medications are withheld for 4 hours.
    d. Patients should be on bed rest for 8 hours before the exam.

15. Physical changes that suggest a severe cardiovascular disorder, such as pulmonary edema and congestive heart failure, include:
    a. peripheral cyanosis of the nails and skin of the nose, lips, and extremities.
    b. pallor.
    c. central cyanosis of the tongue and buccal mucosa.
    d. xanthelasma.

16. Angiotensin-converting enzyme inhibitors are contraindicated in patients with:
    a. hypertension.
    b. diabetes mellitus.
    c. heart failure.
    d. renal failure.

17. A patient on mechanical ventilation who is retaining carbon dioxide is at risk for:
    a. metabolic acidosis.
    b. respiratory acidosis.
    c. metabolic alkalosis.
    d. respiratory alkalosis.

18. Sexual activity after recovery from a myocardial infarction (MI) can be considered:
    a. low risk as sexual activity provides physical and psychological benefits.
    b. high risk as sexual activity could precipitate another MI.
    c. very high risk, especially in patients who also use nitroglycerine for angina.
    d. no risk as sexual activity has no effect on cardiovascular disease

19. When wearing a Holter monitor, a patient should:
    a. refrain from taking cardiac medications.
    b. restrict activities.
    c. maintain an activity diary.
    d. turn it off during the night.

20. The best approach to be used with a 35-year old woman who has Marfan syndrome as well as severe mitral valve prolapse and heart failure is to:
    a. delay surgery as long as possible.
    b. repair the valve rather than replace it.
    c. replace the valve rather than repair it.
    d. avoid surgery because of life-threatening complications.

21. When a person believes that a health action will prevent a negative outcome and then takes that action, what behavioral change model can be applied to this behavior?
   a. Theory of reasoned action
   b. Theory of planned behavior
   c. Stress appraisal and coping theory
   d. Health belief model

22. When assessing nicotine dependence, which action listed below indicates a serious dependence?
   a. Smoking even if bedridden with illness
   b. Smoking the first cigarette within 5 minutes of awakening
   c. Smoking 11–20 cigarettes daily
   d. Smoking in places where it is prohibited

23. Which teaching method listed below is probably the most effective and efficient for teaching a group of patients about lifestyle modifications related to hypertension?
   a. Computer-assisted instruction
   b. Group lectures only
   c. Group lectures and discussion
   d. One-on-one instruction

24. The "dietary approaches to stop hypertension" (DASH), sponsored by the National Institutes of Health and the National Heart, Lung, and Blood Institute, include a 2100-calorie diet. What percentage of this diet is total fat?
   a. 27%
   b. 55%
   c. 18%
   d. 6%

25. Absolute hypovolemic shock is characterized by:
   a. vasodilation.
   b. external loss of fluid only.
   c. internal shifting of fluid or external loss of fluid.
   d. decreased colloidal osmotic pressure.

26. Which educational tool listed below is appropriate for a patient who speaks English but is illiterate?
   a. A children's book.
   b. Handouts prepared at a third-grade level.
   c. Computerized instruction.
   d. Video.

27. A patient spends half the year in one state and half in another state but wants to complete an advance directive. The best approach is to:
   a. complete separate advance directives to comply with each state's regulations.
   b. complete one advance directive as all states have the same regulations.
   c. inform family members of specific wishes only so an advance directive is not necessary.
   d. store the original advance directive in a safety deposit box.

28. Which blood pressure (BP) listed below poses the greatest risk of cardiovascular disease for people over 50 years of age?
    a. Diastolic pressure > 80 mm Hg.
    b. Increased BP after exercise.
    c. Systolic pressure > 140 mm Hg.
    d. Pulse pressure of 40 mm Hg.

29. A patient who has been treated with unfractionated heparin over 5 days develops a sudden drop in platelets from 120,000 mm3 to 45,000 mm3, suggesting heparin-induced thrombocytopenia, which places this patient at risk for:
    a. hemorrhage.
    b. thrombosis and vessel occlusion.
    c. shock.
    d. infection.

30. A nursing team leader delegates a task to an unlicensed assistant. Who is responsible for the patient outcome of this task?
    a. The unlicensed assistant who completes the task
    b. Both the team leader and the unlicensed person who complete the task
    c. The team leader who delegates the task
    d. The administrative staff

31. Endothelial dysfunction is associated with:
    a. cardiac dysrhythmias.
    b. cardiac arrest.
    c. hypertension.
    d. vasodilation.

32. The goal of an exercise stress test is to raise the heart rate to what percentage predicted for age and gender?
    a. 200%
    b. 50%
    c. 80%–90%
    d. >100%

33. Janeway lesions, splinter hemorrhages, and Roth's spots are immunological responses associated with:
    a. endocarditis.
    b. pericarditis.
    c. myocarditis.
    d. aortic valve dysfunction.

34. The best determinant of the effectiveness of patient education is the:
    a. patient's satisfaction.
    b. patient's ability to demonstrate procedure.
    c. patient's ability to explain procedure and demonstrate understanding.
    d. patient's behavior modification and compliance rates.

35. Which of the following treatments is considered appropriate palliative care?
    a. Chemotherapy for cancer
    b. Intubation with mechanical ventilation for respiratory failure
    c. Radiotherapy to relieve pain associated with bone cancer
    d. Total parenteral nutrition for patients who cannot eat.

36. Electrocardiograph changes characteristic of hypokalemia include:
    a. tall peaked T waves with widening and increased amplitude of QRS and prolongation of the QT interval.
    b. a U wave more than 1 mm high after the T wave, AV block, and flat or inverted T waves.
    c. dysrhythmias with prolonged PR and QT intervals and broad flat T waves.
    d. non-specific changes.

37. The metabolic syndrome is characterized by:
    a. abdominal obesity, decreased triglyceride level, increased high-density lipoprotein (HDL) level, and hypertension.
    b. Hypertension, abdominal obesity, and increased HDL level.
    c. Abdominal obesity, increased triglycerides, decreased HDL level, elevation of blood pressure, and increased fasting blood glucose.
    d. Hypotension, decreased fasting blood glucose, increased triglycerides, and decreased HDL level.

38. According to the Nursing Code of Ethics of the American Nurses Association, nurses must support a patient's autonomy and self-determination. If a 24-year old Asian woman states a treatment preference but plans to leave the decision to family members, the nurse should:
    a. try to convince the patient to assert herself.
    b. respect the patient's right to be guided by family.
    c. tell the family that the patient should be the one to make the decision.
    d. ask the ethics committee to intervene so that the patient is properly treated.

39. A patient has an atrioventricular (AV) block in which there are more P waves than QRS complexes with no clear relationship between them and an atrial rate two to three times the pulse rate; there is also an irregular PR interval. What type of AV block is this patient likely to have?
    a. First-degree AV block
    b. Second-degree AV block, Mobitz type I
    c. Second-degree AV block, Mobitz type II
    d. Third-degree AV block

40. Cor pulmonale is characterized by changes in the:
    a. left atria.
    b. left ventricle.
    c. right atria.
    d. right ventricle.

41. The primary reason for completing professional development courses is to:
    a. comply with state requirements for licensure.
    b. remain current in the field of nursing.
    c. meet institutional requirements for employment.
    d. fulfill requirements for a salary increase.

42. Cognitive changes associated with aging affect learning in which of the following ways?
    a. Patients are better able to focus attention because their lives have fewer distractions (kids, jobs).
    b. Explicit memories (facts) decline, but implicit memories (skills) often stay the same.
    c. Older adults have the same ability to learn as young adults.
    d. Patients have less difficulty with complex tasks.

43. What adverse effects are related to immunosuppression with high doses of tacrolimus after a heart transplant?
    a. Facial dysmorphism
    b. Hypertension
    c. Hirsutism and acne
    d. Nephrotoxicity

44. The automatic implantable cardioverter defibrillator (AICD) delivers which of the following impulses?
    a. Continuous (asynchronous) electrical impulses to control pulse rate
    b. Dual-chamber sequential electrical impulses
    c. On-demand (synchronous) electrical impulses when the pulse increases to a preset rate
    d. On-demand electrical impulses when the pulse rate decreases to a preset rate

45. An episode of syncope associated with exertional exercise is a manifestation of:
    a. aortic regurgitation
    b. aortic stenosis.
    c. mitral valve prolapse.
    d. endocarditis.

46. A patient with a dissecting descending thoracic aortic aneurysm will most likely complain of:
    a. severe, dull pain that builds in intensity in the anterior chest and nausea and vomiting.
    b. severe, tearing, knife-like pain that builds in intensity in the anterior chest and nausea and vomiting.
    c. dull, aching pain posteriorly below the scapula and nausea and vomiting.
    d. severe, intense, tearing, knife-like pain posteriorly between the scapulae and nausea and vomiting.

47. A patient who is receiving digoxin (Lanoxin) and furosemide (Lasix) daily is also prescribed tetracycline for rosacea and subsequently develops nausea, vomiting, and tachycardia. The most likely cause is:
    a. digitalis toxicity.
    b. allergic response to tetracycline.
    c. drug interaction.
    d. superinfection.

48. A patient is receiving warfarin (Coumadin) along with other treatment for non-valvular atrial fibrillation. The international normalized ratio range should be:
    a. 1.5–2.
    b. 2–3.
    c. 3–4.
    d. >4.

49. A patient with the recent implantation of a pacemaker develops severe hiccups, which indicates:
   a. irritation of the ventricular wall.
   b. phrenic nerve or muscle stimulation from dislocation of leads.
   c. impending cardiac tamponade.
   d. allergic response to medications.

50. A patient is being considered for thrombolytic therapy with alteplase tissue-type plasminogen activator (t-PA). Contraindications to thrombolytic therapy include which of the following?
   a. The patient has a 3.5 cm aortic aneurysm.
   b. It has been 2 hours since the onset of symptoms.
   c. The patient's blood pressure has been 180/90 mm Hg but is now controlled by medication.
   d. The patient had an ischemic stroke 6 months previously.

51. Which of the following medications should be discontinued for a minimum of 48 hours before cardioversion?
   a. Digoxin
   b. Warfarin
   c. Cardizem
   d. Insulin

52. A patient with heart failure has no symptoms at rest, but symptoms appear with physical exertion and cause some limitations of activities of daily living and slight pulmonary edema. This heart failure is classified as:
   a. class I.
   b. class II.
   c. class III.
   d. class IV.

53. The treatment of choice for significant pulmonary stenosis is:
   a. closed valvotomy.
   b. open valvotomy.
   c. balloon valvuloplasty.
   d. valve replacement with homograft valve.

54. Which of the following medications may be used after cardiac surgery to treat low cardiac output?
   a. Nitroprusside
   b. Dobutamine
   c. Dopamine
   d. Isoproterenol

55. When preparing written materials for patients, what reading level would be appropriate for a homogeneous group of adults in an affluent area?
   a. Grade 3 level
   b. Grade 6 level
   c. Grade 9 level
   d. Grade 12 level

56. Monitoring a patient for acute rejection after cardiac transplantation is primarily done by:
    a. reviewing clinical symptoms.
    b. blood testing.
    c. biopsy.
    d. electrocardiogram.

57. When examining the chest, where is the apex beat (pulsation) usually observed?
    a. It cannot be observed, only palpated
    b. Around the third intercostal space on the left mid-clavicular line
    c. Around the fourth intercostal space on the left mid-clavicular line
    d. Around the fifth intercostal space on the left mid-clavicular line

58. First-line drugs for the treatment of stage I hypertension are:
    a. loop diuretics.
    b. thiazide diuretics.
    c. angiotensin-converting enzyme inhibitors.
    d. calcium channel blockers.

59. Which immunizations are routinely ordered for adults 60–65 years of age and older?
    a. Influenza vaccine only
    b. Pneumococcal polysaccharide-23, influenza vaccine, and herpes zoster vaccine
    c. Hepatitis A and B vaccines
    d. Influenza and hepatitis C vaccines.

60. Which medication order below is written correctly?
    a. Maalox 30 cc PO qhs
    b. Lasix 40.0 mg PO daily
    c. MS 4.0 mg IV q 4 hr prn
    d. Synthroid 0.88 mg PO daily at 0700.

61. The nurse attempts to start an intravenous (IV) line on an elderly patient, but the patient refuses to cooperate. The nurse tells the patient that the nursing assistant will be called to hold him down if he does not cooperate. This nurse's response is best characterized as:
    a. coercion.
    b. non-therapeutic communication.
    c. abuse.
    d. poor judgment.

62. Sexual dysfunction after a heart transplant is primarily caused by:
    a. immunosuppressive drugs.
    b. anxiety.
    c. weakness and malaise.
    d. antihypertensive drugs.

63. A 62-year old male patient has a regular pulse of over 100 bpm with P waves occurring before the QRS complex and sometimes preceding the T wave. The QRS complex is a normal shape and duration. The PR interval is 0.12–0.20 sec, and the P:QRS ratio is 1:1. Based on these findings, the cardiac diagnosis is:
    a. sinus bradycardia.
    b. sinus tachycardia.
    c. sinus arrhythmia.
    d. premature atrial contractions.

64. A patient receives daily warfarin (Coumadin) after treatment for atrial fibrillation. Which of the following substances may interfere with the drug's effectiveness?
    a. One 4-ounce glass of red wine daily
    b. Caffeinated beverages
    c. A daily multivitamin
    d. Milk products

65. Using transesophageal Doppler ultrasonography to measure cardiac output, a short waveform with a rounded apex may indicate:
    a. decreased preload.
    b. increased preload.
    c. increased systemic vascular resistance.
    d. left ventricular failure.

66. Which enzyme test should be measured 8–12 hours after onset of symptoms for the diagnosis of myocardial infarction?
    a. Troponin T and I
    b. Myoglobin
    c. Lactic dehydrogenase
    d. Creatinine kinase /creatinine-myoglobin

67. A 48-year old male patient is referred to a cardiac care center for cardiac rehabilitation after a myocardial infarction. The cardiac care center provides:
    a. primary care.
    b. secondary care.
    c. tertiary care.
    d. quaternary care.

68. An absolute indication for stopping an exercise test is a:
    a. patient complaint of dyspnea that is not noticeable to the observer.
    b. downsloping ST segment depression.
    c. decrease in systolic blood pressure (BP) of10 mm Hg or less from baseline despite an increased workload but absent evidence of ischemia.
    d. decrease in systolic BP of 10 mm Hg or more from baseline despite an increased workload and with evidence of ischemia.

69. A 76-year old woman with end-stage heart failure was placed on hospice care by her physician 6 months earlier (two 90-day periods), but she is still alive. Her family asks the nurse if the patient will be removed from hospice care. Which response by the nurse is best in this situation?
  a. "She will be removed from hospice care until her condition worsens because she has exceeded the 6-month period."
  b. "She has exhausted all of her hospice care benefits and will be removed from hospice care."
  c. "She can continue with hospice care as long as the physician authorizes the care every 60 days."
  d. "She can continue with hospice care if the physician continues to authorize care every 90 days."

70. Thirty hours after valvular surgery that required cardiopulmonary bypass, a 75-year-old patient, who has been apathetic and forgetful for the previous 12 hours, becomes very disoriented, confused, and combative, pulling out his intravenous lines. He is most likely suffering from:
  a. post-pump delirium and psychosis.
  b. ischemic stroke.
  c. a reaction to drugs.
  d. hypoxia.

71. A patient with a total cholesterol of 206, triglycerides of 105, high-density lipoprotein (HDL) of 35, and low-density lipoprotein (LDL) of 150 should have treatment with a goal to:
  a. lower total cholesterol and triglyceride levels.
  b. lower total cholesterol and HDL levels.
  c. lower total cholesterol and raise LDL levels.
  d. lower total cholesterol and LDL levels and raise HDL levels.

72. Which rhythm disturbance is most common after cardiac surgery?
  a. Ventricular fibrillation
  b. Ventricular tachycardia
  c. Premature ventricular contractions
  d. Atrial fibrillation, flutter, and tachycardia

73. Which self-monitoring skill is essential for a patient with heart failure?
  a. Intake of fats
  b. Daily weight
  c. Degree of edema
  d. Exercise

74. A frail 80-year old patient who lives alone requires long-term intravenous (IV) antibiotic therapy for prosthetic valve endocarditis from Staphylococcus epidermidis. His condition is stable at present. The most effective care plan includes:
  a. keeping the patient in the acute care hospital until therapy is completed.
  b. sending the patient home and having home health nurses provide home intravenous antibiotic therapy.
  c. instructing the patient to self-administer the antibiotic therapy.
  d. transferring the patient to an extended care facility for continued treatment.

75. A patient with severe pain is receiving pain medication routinely every 6 hours but usually complains of breakthrough pain in 4 hours, requiring an additional injection, which indicates that:
 a. the patient has a low pain tolerance and may need to be distracted.
 b. the routine pain medication may need to be given every 4 hours or the dosage changed.
 c. pain control is adequate with the additional medication.
 d. pain may be intractable and cannot be controlled.

76. Adequate perfusion requires a mean arterial pressure (MAP) of:
 a. >40 mm Hg.
 b. >50 mm Hg.
 c. >60 mm Hg.
 d. >70 mm Hg.

77. Patients with peripheral arterial disease and aspirin intolerance should be prescribed:
 a. clopidogrel.
 b. warfarin.
 c. unfractionated heparin.
 d. low-molecular-weight heparin.

78. According to the AHA/ACC Guideline for the Management of Patients with Non–ST-Elevation Acute Coronary Syndromes, for early risk stratification of patients presenting in the ED with chest pain or other symptoms indicative of acute coronary syndrome, a 12-lead ECG should be done within:
 a. 5 minutes.
 b. 10 minutes.
 c. 15 minutes.
 d. 20 minutes.

79. For a patient receiving a calcium channel blocker, such as diltiazem, which type of supplement may reduce effectiveness?
 a. Vitamin C.
 b. B-complex vitamins.
 c. Potassium.
 d. Calcium.

80. A patient preparing for discharge has been advised to make multiple lifestyle changes related to diet, medications, habits, and exercise, but the patient is upset about the changes and states repeatedly that the physician is expecting too much. The best response is:
 a. "It will get easier with time."
 b. "It's difficult to make all of these changes."
 c. "Let me help you map out a plan."
 d. "Just take one day at a time."

81. If a patient has a base normal control prothrombin time (PT) of 10 seconds, the maximum target PT with warfarin therapy is usually:
 a. 15 seconds.
 b. 20 seconds.
 c. 25 seconds.
 d. 30 seconds.

82. If a patient is taking a bile acid sequestrant, such as cholestyramine, to lower low-density lipoprotein (LDL), how long after taking the drug should the patient wait before taking other medications?
    a. Waiting is not necessary.
    b. 1 to 2 hours.
    c. 2 to 4 hours.
    d. 4 to 6 hours.

83. Which of the following antiplatelet drugs poses the least risk of bleeding?
    a. aspirin (ASA).
    b. clopidogrel.
    c. abciximab.
    d. eptifibatide.

84. Which of the following conditions is an indication for thrombolytic therapy?
    a. NSTEMI.
    b. STEMI.
    c. Unstable angina.
    d. Stable angina.

85. If a patient has undergone fibrinolytic therapy per accelerated infusion of alteplase 100 mg for an acute myocardial infarction and shows 20% reduction in ST elevation after 90 minutes, the cardiac/vascular nurse anticipates:
    a. further monitoring.
    b. additional thrombolysis.
    c. angiography/rescue percutaneous coronary intervention (PCI).
    d. administration of fondaparinux.

86. Which of the following patients may be an acceptable candidate for catheter-directed thrombolysis (CDT) for peripheral arterial occlusion?
    a. Patient with non–life-threatening limb ischemia of 12 days.
    b. Patient with limb-threatening ischemia, unknown duration.
    c. Patient with non–life-threatening limb ischemia for 21 days.
    d. Patient with limb-threatening ischemia of 3 days.

87. On the ECG recording, a normal sinus rhythm is characterized by a PR interval of:
    a. 0.04 to 0.1 seconds.
    b. 0.12 to 0.2 seconds.
    c. 0.16 to 0.24 seconds.
    d. 0.2 to 0.28 seconds.

88. If a patient exhibits a ventricular rate of 150 bpm, the most likely cause of dysrhythmia is:
    a. accelerated idioventricular rhythm.
    b. junctional tachycardia.
    c. atrial fibrillation.
    d. atrial flutter.

89. After administering sublingual nitroglycerin to a patient for angina, the cardiac/vascular nurse should expect a reduction in pain within:
    a. 30 seconds to 1 minute.
    b. 1 to 2 minutes.
    c. 3 to 4 minutes.
    d. 5 to 8 minutes.

90. Beta-blockers are generally contraindicated for patients with a history of:
    a. liver disease
    b. asthma.
    c. stroke.
    d. kidney disease.

91. *Rest potentiation* of the heart refers to:
    a. faster rate of stimulation resulting in stronger contraction.
    b. slower rate of stimulation resulting in weaker contraction.
    c. pause resulting in stronger ensuing contraction.
    d. extra beat resulting in stronger ensuing contraction.

92. In order to modify risk of cardiovascular disease for patients with peripheral arterial disease (PAD), the primary lifestyle change should be:
    a. emotional support.
    b. improved diet.
    c. increased exercise.
    d. smoking cessation.

93. At what heart rate is diastolic filling so reduced that stroke volume is diminished and coronary ischemia occurs?
    a. >140 bpm.
    b. >160 bpm.
    c. >180 bpm.
    d. >200 bpm.

94. Which of the following is a risk factor for coronary artery disease?
    a. Sister diagnosed with coronary artery disease at age 63.
    b. Father diagnosed with coronary artery disease at age 60.
    c. Mother diagnosed with coronary artery disease at age 65.
    d. Brother diagnosed with coronary artery disease at age 56.

95. When conducting the NIH Stroke Scale and evaluating "best gaze," the cardiac/vascular nurse notes a forced deviation to the side of the stroke and the patient is unable to follow the nurse's moving finger with the eyes, so the nurse carries out the oculocephalic maneuver. A normal response is:
    a. no eye movement during the maneuver.
    b. eyes deviate to the side the head is turned to and then returns to midline.
    c. eyes deviate vertically as the head is turned and then return to previous position.
    d. eyes deviate to opposite side the head is turned to and then return to midline.

96. When assessing the adequacy of a patient's diet, the cardiac/vascular nurse recognized that, for an elderly adult weighing 70 kg (154 lb), the average caloric requirement per day is about:
    a. 1400.
    b. 1750.
    c. 2000.
    d. 2200.

97. Which of the following actions by a patient most indicates a lack of readiness to learn about his heart disease and lifestyle management techniques?
    a. Patient states that the medication regimen is too confusing.
    b. Patient has not read any of the written educational material left at bedside.
    c. Patient turns on the TV to watch a football game when the nurse is instructing.
    d. Patient remains passive, asks no questions, and shows no interest in instruction.

98. According to the AHA/ACC Guideline for the Management of Patients with Non–ST-Elevation Acute Coronary Syndromes, patients presenting in the ED with chest pain or symptoms indicative of acute coronary syndrome should receive oxygen:
    a. in all situations.
    b. if anxious and frightened.
    c. with oxygen saturation <90%.
    d. with oxygen saturation <94%.

99. According to the Protection Motivation Theory, action to bring about change is precipitated by:
    a. threat.
    b. education.
    c. fear.
    d. motivation.

100. Considering health literacy, the cardiac/vascular nurse should expect that the average reading level of the US population is:
    a. ≤4th grade.
    b. ≤5th grade.
    c. ≤6th grade.
    d. ≤8th grade.

101. When administering the Tinetti Gait and Balance Instrument to an older adult, the balance assessment begins with the patient:
    a. standing in front of a chair.
    b. sitting in an armed chair.
    c. sitting in an armless chair.
    d. standing with eyes closed.

102. If an older adult with aortic stenosis undergoes percutaneous balloon valvuloplasty, restenosis often occurs within:
    a. 6 months.
    b. 1 to 2 years.
    c. 2 to 4 years.
    d. 5 to 10 years.

103. A patient with hypertension and diabetes mellitus had been a heavy smoker for 40 years before having a myocardial infarction; however, she has continued to smoke even though she states, "I know I should quit." The best response is:
    a. "Tell me about that."
    b. "Your life may depend on quitting."
    c. "You should join a support group."
    d. "You could try the nicotine patch."

104. Which of the following educational programs might best be conducted as a webinar?
    a. Video series regarding cardiac anatomy and physiology.
    b. Orientation program for newly hired cardiac/vascular nurses.
    c. Online course for cardiac/vascular nurse continuing education.
    d. Interactive discussion about new techniques in cardiac rehabilitation.

105. If a cardiac/vascular nurse working in a semi-rural area proposes a mobile clinic to better monitor, screen, and counsel patients who often cannot or do not seek medical care, the most likely impediment is:
    a. patient acceptance.
    b. cost-effectiveness.
    c. staffing needs.
    d. clinician resistance.

106. According to the Seventh Report of the Joint National Committee on Prevention, Detection, Evaluation, and Treatment of High Blood Pressure, systolic blood pressure is a greater cardiovascular risk factor than diastolic blood pressure after age:
    a. 40.
    b. 45.
    c. 50.
    d. 60.

107. A low score on the Care Transitions Measure (CTM-15) is predictive of:
    a. rehospitalization or return to emergency department.
    b. stable transition to a different level of care.
    c. increased risk of nonadherence to medical regimen.
    d. patient adherence with medical regimen.

108. According to Healthy People 2020 initiatives, which of the following patients should be screened for peripheral arterial disease with the ankle-brachial index (ABI)?
    a. 65-year-old obese female patient.
    b. 55-year-old diabetic male patient with leg pain.
    c. 60-year-old male patient after myocardial infarction.
    d. 35-year-old female patient with C-6 spinal cord injury.

109. According to the ACCF/AHA Guideline for the Management of ST-Elevation Myocardial Infarction, the pain medication of choice for patients with STEMI and acute pulmonary edema is:
    a. COX-2 inhibitors.
    b. NSAIDs.
    c. meperidine.
    d. morphine sulfate.

110. A patient with stage 2 Alzheimer disease and coronary artery disease can function fairly well in her home environment but has increasing short-term memory loss and often forgets to take her medications even though her daughter calls to remind her. The best solution is likely:
    a. providing an electronic medication dispenser.
    b. providing daily home health care for medication administration.
    c. arranging for a neighbor to administer the medications.
    d. moving patient to an assisted living facility.

111. A normal value for the activated partial thromboplastin time (aPTT) is:
    a. 7 to 12 seconds.
    b. 10 to 14 seconds.
    c. 21 to 35 seconds.
    d. 30 to 45 seconds.

112. According to the ACC/AHA Guideline on the Treatment of Blood Cholesterol to Reduce Atherosclerotic Cardiovascular Risk in Adults, the goal for LDL cholesterol reduction with treatment with high-intensity statin is:
    a. 30% to 40%.
    b. ≥50%.
    c. 30% to <50%.
    d. 40% to 50%.

113. If a patient with mechanical prosthetic heart valve is on warfarin therapy and has an INR of 3.2, this probably indicates:
    a. inadequate anticoagulation.
    b. slightly excess anticoagulation.
    c. emergent risk of bleeding.
    d. normal INR for this patient.

114. When monitoring a patient's 12-lead ECG, the cardiac/vascular nurse would expect a lead facing an injured area of the heart to show:
    a. ST-segment elevation.
    b. ST-segment inversion.
    c. T-wave deflection upward.
    d. R-wave regression.

115. If C-reactive protein (CRP) is 8 mg/L in a patient with normal lipid values, this may indicate:
    a. decreased risk of cardiovascular disease.
    b. increased risk of cardiovascular disease.
    c. presence of myocardial injury.
    d. presence of myocardial ischemia.

116. When baroreceptors in the aortic arch and carotid arteries sense volume overload, the usual response is:
    a. decreased heart rate and vasoconstriction.
    b. increased heart rate and vasoconstriction.
    c. decreased heart rate and vasodilation.
    d. increased heart rate and vasodilation.

117. Which of the following is a common age-associated change in the cardiovascular system?
    a. Systolic blood pressure decreased.
    b. Cardiac valves thin.
    c. Cardiac reserve increased.
    d. Pacemaker cells decreased in number.

118. If a patient with hypertension has been prescribed the DASH diet, how many servings of sweets and added sugars may the patient have per week?
    a. ≤5.
    b. ≤10.
    c. ≤15.
    d. ≤20.

119. Which of the following services can a patient expect from Mended Hearts?
    a. Financial assistance.
    b. Visiting program (in-hospital).
    c. In-home care.
    d. Transportation assistance.

120. Which of the following is part of exclusion criteria for therapeutic hypothermia for a patient who experienced sudden cardiac arrest and resuscitation?
    a. Chemical thrombolysis.
    b. Sudden cardiac arrest 3 hours previously.
    c. Major surgery 1 week previously.
    d. Maintenance of systolic BP of 92 to 94 mm Hg after CPR.

121. If the cardiac/vascular nurse is serving as a preceptor for a nursing student and feels that the student lacks essential skills, the cardiac/vascular nurse should first:
    a. terminate the preceptor relationship.
    b. report the student to the nursing program director.
    c. ask other preceptors for advice.
    d. meet with the student to outline concerns.

122. The primary treatment focus for patients with dilated cardiomyopathy is:
    a. promoting activity.
    b. controlling heart failure.
    c. preparing for heart transplant.
    d. preventing sudden death.

123. A physician with whom the staff is very friendly is admitted to the cardiac unit with a myocardial infarction, and a number of nurses, who are not assigned to the patient, review his laboratory findings by reading over the shoulder of the physician's assigned nurse. This is primarily a(n):
    a. HIPAA violation.
    b. standard procedure.
    c. minor violation of privacy.
    d. unprofessional activity.

124. A patient experienced a severe adverse reaction to a drug while left unattended because of suboptimal staffing. This problem will likely be referred to:
    a. district attorney.
    b. risk management.
    c. nurses' union.
    d. attorneys for the organization.

125. A patient, Ms. Jones, who has had recent cardiac catheterization and angioplasty, presents with increasing shortness of breath, cough, and chest pain, pulse of 130, BP of 140/60, and respirations 32 per minute. Using the SBAR communication technique, how will the cardiac/vascular nurse begin the report to the physician?
    a. "I believe Ms. Jones may have a pulmonary embolism or cardiac event."
    b. "Ms. Jones has a pulse of 130, BP 140/60, and respirations of 32 per minute."
    c. "Ms. Jones has increasing shortness of breath, cough, and chest pain for the past hour."
    d. "Ms. Jones recently had cardiac catheterization and angioplasty.

126. If the cardiac/vascular nurse overhears another nurse berating a patient, telling the patient that she is "lazy and unmotivated," and refusing to assist the patient to the bathroom, the best initial response is to:
    a. immediately intervene.
    b. report the other nurse to a supervisor.
    c. confront the other nurse later.
    d. assume the other nurse is acting in the patient's best interests.

127. A patient is awaiting surgical intervention for a dissecting aortic aneurysm. Prior to surgery, the patient's systolic BP should be maintained at:
    a. 90 to 100 mm Hg.
    b. 100 to 110 mm Hg.
    c. 110 to 120 mm Hg.
    d. 120 to 130 mm Hg.

128. If the cardiac/vascular nurse proposes forming an interdisciplinary team to work on process improvement, the best members are likely to be those who:
    a. are personal friends.
    b. work well with others.
    c. volunteer to participate.
    d. have needed knowledge/skills.

129. Which of the following would disqualify a patient for home health care under Medicare?
    a. The patient walks 1 mile daily in her neighborhood.
    b. The patient attends a cardiac rehabilitation program weekly.
    c. The patient attends church with her daughter each week.
    d. The patient attends an adult daycare program while her daughter works.

130. A close personal friend of the cardiac/vascular nurse is a patient on the cardiac unit, and the cardiac/vascular nurse trades assignments with another nurse in order to be assigned to the patient. This constitutes a(n):
    a. HIPAA violation.
    b. unprofessional act.
    c. professional boundary violation.
    d. acceptable procedure.

131. A patient with bradycardia of 30 bpm is to have a temporary transcutaneous pacemaker (TCP) until a transvenous catheter can be inserted and the cause of the bradycardia determined. In preparation for the TCP, the nurse should advise the patient to expect:
    a. no discomfort.
    b. slight discomfort with pacing.
    c. sharp constant chest pain.
    d. muscle contractions and discomfort with pacing.

132. Osler's nodes may be found with:
    a. endocarditis.
    b. heart failure
    c. pericarditis.
    d. myocarditis.

133. The mother of an 18-year-old patient with hypertrophic cardiomyopathy has been scheduled twice to attend CPR classes before her son is discharged but has failed to attend the classes, stating that the CPR class is "not necessary" and "a waste of time." According to Kübler-Ross's stages of grief, the mother is probably experiencing:
    a. depression.
    b. denial.
    c. anger.
    d. acceptance.

134. If a patient states, "The doctor promised that I didn't have to exercise today," and the cardiac/vascular nurse knows the physician told the patient to exercise more, the best response is:
    a. "You know that is not true."
    b. "I don't believe the doctor said that at all."
    c. "Why are you insisting you don't need to exercise when the doctor says you need to?"
    d. "That's surprising because the doctor wrote an order for you to walk twice today."

135. The ECG shows a heart rate of 80 bpm with regular rhythm and normal P waves and QRS complex. The PR interval is 0.5 seconds. This finding is characteristic of:
    a. first-degree atrioventricular block.
    b. second-degree atrioventricular block, type I.
    c. second-degree atrioventricular block, type II.
    d. third-degree atrioventricular block.

136. The primary difference between partnership councils and other forms of shared governance is that partnership councils usually include:
    a. only nursing personnel.
    b. only one level of an organization.
    c. all disciplines in an organization.
    d. only physicians and nursing personnel.

137. If a Middle Eastern female patient leaves all medical decisions about her treatment to her husband, this probably represents:
    a. a cultural norm.
    b. an abusive relationship.
    c. low health literacy.
    d. apathy.

138. A patient has coronary artery disease, and the patient's list of medications shows that the patient is currently taking clopidogrel 75 mg daily, omeprazole 20 mg daily, metoprolol 50 mg twice daily, docusate sodium 1 capsule daily, and atorvastatin 80 mg daily. Which drug poses the greatest risk of drug-drug interactions?
    a. clopidogrel.
    b. atorvastatin.
    c. metoprolol.
    d. omeprazole.

139. If a nursing diagnosis is "ineffective self-health management associated with lack of knowledge about condition and therapy," an appropriate patient goal is:
    a. "Patient exhibits improved self-health management and positive attitude toward health."
    b. "Patient identifies personal needs in relation to health management."
    c. "Patient can describe key elements of the disease process and therapeutic regimen."
    d. "Patient expresses a willingness to undergo lifestyle changes."

140. The primary advantage of PCI with drug-eluting stents or bare-metal stents compared with balloon angioplasty alone is:
    a. Decreased restenosis.
    b. Decreased need for postoperative medications
    c. Decreased mortality rates.
    d. Decreased particle embolization.

141. A patient with an automatic implantable cardioverter defibrillator (AICD) should generally be advised to avoid:
    a. microwave ovens.
    b. MRIs.
    c. metal detectors.
    d. anti-theft devices.

142. For a patient with an Unna boot, the most important factor in promoting adequate compression is:
    a. elevation of the foot.
    b. proper application.
    c. concurrent medications.
    d. ambulation.

143. According to the ACCF/AHA/HRS Focused Update on the Management of Patients with Atrial Fibrillation, the goal for patients with atrial fibrillation is generally a ventricular rate at rest of:
    a. 60 to 80.
    b. 80 to 100.
    c. 90 to 115.
    d. 115 to 125.

144. According to the AACVPR's *Guidelines for Cardiac Rehabilitation and Secondary Prevention Programs*, patients should be referred to a cardiac rehabilitation program if:
    a. the patient has adequate insurance coverage for rehabilitation.
    b. the patient's mobility was limited by an acute cardiovascular event.
    c. the patient is unable to adequately exercise independently.
    d. the patient experienced an acute cardiovascular event.

145. A patient has been admitted to the cardiac care unit with chest pain and atrial fibrillation. Which of the following tasks is appropriate to delegate to unlicensed assistive personnel?
    a. apical/radial pulse rate.
    b. monitoring the IV fluids.
    c. daily weight.
    d. response to analgesia.

146. A patient is being treated for acute heart failure. Which of the following tasks has priority?
    a. Monitor response to medications.
    b. Check patient's skin for lesions.
    c. Instruct patient in low-sodium diet.
    d. Check that call light is within reach.

147. Lidocaine is used primarily for treatment of:
    a. PVC suppression.
    b. VT/VF.
    c. Atrial fibrillation.
    d. PAC suppression.

148. A patient receiving IV morphine for treatment of severe chest pain develops opioid-induced hypotension. The best approach to treating the hypotension is:
    a. administer naloxone (Narcan).
    b. administer antihistamine.
    c. administer crystalloid bolus and continue morphine.
    d. hold morphine and administer crystalloid bolus.

149. Which of the following is a characteristic of non–Q-wave myocardial infarction?
    a. MI is usually transmural.
    b. Coronary occlusion complete in 80% to 90% of patients.
    c. Contraction necrosis associated with reperfusion is common.
    d. Peak CK levels occur in about 24 hours.

150. If a patient is classified as having NYHA class I heart failure, the type of symptoms the patient should expect with activities includes:

    a. no symptoms.
    b. slight shortness of breath.
    c. marked dyspnea and/or angina on exertion.
    d. Severe symptoms even at rest.

Answers and Explanations

1. A: The most common initial treatment of acute pulmonary edema is oxygen to relieve dyspnea, nitroglycerine to reduce preload, loop diuretics (usually furosemide-Lasix) to promote diuresis and venodilation, and morphine to reduce associated anxiety (although some physicians avoid morphine because of side effects). Angiotensin-converting enzyme inhibitors are also sometimes used to reduce afterload, but thiazide diuretics are not used to treat acute pulmonary edema. Calcium channel blockers may induce acute pulmonary edema if used with tocolytics.

2. D: The daughter should be advised that cardiopulmonary resuscitation must be withheld in accordance with the advance directive and desires of the mother. A valid do-not-resuscitate order is in place and does not require verification. Family members often panic at the time of death and want to institute life-saving measures against the wishes of the patient, but this does not override the patient's explicit directions. The staff should provide emotional support for the family. While this is an ethical issue, there is no time to contact an ethics committee.

3. B: Emergency defibrillation is usually performed in patients with ventricular tachycardia (VT) who are also unconscious. Ventricular tachycardia is characterized by three premature ventricular contractions or more in a row and a ventricular rate of 100–200 bpm. The rapid rate of contractions makes VT dangerous as the ineffective beats may render the person unconscious with no palpable pulse. A detectable rate is usually regular and the QRS complex is ≥ 0.12 second and (often) abnormally shaped. The P wave may be undetectable with an irregular PR interval if the P wave is present. The P:QRS ratio is difficult to ascertain if the P wave is missing.

4. C: Cardiac tamponade may result in decreased chest tube drainage, muffled heart sounds, tachycardia, pulsus paradoxus, and decreased urinary output. The pulmonary artery wedge pressure, central venous pressure, and pulmonary artery diastolic pressure equalize. The cause is fluid accumulating in the pericardial sac, compressing the heart. In some cases, it can be caused by kinks or obstructions in the drainage tube. These tubes may be gently milked to remove obstructions, but the nurse should avoid the creation of negative pressure (through stripping), which can damage the surgical site.

5. B: Ischemia is characterized by inverted T waves. As the cardiac muscle is damaged, the ST segment is elevated with elevated symmetrical T waves. With a Q-wave myocardial infarction, Q or QS waves develop as repolarization is altered or absent. Changes in the Q waves are usually permanent, so an old myocardial infarction (MI) is evidenced by abnormal Q waves or decreased elevation of the R waves without alterations of ST and T waves. A non-Q-wave MI does not cause Q-wave changes.

6. D: The sudden onset of intermittent substernal pain that is referred to the neck, arms, and back is typical of pericarditis. Angina pain, usually related to exertion, lasts 5–15 minutes and is substernal or retrosternal, radiating across chest and sometimes to the inside of the arm, neck, or jaw. Myocardial pain lasts over 15 minutes and occurs spontaneously or after an episode of unstable angina. It is substernal or over the pericardium. It may spread across the chest and into shoulders and hands. Anxiety pain lasts 2–3 minutes and tends to occur across the chest but does not radiate; however, some patients complain of numbness of the hands and mouth.

7. A: An ankle systolic pressure of 90 divided by a brachial systolic pressure of 120 equals 0.75. Blood pressure at the ankle should be equal to or slightly higher than that of the arm. With peripheral arterial disease, the ankle pressure falls. The degree of disease relates to the score:
- 1.3: Abnormally high, may indicate calcification of vessel wall
- 1 to 1.1: Normal
- < 0.05: Narrowing of one or more leg blood vessels
- < 0.8: Moderate, associated with intermittent claudication
- < 0.6 to 0.8: Borderline perfusion
- 0.5 to 0.75: Severe disease, ischemia
- < 0.5: Pain even at rest. Limb threatened
- 0.25: Critical limb-threatening condition

8. D: S4 is an extra beat (atrial gallop), occurring just before S1 and producing a triple "Tennessee" rhythm. It is often associated with left ventricular hypertrophy, hypertension, or aortic stenosis. S1 and S2 are normal heart sounds. S1 indicates the onset of systole with closure of both the tricuspid and mitral valves. S2 is the end of systole and indicates closure of the pulmonary and aortic valves. S3 is an extra beat, producing a triple rhythm ("Kentucky"), and indicates decreased ventricular compliance, often related to left ventricular failure and mitral regurgitation.

9. C: Anticoagulation therapy is given before direct current cardioversion and also before chemical cardioversion in most cases. There is no time to start anticoagulation when emergency defibrillation is needed. With fibrillation, blood clots may form within the heart, and when the pulse rate converts to normal, these clots can travel, increasing the risk of heart attack or stroke; thus, the patient is usually maintained on anticoagulation (commonly warfarin [Coumadin]) for up to 6 months after cardioversion.

10. D: Drinking heavily on only one occasion can result in cardiovascular impairment. While the affect of alcohol on the heart is more severe if there is underlying cardiac disease, an overdose of alcohol even with no underlying disorder weakens cardiac contractions, causing the heart rate to increase. Alcohol depresses the autonomic nervous system, which can lead to heart failure, cardiac dysrhythmias (most commonly atrial fibrillation), and cardiac arrest. Chronic drinking can severely damage the heart and blood vessels, resulting in hypertension and cardiomyopathy.

11. B: Urinary output after surgery varies, according to fluid intake, but should be more than 25 mL/hr. Urinary output less than 25 mL/hr indicates decreased renal function. Urine specific gravity should be maintained at 1.105–1.025, indicating the ability of the kidneys to concentrate urine in the renal tubules. Blood urea nitrogen, creatinine, urine, and serum electrolytes are monitored to ensure that the kidneys can excrete waste products. Urinary output is usually monitored every half hour while the patient is in the critical care unit.

12. A: Most cocaine users typically demonstrate hypertension and an increased heart rate. Chest pain may mimic a myocardial infarction. Vasoconstriction occurs both within the coronary arteries and the peripheral circulation, resulting in hypertension and episodes of cardiac ischemia that may cause infarcts. In some cases, multiple infarcts may occur even with normal coronary arteries. Cardiomyopathy with enlargement of the left ventricular muscle is common in chronic users.

13. B: Venous ulcers are typically superficial irregular ulcers on the medial or lateral malleolus and sometimes the anterior tibial area and cause varying degrees of pain. Surrounding skin often has a brownish discoloration. Edema is moderate to severe. Arterial ulcers are painful, deep, circular,

often necrotic ulcers found on toe tips, toe webs, heels or other pressure areas. There is often rubor on dependency but pallor on foot elevation, and skin is pale, shiny, and cool. Edema is minimal.

14. A: No special preparation is needed for a radionuclide ventriculogram. A sample of blood is withdrawn, labeled with a technetium 99m radionuclide and then is injected back into the patient. With electrocardiogram (ECG) guidance, images are obtained during the cardiac cycle. The video display provides images similar to that of a contrast angiogram. The radionuclide ventriculogram is used to evaluate diastolic and systolic function for patients with heart failure from valvular heart disease or to monitor the toxic effects of chemotherapeutic drugs.

15. C: Central cyanosis of the tongue and buccal mucosa indicates severe cardiovascular disease, such as pulmonary edema or congestive heart failure. Pallor is the result of decreased levels of oxyhemoglobin, usually resulting from anemia or decreased perfusion. Peripheral cyanosis of the nails, nose, and extremities indicates decreased circulation and can occur with heart failure or other causes of vasoconstriction (e.g., cold). Xanthelasma is a yellowish plaque, usually on the eyelids, indicating high levels of cholesterol.

16. D: Angiotensin-converting enzyme (ACE) inhibitors are contraindicated in patients with renal failure, as one of the most serious side effects of these drugs is renal impairment, especially in patients also taking diuretics and non-steroidal anti-inflammatory drugs. The ACE inhibitors are commonly used to treat hypertension and heart failure. They are often combined with diuretics, such as the thiazide diuretics (hydrochlorothiazide) for hypertension or furosemide (Lasix) for heart failure. The ACE inhibitors are sometimes given to patients with diabetes mellitus to prevent diabetic neuropathy.

17. B: Mechanical ventilation can cause hypoventilation and carbon dioxide retention, resulting in respiratory acidosis. Renal compensatory actions include retention of bicarbonate (HCO3) and increased excretion of hydrogen (H). Serum pH and PCO2 are decreased. Symptoms include flushed skin, ventricular fibrillation, and hypotension. Patients may develop drowsiness, headaches, disorientation, seizures, and coma.

18. A: The risks associated with sexual activity after recovery from a myocardial infarction are very low, and most heart recovery programs encourage exercise. However, before a sexual encounter, it is important to consider the following:
- The person should be well rested.
- The person should wait 1–3 hours after eating.
- A comfortable position should be used to minimize stress.
- Foreplay is important so that the heart rate increases and strengthens in preparation for intercourse.
- If the person takes nitroglycerine for angina, this medication should be taken before sexual activity.

19. C: While wearing a Holter monitor, patients should maintain an activity diary so that any abnormality can be linked to this activity. Conversely, the diary may demonstrate that no abnormality occurs with certain activities. Patients should continue with prescribed medications and carry out normal activities since the primary purpose of a Holter monitor is to assist in diagnosis and to determine triggers for abnormal electrocardiogram readings. The monitor should be used during the night as some cardiac abnormalities may occur during sleep.

20. B: The best approach for severe mitral valve prolapse with heart failure is to repair the valve rather than to replace it because of the connective tissue abnormalities associated with Marfan syndrome. These abnormalities may result in dehiscence when prosthetic valves are used. Severe mitral valve prolapse can result in complications, such as heart failure, endocarditis, and cardiac arrest, so delaying surgery increases the risk; therefore, delaying surgery and not operating are options only for mild cases of mitral valve prolapse.

21. D: The health belief model is used to predict health behavior when a person takes a health action to avoid negative consequences if the person believes the action will prevent a negative outcome. The theory is based on six basic perceptions:
- Susceptibility, the belief that a person may get a negative condition
- Severity, an understanding of how serious a condition is
- Benefit, a belief that action will reduce risk
- Barriers, such as direct or psychological costs
- Action cues or strategies, such as education, to encourage action
- Self-efficacy, the confidence in the ability to take action and to achieve positive results

22. B: Smoking the first cigarette within 5 minutes of awakening is one of the primary signs of a high level of nicotine dependence as is smoking 31 or more cigarettes daily. Patients who are dependent on cigarettes also often smoke in areas where it is prohibited (e.g., at work) and smoke even if they are extremely ill. Patients may benefit from keeping a smoking diary to help to identify their smoking patterns

23. C: The most effective and efficient method of teaching a group about lifestyle changes is the group lecture and discussion. These allow the nurse to provide information and for people with shared concerns to interact and discuss issues. Computer-assisted instruction is not effective for all patients, especially older adults, and lectures only may not address specific concerns of the patients. One-on-one instruction is good for teaching specific processes or information, but it does not allow patients to share their concerns with others.

24. A: The goals of the 2100-calorie DASH diet include:
- Total fat: 27%.
- Saturated fat: 6%.
- Protein: 18%
- Carbohydrates: 55%.

Cholesterol is limited to 150 mg/day and sodium to 1500–2300 mg/day. People are encouraged to eat six to eight servings of whole grains, four to five servings of fruit and vegetables, 30 g of fiber, and 6 oz of lean meat daily as well as four to five servings of nuts, seeds, or legumes each week. Sweets and added sugars are limited to five or fewer servings each week.

25. C: Hypovolemic shock occurs when there is inadequate intravascular fluid. The loss is absolute if caused by internal shifting of fluid or external loss of fluid, such as with massive hemorrhage, thermal injuries, severe vomiting and diarrhea, or a ruptured spleen. The loss is relative if related to vasodilation, increased capillary membrane permeability from sepsis or injuries, and decreased colloidal membrane permeability from loss of sodium or from diseases, such as hypopituitarism or cirrhosis.

26. D: Videos are appropriate educational tools for illiterate patients. Material should be at an adult level, so a children's book is not appropriate, and material at a third-grade level may be too difficult for someone who cannot read. Computerized instruction almost always involves some reading for instructions, so this also may not be appropriate. Allowing patients and their families to watch a video demonstration can help them to grasp the fundamentals before they must apply them. Videos are much more effective than written materials for those with low literacy or poor English skills.

27. A: Each state has separate regulations regarding advance directives, so the patient should check state regulations and fill out two advance directives if necessary. Most require two witnesses, but some do not. Some states invalidate an advance directive if the person is pregnant. Telling family members is not adequate as these people may not be available or may be unwilling to carry out the patient's wishes. Advance directives should not be placed in a safety deposit box where access is limited.

28. C: The greatest risk of cardiovascular disease for people over 50 years of age is from a systolic blood pressure (BP) of 140 mm Hg or more rather than an increased diastolic pressure. However, increased diastolic pressure (> 80 mm Hg) is a greater risk factor for people younger than 50 years of age. Pulse pressure of 40 mm Hg is normal for people at rest. Patients should avoid caffeine, exercise, and smoking for 30 minutes before a BP examination:
- Normal BP: < 120/80 mm Hg
- Pre-hypertension: 120–130/80–90 mm Hg
- Stage 1 hypertension: 140–159/90–99 mm Hg
- Stage 2 hypertension: ≥ 160/100 mm Hg

29. B: Heparin-induced thrombocytopenia can cause a thrombosis syndrome that increases the patient's risk for thrombosis and vessel occlusion rather than hemorrhage. A platelet count below 50,000 mm3 indicates a type II reaction (rather than transient type I reaction), an autoimmune reaction to heparin; the reaction causes heparin-antibody complexes to form and a release of platelet factor 4, which, in turn, attracts heparin molecules that adhere to platelets and endothelial lining, stimulating thrombin and platelet clumping. Discontinuation of the heparin and treatment with direct thrombin inhibitors (lepirudin [Refludan], argatroban [Argatroban]) are indicated.

30. C: A nurse who delegates a task to an unlicensed assistant is accountable for patient outcomes and for supervision of the person to whom the task was delegated. The scope of nursing includes delegation of tasks to unlicensed assistive personnel, providing those personnel have adequate training and knowledge. Delegation can be used to manage the workload and to provide adequate and safe care. Delegation should be done in a manner that reduces liability by providing adequate communication.

31. C: Endothelial dysfunction is a key factor in the development of atherosclerosis and hypertension. The ability of arteries and arterioles to dilate is impaired. As the impairment of the endothelium becomes greater, the blood pressure rises. The endothelium mediates hemostasis, coagulation, fibrinolysis, cell proliferation, and cell wall inflammatory mechanisms. Endothelial dysfunction is associated with hyperlipidemia, smoking, diabetes, and lack of exercise. Research has not yet indicated if endothelial dysfunction is the direct cause of hypertension or the result.

32. C: The goal of the exercise stress test is to raise the heart rate to 80%–90% of that predicted for age and gender. Cardiac stress testing is done to determine if the coronary arteries dilate adequately during exercise. Normal coronary arteries dilate four times the resting diameter when under stress, so testing when exercising is more accurate than when resting to determine if there is

compromised blood flow. The Bruce protocol, in which the speed and grade of the treadmill increases every 3 minutes, is most common. Chemical stress tests, using adenosine or dipyridamole (Persantine), may be used for those who cannot exercise.

33. A: Janeway lesions, splinter hemorrhages, Roth's spots, petechiae on oral mucosa, and glomerulonephritis are immunological responses associated with endocarditis, which is an infection of the endothelial surface and valves of the heart caused by invasion of the tissue by a pathogen, usually after surgery, intravenous (IV) catheterization, or IV drug abuse. Other manifestations include low-grade fever, anorexia, weight loss, malaise, splenomegaly, and anemia. Patients with pericarditis present with chest pain, mild fever, increased erythrocyte sedimentation rate, white blood cell count, and friction rub. It may cause aortic valve dysfunction or mitral valve insufficiency. Patients with myocarditis may present asymptomatically or with fatigue, dyspnea, and palpitations but also with sudden cardiac arrest.

34. D: Behavior modification and compliance rates are the best determinants of the effectiveness of patient education. Patients may be satisfied, may understand, and may be able to provide a demonstration, but if they do not use what they have learned, the education has not been effective. Behavior modification involves thorough observation and measurement, identifying behavior that needs to be changed, and then planning and instituting interventions. Compliance rates should be determined by observation on multiple occasions.

35. C: Palliative care provides comfort rather than curative treatment although sometimes treatment that may be considered curative—such as radiotherapy—may be used to relieve pain or symptoms. Palliative care is meant to improve the quality of life and relieve suffering but to neither prolong life nor hasten death. Palliative care provides adequate pain management and relief of symptoms (nausea, shortness of breath). Chemotherapy, intubation, ventilation, and total parenteral nutrition are not generally considered palliative care.

36. B: Changes on an electrocardiogram (ECG), such as a U wave more than 1 mm high after the T wave, AV block, and flat or inverted T waves, are characteristic of hypokalemia. Tall peaked T waves with widening and increased amplitude of QRS and prolongation of the QT interval are characteristic of hyperkalemia. Dysrhythmias with prolonged PR and QT intervals and broad flat T waves are characteristic of hypomagnesemia. Other electrolyte imbalances are not reflected by specific ECG changes although hypermagnesemia can lead to cardiac arrest, and hypercalcemia can cause dysrhythmias (similar to those of digitalis toxicity).

37. C: The metabolic syndrome (insulin resistance) puts people at risk for the development of diabetes mellitus and cardiovascular disease; it is characterized by abdominal obesity (> 35 inches in women and > 40 inches in men), increased triglycerides (≥ 150), decreased HDL level (< 40 in men and < 50 in women), elevation of blood pressure ($\geq 130/85$ mm Hg), and increased fasting glucose (≥ 110). Other indicators include elevation of C-reactive protein, evidence of a proinflammatory state, high levels of fibrinogen, and evidence of a prothrombotic state.

38. D: Under the Nursing Code of Ethics of the American Nurses Association, autonomy and self-determination are viewed within the broader context of diverse cultures. The idea of individualism is less important in some cultures, so the nurse must respect and appreciate the patient's right to be guided by her family. Trying to convince the patient to assert herself may just lead to emotional conflict. This is not an appropriate concern for the ethics committee, as the woman is not being forced to comply with family decisions but chooses to do so.

39. D: In third-degree atrioventricular (AV) block, there are more P waves than QRS complexes with no clear relationship between them and an atrial rate two to three times the pulse rate, with an irregular PR interval. If the sinoatrial node malfunctions, the AV node fires at a lower rate, and if the AV node malfunctions, the pacemaker site in the ventricles takes over at a bradycardic rate: thus, with complete AV block, the heart still contracts but often ineffectually. The atrial P (sinus rhythm or atrial fibrillation) and the ventricular QRS (ventricular escape rhythm) are stimulated by different impulses, so there is AV dissociation. The heart cannot compensate with exertion.

40. D: Cor pulmonale (also known as pulmonary heart disease) is characterized by changes in the right ventricle because of a pulmonary disorder, such as chronic obstructive pulmonary disease. Cor pulmonale begins with endothelial dysfunction, resulting in vasoconstriction and vessel wall thickening, with sustained pulmonary hypertension, resulting in right ventricular hypertrophy in chronic cor pulmonale and right ventricular dilation in acute cor pulmonale. The end result is right-sided heart failure.

41. B: The primary reason for completing continuing education courses is to remain current in the field of nursing. It is every nurse's responsibility to be informed and aware of changes in practice. Many states require continuing education for licensure, and some institutions require continuing education for employment. Taking courses to meet requirements for salary increase is a personal reason that does not obviate professional responsibility for learning.

42. B: Cognitive changes associated with aging may result in the decline of explicit memories (facts) while implicit memories (skills) remaining intact. Older adults may have difficulty in completing complex tasks that require processing of new information and may become easily distracted and less able to focus attention. Working memory declines, making it more difficult for older adults to complete mental processes that require keeping facts in memory (e.g., calculating costs); they may also have difficulty retrieving words, such as the names of people or objects.

43. D: High doses of tacrolimus (an immunosuppressive macrolide antibiotic) can result in nephrotoxicity (similar to cyclosporine) with elevated blood urea nitrogen and creatinine. Other effects include hyperkalemia, insomnia, and malaise. Tacrolimus is often used instead of cyclosporine because it is generally well tolerated and is also effective for rescue therapy during cardiac rejection. Hypertension is an adverse effect of cyclosporine and corticosteroids. Facial dysmorphism is related to cyclosporine use. Hirsutism and acne are common adverse effects of corticosteroids.

44. C: The automatic implantable cardioverter defibrillator (AICD), used to control tachycardia and fibrillation, provides on-demand (synchronous) small electrical impulses to the atrial or ventricular myocardium to slow the heart when the pulse rate increases to a preset rate. If fibrillation occurs, a high-energy shock is delivered. It takes 5–15 seconds for the device to detect abnormalities in the pulse rate, and more than one shock may be required, so fainting may occur. Some devices can function as both a pacemaker and an ICD for patients with episodes of both bradycardia and tachycardia.

45. B: Syncope associated with exertional exercise is a manifestation of aortic stenosis. With aortic stenosis, exercise results in reduced cerebral blood flow because of peripheral dilation without increased cardiac output. In some cases, the hypotension related to syncope may result in ventricular fibrillation or ventricular tachycardia and death. Syncope, a sudden brief loss of consciousness, may also be caused by carotid sinus sensitivity (vasovagal syndrome), dysrhythmias

(tachycardia, bradycardia). In older adults, syncope often occurs with postural hypotension, sometimes related to medications or alcohol.

46. D: Symptoms typical of a dissecting descending aortic aneurysm include severe, intense, knife-like pain posteriorly between the scapulae and nausea and vomiting. In addition, patients may be cold and clammy. Dissection of the ascending thoracic aorta results in similar symptoms, but the pain is in the anterior chest. Pain with dissection does not generally increase in intensity, as it is severe at onset when the tearing occurs. Peripheral arteries may be involved, which can cause numbness, tingling, and evidence of vascular insufficiency in the affected limb.

47. A: The most likely cause of nausea, vomiting, and tachycardia is digitalis toxicity. Most cases of digitalis toxicity can be traced to drug interactions. In this case, both furosemide (Lasix) and tetracycline can cause digitalis toxicity when taken with digoxin (Lanoxin). Digoxin levels should be monitored to ensure that therapeutic levels (0.5–2.0 ng/mL) are maintained. Early signs of digitalis toxicity include fatigue, lethargy, depression, nausea, and vomiting. Sudden changes in heart rhythm, atrioventricular or sinoatrial block, new ventricular dysrhythmias, or tachycardia may occur. Digoxin immune FAB (Digibind) may be given to inactivate digoxin, if necessary.

48. B: While the international normalized ratio (INR) is individualized, depending on baseline readings, a normal INR is usually about 1. Patients receiving warfarin (Coumadin) for atrial fibrillation are usually maintained at an INR of 2–3. The INR for prophylaxis for deep vein thrombosis is 1.5–2 and for pulmonary emboli and mechanical heart values is 3–4. The higher the number, the greater the anticoagulation effect, so a level over 4 may put the patient at risk for hemorrhage.

49. B: Hiccups are an indication that a pacemaker lead has become dislodged and is causing phrenic nerve or muscle stimulation. Other complications include infection; bleeding; hematoma; puncture of the subclavian vein or internal mammary artery, causing hemothorax; irritation of the ventricular wall by the endocardial electrode, causing ectopic beats or tachycardia; malfunction or perforation of the myocardium from dislodgement of a transvenous lead; and cardiac tamponade, resulting from removal of epicardial wires used for temporary pacing.

50. A: Contraindications to thrombolytic therapy include an aortic aneurysm, hemorrhagic stroke, recent surgery, or bleeding. While ideally, thrombolytic therapy should be administered within 90 minutes of the onset of symptoms, some thrombolytics (tenecteplase) may be given within 6 hours and some within 12 hours. A history of any type of stroke within 2 months precludes thrombolytic therapy. Severe hypertension (> 210/130 mm Hg) that is uncontrolled by medications or that occurs with retinal-vascular disease is also a contraindication. Relative contraindications include age over 75 years, pregnancy, pericarditis, and endocarditis.

51. A: Digoxin should be withheld for a minimum of 48 hours before cardioversion. Anticoagulation, usually with warfarin (Coumadin), is prescribed at least 3 weeks before cardioversion to prevent emboli. Sometimes drug therapy is used in conjunction with cardioversion: for example, antiarrhythmics (Cardizem, Cordarone) may be given before the procedure to slow the heart rate. Insulin should not be withheld for 48 hours, but the patient must fast before cardioversion and may be asked to delay the insulin injection on the morning of the procedure.

52. B: Symptoms that do not occur with rest but with physical exertion, limitations with the activities of daily living (ADLs), and slight pulmonary edema are typical of class II heart failure:

- Class I: Asymptomatic during normal activities and no pulmonary congestion or peripheral hypotension. Prognosis is good.
- Class II: No symptoms at rest but symptoms appear with physical exertion, limiting ADLs. Slight pulmonary edema may be evident. Prognosis is good.
- Class III: Obvious limitations of ADLs and discomfort on any exertion. Prognosis is fair.
- Class IV: Symptoms are present. Prognosis is poor.

53. C: Balloon valvuloplasty is the treatment of choice for significant pulmonary stenosis, resulting in a narrowing of the valve or the area above or below the valve. Closed valvotomy (without cardiopulmonary bypass) is no longer done, but open valvotomy with cardiopulmonary bypass may be needed if the balloon valvuloplasty is unsuccessful and symptoms recur. Valve replacement with a homograft valve is sometimes required, usually as an intervention after previous failure to correct the disorder.

54. B: Dobutamine is used to treat low cardiac output after cardiac surgery. Nitroprusside decreases blood pressure and afterload. Dopamine is used to treat shock and hypotension for patients who require volume resuscitation. Isoproterenol is used to stimulate the heart in patients with severe bradycardia. Other drugs include nitroglycerine, which is used to prevent spasm in arterial grafts and to reduce preload and afterload, and epinephrine, which is used to treat low cardiac output related to shock. Milrinone is also used to treat low cardiac output. Phenylephrine, norepinephrine, and vasopressin increase systemic vascular resistance and blood pressure and are used to treat shock.

55. B: The best reading level for a group of adults from an affluent area is grade six. The average American reads effectively at the sixth- to eighth-grade level, regardless of education achieved, and research shows that even people with high reading skills learn health information most effectively when the material is presented at the sixth- to eighth-grade reading level. Grade-three reading level is too simple for native English speakers but might be appropriate for an immigrant population with limited English.

56. C: While clinical symptoms, blood tests, and electrocardiogram monitoring are all important, biopsy remains the primary tool to diagnose acute rejection after cardiac transplantation. Acute rejection can occur with few clinical symptoms even when using cyclosporine or tacrolimus to prevent rejection, so routine biopsies are done for the first 3 months after surgery. The first biopsy is generally done in 2 weeks and then once weekly for the first month; biopsies are then tapered to every other week and then once monthly after the initial 3-month period and then every 4–12 months, depending on the institutional protocol.

57. D: The apex beat (pulsation) can be observed in about half of patients at about the fifth intercostal space along the left mid-clavicular line. The pulsation is caused by thrusting of the left ventricle. The pulsation is easy to observe in patients with thin chest walls. If the heart is enlarged, the pulsation may be observed at the second intercostal space. Aiming a flashlight at a tangential angle across the chest can help cast a shadow that facilitates observation. If no pulsation is evident, the apex beat can be palpated in the same area.

58. B: Thiazide diuretics are the first-line drugs used to treat stage I hypertension. Stage II hypertension is usually treated with a two-drug combination of a thiazide diuretic with an angiotensin-converting enzyme (ACE) inhibitor, ARB, beta-blocker, or calcium-channel blocker. If

there are compelling indications, such as heart failure, post–myocardial infarction, coronary disease risk, diabetes, or chronic kidney disease, then a wide range of drugs may be needed, including diuretics, beta-blockers, ACE inhibitors, ARB, calcium channel blockers, or aldosterone antagonists, depending on the condition.

59. B: Pneumococcal polysaccharide-23 (single dose), influenza (annual), and herpes zoster (single dose) immunizations are recommended for all adults 60–65 years of age and older. Hepatitis B is recommended for older adults with end-stage renal disease (including those receiving dialysis), chronic liver disease, or HIV/AIDS and those in correctional facilities or substance abuse facilities. Hepatitis A is recommended for those at risk because of lifestyle (e.g., men who have sex with men, substance abusers) or medical conditions (e.g., liver disease). International travelers may receive hepatitis A and B vaccines, depending on the destination. There is no hepatitis C vaccine.

60. D: Synthroid 0.88 mg PO daily at 0700 is the correct medication order because of the following: (1) the medication is spelled out; (2) the decimal has a leading zero; (3) PO is clearly written; and (4) "daily" is used instead of "qd," which can be misinterpreted as qid if the nurse uses periods or does not write clearly. Additionally, a 24-hour time designation is used. "Maalox 30 cc" should be "Maalox 30 mL" because "cc" may be misread as "U" for unit. Instead of "qhs," which can be misread as "qhr," "nightly" should be used. "Lasix 40.0 mg" should be "Lasix 40 mg" because the trailing zero may cause someone to read the order as "400 mg." "MS" could be misread as magnesium sulfate.

61. A: Threatening to force a patient to undergo a treatment is a form of coercion. Nurses can easily intimidate patients into having procedures or treatments they do not want. Regardless of age, patients have the right to choose and refuse treatment. Forcing patients to do something against their will can be considered as borderline abuse. Furthermore, this can sometimes degenerate into actual abuse if physical coercion is involved. If patients are cognitively impaired, other family members may be designated to make decisions, but every effort should be made to gain the patient's cooperation.

62. D: Sexual dysfunction, including impotence, is quite common after heart transplant surgery and most often relates to antihypertensive drugs. Hypertension is a chronic problem after a heart transplant, especially with some immunosuppressive drugs, such as cyclosporine, and patients may require two or more drugs to control blood pressure. The patient should be given assistance or counseling to deal with sexual dysfunction, both before and after surgery. In some cases, alternative drugs may be used.

63. B: Sinus tachycardia is characterized by a pulse of 100 bpm and above. The rapid pulse decreases diastolic filling time and reduces cardiac output with resultant hypotension and pulmonary edema. Bradycardia is characterized by a pulse of 60 bpm and less. Sinus arrhythmia is characterized by cyclic changes in pulse during respiration and is common in children and young adults; however, it may also occur with vagal stimulation from suctioning, vomiting, or defecating. Premature atrial contractions are essentially extra beats caused by an electrical impulse to the atrium before the sinus node impulse, resulting in an irregular pulse.

64. B: Caffeinated beverages (e.g., tea, coffee, hot chocolate) may increase the effects of warfarin (Coumadin). Alcohol intake should be limited to no more than three drinks daily. A daily multivitamin should not affect warfarin, but some herbal medications can affect clotting time. Milk products should not affect warfarin, but foods that are high in vitamin K (e.g., broccoli; green leafy vegetables, such as kale, turnip greens, beet greens; cauliflower; legumes; soybean oil; canola oil) may affect the medication and should be limited.

65. D: Using transesophageal Doppler ultrasonography to measure cardiac output, a short waveform with a rounded apex may indicate left ventricular failure. Decreased preload (hypovolemia) is indicated by a pointed wave with a narrow base. As preload increases with fluid administration, the base widens. Increased systemic vascular resistance (high afterload) is indicated by a pointed short waveform with a narrow base, with both height and base increasing with vasodilation, which reduces afterload.

66. A: Troponin levels (cTnT and cTnI) should be measured 8–12 hours after the onset of symptoms. Earlier testing may result in false negatives. Levels rise within 3–4 hours and peak at 4–24 hours but do not return to normal for 1–3 weeks. Myoglobin (MB) begins to rise within 1–3 hours and peaks at 4–12 hours, returning to normal usually in about 12– 36 hours, but it is nonspecific for cardiac damage. Measurement of low-density lipoprotein levels is not usually ordered because troponin tests are more specific. Creatinine kinase (CK) levels rise in 3–6 hours, peaking at 24–36 hours, and return to normal in 3 days. The more specific CK-MB (found only in cardiac cells) increases at 4–8 hours and peaks at 12–24 hours, returning to normal in 3–4 days. CK/CK-MB should be tested on admission and in 24 hours.

67. C: A cardiac care center provides tertiary care, as it is a specialized center with a variety of programs to meet the needs of the cardiac patient. Primary care is usually provided by the first physician the patient sees, such as a general practitioner or an internist. Secondary care is provided by a specialist, such as a cardiologist, to whom the patient is referred. Quaternary care is provided by those who are highly specialized in very specific and limited areas of medicine or involved in special experimental programs.

68. D: The absolute indication for stopping an exercise test is a decrease in blood pressure of 10 mm Hg or more from baseline despite increased workload with evidence of ischemia. The other choices are relative indications and depend upon the patient's general condition and the assessment of the observer. Other absolute indications include moderate-to-severe angina, cyanosis or pallor, nervous system symptoms (dizziness, ataxia), sustained ventricular tachycardia, ST segment elevation of 10 mm or more in leads without Q waves (other than V1 or VR), and the patient's wish to stop the test.

69. C: Initially, a physician must certify that a patient who is eligible for Medicare A is terminal with a life expectancy 6 months or less (two 90-day periods), but if the patient remains alive, the physician can extend coverage by authorizing care every 60 days. The goal is to maintain the patient in the home environment with home health aides, homemakers, durable goods, pain management, case management, counseling, and social worker assistance. Routine intermittent home care must comprise 80% of the total care with in-home continuous care and in-patient hospice care available for short periods.

70. A: The patient described in the question is demonstrating symptoms of post-pump delirium psychosis (PPD). Patients may exhibit symptoms ranging from memory loss, alterations of personality, and apathy to clinical psychosis. Risk factors include increasing age, poor cardiac status preoperatively or postoperatively, co-morbidities, hypoxia, sepsis, CPB for more than 2–3 hours, and valvular surgery. Postoperative infection, sleep deprivation, and medications can also be factors. Usually, PPD occurs 48 hours or less postoperatively and lasts 2–5 days.

71. D: The treatment goal would be to lower total cholesterol to 200 or less and LDL to 130 or less and raise the HDL to 40 or more. Treatment usually includes an increase in exercise, such as daily

walking; dietary modifications, such as a decrease in saturated fats; and anti-lipid medications, such as the statins. Normal cholesterol ranges include:
- Total cholesterol: 120–200 mg/dL; borderline high is 200–239 mg/dL.
- Triglyceride: 0–150 mg/dL; borderline high is 150–199 mg/dL.
- HDL: 40–70 mg/dL. This is the "good" cholesterol.
- LDL: 50–129 mg dL; borderline high is 130–159 mg/dL. This is the "bad" cholesterol.

72. D: Atrial arrhythmias, including fibrillation, flutter, and tachycardia, are very common after cardiac surgery, occurring in over half of patients with valvular surgery. Arrhythmias occur usually in the first 2–3 postoperative days and are often transient but may recur. Arrhythmias are usually related to surgical manipulation. Treatment includes digoxin, β-blockers, calcium channel blockers, and amiodarone (often given preoperatively for 7 days to reduce the incidence of postoperative arrhythmias. Electrical cardioversion may be indicated after 24 hours if sinus rhythm remains abnormal.

73. B: The self-monitoring skill that is most essential for a patient with heart failure is daily weight as increased weight can indicate fluid overload and edema before it becomes evident (usually after about 5 L of retained fluid or a 10-pound weight increase). Patients may also need to monitor sodium intake. Self-management skills require an initial discussion of needs and presentation of scenarios to help the patient determine appropriate responses and practice self-management.

74. D: While home intravenous (IV) antibiotic therapy is appropriate for many patients, the patient in the question is frail and elderly and not a good candidate for home treatment, so transferring the patient to an extended care facility is probably the best option. Extended treatment in an acute hospital is probably not necessary since the patient's condition is stable. A few patients may be able to self-administer IV medications if they have adequate instruction and family or other support, but the patient in the question is frail, elderly, and lives alone.

75. B: If a patient asks for pain medication after 4 hours when it has been prescribed for every 6 hours, the pain control is not adequate to prevent breakthrough pain, and the routine medication may need to be increased in dosage or frequency. While tolerance to pain varies, pain is what the individual perceives it to be, and distraction is rarely effective in relieving severe pain. Since breakthrough pain commonly occurs, this most likely reflects inadequate control. Patients have a right to pain control, and almost all pain can be controlled with proper analgesia.

76. C: Adequate perfusion requires a mean arterial pressure (MAP) of >60 mm Hg because ischemia of the internal organs will occur if the MAP falls below this level for an extended period. MAP is the average pressure within the arterial system. Because the duration of diastole is about twice that of systole, the formula to calculate the MAP is systolic BP plus 2 times the diastolic BP divided by 3:
- MAP = systolic + 2(diastolic) / 3

77. A: Patients with peripheral arterial disease and aspirin intolerance should be prescribed clopidogrel. Antiplatelet therapy is essential to reducing the risk of cardiovascular disease events, but heparin and warfarin are not recommended as preventive medications. Clopidogrel requires activation by CYP2C19, and tests are available to determine if patients have normal CYP2C19 function. NSAIDs should be avoided with clopidogrel as the combination may increase risk of GI bleeding. Platelet aggregation does not return to normal after discontinuation of clopidogrel for about 5 days.

78. B: According to the AHA/ACC Guideline for the Management of Patients with Non–ST-Elevation Acute Coronary Syndromes, for early risk stratification of patients presenting in the ED with chest pain or other symptoms indicative of acute coronary syndrome, a 12-lead ECG should be done within 10 minutes of arrival at the ED. If this initial ECG is negative and the symptoms persist, then repeat 12-lead ECGs should be done every 15 to 30 minutes for the first hour. Additionally, serial troponin I or T (with contemporary assay) should be completed every 3 to 6 hours.

79. D: For a patient receiving a calcium channel blocker (CCB), such as diltiazem, calcium supplements may reduce effectiveness. CCBs are class IV antidysrhythmics, primarily used for SVT but also frequently used to reduce hypertension and to relieve angina. CCBs block the inward flow of calcium ions into the calcium channels in the heart's conduction tissue. Patients must be advised to avoid calcium supplements and calcium-based antacids, such as Tums. Vitamin D supplements may also interfere with absorption.

80. B: If a patient preparing for discharge has been advised to make multiple lifestyle changes in relation to diet, medications, habits, and exercise but the patient is upset about the changes and states repeatedly that the physician is expecting too much, the best response is: "It's difficult to make all of these changes." When a patient is venting and upset, often the best response is to be empathetic, showing that the person's concerns are understood and appreciated. Giving advice to a patient when they are in a resistant frame of mind could merely further resistance.

81. C: If a patient has a base normal control prothrombin time (PT) of 10 seconds, the maximum target PT with warfarin therapy is usually 25 seconds. The normal time is 10 to 14 seconds, and with warfarin, the PT should be 1 to 2.5 times the base control value. Prothrombin (factor II) is produced by the liver, and the PT can be used to evaluate extrinsic coagulation factors (V, VII, and X), fibrinogen, and prothrombin, and may be used to monitor oral anticoagulation therapy as well.

82. D: If a patient is taking a bile acid sequestrant, such as cholestyramine, to lower LDL, a patient should wait 4 to 6 hours after taking the drug before taking other medications because pronounced drug interactions with multiple drugs may occur. Alternately, other medications may be taken 1 to 2 hours prior to the bile acid sequestrant. Cholestyramine especially poses a problem because it may be prescribed twice daily. The drug is administered in powdered form and must be mixed with liquid and should be taken with a meal.

83. A: While all antiplatelet drugs pose some risk of bleeding, ASA poses the least risk but can result in gastrointestinal bleeding, a risk somewhat mitigated by taking ASA with food or using enteric-coated formulations. Clopidogrel poses a greater risk of gastrointestinal bleeding and intracranial bleeding. The drugs with the greatest risk are the intravenous glycoprotein IIb/IIIa inhibitors, including abciximab, tirofiban, and eptifibatide. All patients should be assessed for risk of bleeding before administration of antiplatelet drugs.

84. B: ST-elevation MI (STEMI) is an indication for thrombolytic therapy as is new left bundle branch block (LBBB). When a vessel is completely occluded for an extended period of time, the thrombin and fibrin become increasingly concentrated, and a STEMI usually develops, characterized by both ST-elevation and T-wave inversion. In about 90% of STEMIs, pathologic Q waves develop. Thrombolysis should ideally be carried out within 30 minutes to be most effective; however, there is benefit within the first 12 hours and in some cases up to 24 hours.

85. C: If a patient has undergone thrombolysis per accelerated infusion of alteplase 100 mg (maximum dose) for an acute myocardial infarction and shows 20% reduction in ST elevation after

90 minutes, the cardiac/vascular nurse anticipates angiography and rescue PCI because ST elevation should decrease by at least 50% within this timeframe. Fibrinolytic therapy is often administered instead of PCI if PCI is not available at the hospital or within an acceptable period of time, so arrangements should be made to transfer the patient to another facility if necessary.

86. A: The patient that may be an acceptable candidate for catheter-directed thrombolysis (CDT) for peripheral arterial occlusion is the one with non–life-threatening limb ischemia of 12 days. Thrombolysis may be indicated (depending on risk factors) if the ischemia has been present for fewer than 14 days. CDT is not indicated for limb-threatening ischemia because lysis of the occluding clot may take between 6 and 72 hours. These patients should undergo emergent embolectomy.

87. B: On the ECG recording, a normal sinus rhythm is characterized by a PR interval of 0.12 to 0.2 seconds. Normal rate is 60 to 100 bpm, with rates below 60 considered bradycardic and rates above 100 considered tachycardic. The PR interval usually remains normal with both sinus bradycardia and sinus tachycardia. P waves should precede each QRS complex and should be consistent in shape. The duration of the QRS complex should range from 0.04 to 0.1 seconds.

88. D: If a patient exhibits a ventricular rate of 150 bpm, the most likely cause of dysrhythmia is atrial flutter. While the atrial rate with atrial flutter may vary from 250 to 450 bpm, around 300 bpm is the most common. The AV node generally blocks about 50% of the atrial impulses in order to prevent too rapid contractions, resulting in a ventricular rate of about 150 bpm. This would be categorized as atrial flutter with 2:1 conduction.

89. C: After administering sublingual nitroglycerin to a patient for angina, the cardiac/vascular nurse should expect a reduction in pain within 3 to 4 minutes. If no relief occurs, the drug may be administered every 5 minutes to a total of 3 doses. Sublingual or buccal preparations are usually given for acute angina because they are absorbed into the bloodstream quickly but IV nitroglycerine may be given in the hospital.

90. B: Beta-blockers are generally contraindicated for patients with a history of asthma and COPD because they may cause bronchospasm and may block the effects of bronchodilators. Some patients may develop cough-variant asthma as an adverse effect of beta-blockers. Other contraindications include severe sinus bradycardia and second- or third-degree heart block because beta-blockers slow conduction. Beta-blockers should also be avoided in the presence of cardiogenic shock or acute heart failure. Beta-blockers may interact with a number of different medications.

91. C: *Rest potentiation* of the heart refers to a pause resulting in a stronger ensuing contraction, assuming an intact organism. After an extra beat, the ensuing contraction is stronger, an effect referred to as *postextrasystolic potentiation*. The force of contraction is influenced by the heart rate, a phenomenon referred to as the Treppe or staircase phenomenon, so the faster the rate of stimulation, the stronger the contraction, and the slower the rate of stimulation, the weaker the contraction.

92. D: In order to modify risk of cardiovascular disease for patients with peripheral arterial disease (PAD), the primary lifestyle change should be smoking cessation. Patients are at high risk for MI, cerebrovascular accident (CVA), and cardiovascular disease–associated death. Smoking cessation is especially important because of the vasoconstrictive and inflammatory properties of tobacco. Because of the addictiveness of tobacco products, patients may require comprehensive assistance, such as medications, education, and support groups, in order to succeed in smoking cessation.

93. C: At a heart rate of >180 bpm, diastolic filling is so reduced that stroke volume is diminished and coronary ischemia occurs. This may occur at much lower rates if heart failure or cardiac pathology is present. Generally, an increased heart rate results in increased cardiac output and the strength of contraction increases with the heart rate. Normal cardiac output is 5.5 L/min (70 kg male patient) but can increase to 18 L/min with exercise in order to meet body demands.

94. A: An increased risk factor for coronary artery disease is a sister who developed the disorder at age 63. Family history of coronary artery disease is a risk factor for developing the disease. Risk increases if a father or brother developed the disease before age 55 or if a mother or sister developed it before age 65, as onset is usually later in females than males. Other risk factors include advanced age, male gender, smoking, hypertension, hyperlipidemia, obesity, lack of exercise, and stress.

95. D: If deviation is present when assessing best gaze, then the oculocephalic maneuver can be carried out to determine if one or both eyes has reflexive movement. The cardiac/vascular nurse must grasp the patient's head on each side and turn it quickly side to side while observing the eyes. A normal response is for the eyes to deviate to the opposite side the head is turned to and then to return toward midline. If there is no movement, then the best gaze is scored as 2 (out of a 0 to 2 range) because the oculocephalic maneuver did not overcome the deviation.

96. B: When assessing the adequacy of a patient's diet, the cardiac/vascular nurse recognized that, for an elderly adult weighing 70 kg (154 lb), the average caloric requirement per day is about 1750 calories. On average, elderly adults require approximately 25 calories per kg of body weight, while a healthy younger adult requires 30 calories per kg. Obese adults who need to lose weight should have an intake ranging from 20 to 25 calories per kg.

97. D: If a patient remains passive, asks no questions, and shows no interest during instruction, then the patient is not exhibiting readiness to learn; the patient is not engaged in any way. If a patient indicates confusion about the medication regimen, this indicates the patient is seeking more information. Patients who are not visual learners or who lack literacy skills may avoid written materials, and if a patient turns on the TV to watch a football game when the nurse is instructing, this may simply indicate that the nurse has not chosen a good time for instruction.

98. C: According to the AHA/ACC Guideline for the Management of Patients With Non–ST-Elevation Acute Coronary Syndromes, patients presenting in the ED with chest pain or symptoms indicative of acute coronary syndrome should receive oxygen with oxygen saturation <90%, respiratory distress, or indications of hypoxemia. Patients should also receive sublingual nitrates every 5 minutes for up to 3 doses, and IV morphine to control pain. NSAIDs other than aspirin should be avoided. Beta-blockers should be started within 24 hours.

99. A: According to the Protection Motivation Theory, action to bring about change is precipitated by a threat, such as hypertension that threatens health. This threat serves as a stimulus for protection motivation. The patient cognitively assesses sources of information (internal and external) and the extent of a threat and develops coping mechanisms that include action to bring about change. According to this theory, protective coping strategies develop based on the patient's perception of the severity of the threat, the probability the threat will occur, the ability of preventive measures to allay the threat, and the degree of self-efficacy.

100. D: In assessing health literacy, the cardiac/vascular nurse should expect that the average reading level of the US population is ≤8th grade. However, almost half of American lack the basic skills in reading and comprehension needed to carry out every day literacy tasks, and many adults read at levels that are 2 to 4 grade levels below their level of completed formal education. Thus, the cardiac/vascular nurse must assess each patient individually and cannot make assumptions based on formal education history alone.

101. C: When administering the Tinetti Gait and Balance Instrument to an older adult, the balance assessment begins with the patient sitting in an armless chair. The patient is assessed for the ability to lean or slide in the chair, arise, stand immediately without stagger, remain standing, stand with feet close together while pushed, stand with eyes closed, turn full circle, and then sit down. The higher the score, the better the performance. Sixteen is the total maximum number of points for the balance portion of the assessment.

102. B: If an older adult with aortic stenosis undergoes percutaneous balloon valvuloplasty, restenosis often occurs within 1 to 2 years. Balloon valvuloplasty is most commonly used for patients who are not candidates for open surgical procedures, but patients must be monitored closely following the valvuloplasty. Complications may include bleeding/hematoma at insertion site (usually the femoral vein), damage to valve leaflets (rare), worsening of condition, embolism (rare), and cardiac abnormalities, such as arrhythmias or ischemia.

103. A: If a patient with hypertension and diabetes mellitus was a heavy smoker for 40 years before suffering a myocardial infarction, but she has continued to smoke even though she states, "I know I should quit," the best response is, "Tell me about that." This is a patient-centered response that encourages the patient to reflect and respects the patient's autonomy. It is clear the patient knows the importance of smoking cessation, so repeating advice to quit or making further suggestions may only engender a negative response—reasons why the patient cannot quit.

104. D: The educational program that might best be conducted as a webinar is the interactive discussion about new techniques in cardiac rehabilitation because the key feature of a webinar is interactivity, so participation is synchronous (in real time). Orientation program and online courses are generally set up as asynchronous so that they can be accessed at any time. A webinar is generally not needed for a video series because videos are not, by nature, interactive.

105. B: If a cardiac/vascular nurse working in a semi-rural area proposes a mobile clinic to better monitor, screen, and counsel patients who often cannot or do not seek medical care, the most likely impediment is cost-effectiveness. While a mobile unit may seem an ideal solution, both the initial cost and ongoing costs are high, and demonstrating cost savings, such as fewer rehospitalizations, can be difficult, especially if the patient population is low. Mobile clinics are often funded by grants to target specific populations.

106. C: According to the Seventh Report of the Joint National Committee on Prevention, Detection, Evaluation, and Treatment of High Blood Pressure, systolic blood pressure is a greater cardiovascular risk factor than diastolic blood pressure after age 50. Before age 50, diastolic hypertension with or without systolic hypertension is the most common but this changes at about age 50 when the diastolic blood pressure stabilizes. However, the systolic blood pressure continues to rise, so controlling systolic blood pressure in patients older than 50 is essential to reducing risk of cardiovascular events/mortality and stroke.

107. A: A low score on the Care Transitions Measure (CTM-15) is predictive of rehospitalization or return to the emergency department. The CTM-15 has 15 statements that patients score using a Likert scale (strongly disagree, disagree, agree, strongly disagree, or don't know/don't remember, not applicable). Statements focus on in-hospital care, discharge planning, follow-up care, and patient medications, and ask patients to rate their understanding, satisfaction, and confidence in their own ability to manage health care.

108. B: According to the Healthy People 2020 initiatives, a 55-year-old diabetic male patient with leg pain should be screened for peripheral arterial disease with the ankle-brachial index (ABI) because the patient is symptomatic (leg pain) and has a disorder that increases risk (diabetes). General screening of the adult population is not recommended in the absence of symptoms because evidence-based research shows no advantage, and false positives may result in increased cost and increased patient anxiety.

109. D: According to the ACCF/AHA Guideline for the Management of ST-Elevation Myocardial Infarction, the pain medication of choice for patients with STEMI and acute pulmonary edema is morphine sulfate, which should relieve the pain, respiratory distress, and associated anxiety. Atropine can be administered if necessary if the morphine induces bradycardia, and naloxone may be necessary if excessive sedation occurs. Both NSAIDs and COX-2 inhibitors increase risk of severe complications, such as reinfarction and death, and should be avoided.

110. A: If a patient with stage 2 Alzheimer disease and coronary artery disease can function fairly well in her home environment but has increasing short-term memory loss and often forgets to take her medications (even though her daughter calls to remind her), the best solution is likely providing an electronic medication dispenser. Some dispensers require filling only once a week or once a month and have various methods to remind patients to take medications, including beeps, alarms, and verbal messages.

111. C: A normal value for the activated partial thromboplastin time (aPTT) is 21 to 35 seconds (may vary somewhat according to reference lab). This test is commonly used to monitor heparin dosage. The aPTT is prolonged with deficiencies of clotting factors, vitamin K deficiency, and administration of unfractionated heparin or direct thrombin inhibitors (hirudin, dabigatran, and argatroban). Warfarin usually only prolongs the aPTT by a few seconds, although with overdose the prolongation may be pronounced.

112. B: According to the ACC/AHA Guideline on the Treatment of Blood Cholesterol to Reduce Atherosclerotic Cardiovascular Risk in Adults, the goal for LDL cholesterol reduction with treatment with high-intensity statin is ≥50% from baseline. For patients treated with moderate-intensity statins, the goal is 30% to <50% reduction from baseline. If baseline is not known, then reduction should generally be <100 mg/dL. Patients should be monitored every 3 to 12 months to assess adherence and lifestyle changes.

113. D: If a patient with mechanical prosthetic heart value is on warfarin therapy and has an INR of 3.2, this probably indicates a normal INR for this patient because patients with mechanical prosthetic heart valves are usually maintained at an INR of 2.5 to 3.5. This is higher than for patients without prosthetic valves because these patients are usually maintained at 2 to 3. The INR is not used for screening purposes but is routinely used to monitor oral anticoagulation therapy.

114. A: When monitoring a patient's 12-lead ECG, the cardiac/vascular nurse would expect a lead facing an injured area of the heart to show ST-segment elevation and those leads facing away from

the injured area to show ST-segment depression. Abnormal variations in the ST segment include elevation of more than 1 mm above the baseline and depression of more than 0.5 mm below the baseline. T-waves may vary for many reasons; very tall or inverted T-waves may indicate myocardial ischemia. Abnormal Q waves commonly occur with myocardial necrosis.

115. B: If C-reactive protein (CRP) is >3 mg/L (especially >10 mg/L) in a patient with normal (or abnormal) lipid values, this may indicate increased risk of cardiovascular and peripheral arterial disease. CRP is a glycoprotein produced in the liver in response to acute inflammation and serves as a nonspecific marker for inflammation. CRP is often ordered along with an ESR. Lowest risk is at <1 mg/L, and moderate risk is at 1 to 3 mg/L. CRP may better predict risk of cardiac disease in females than LDL levels.

116. C: When baroreceptors in the aortic arch and carotid arteries sense volume overload or increased pressure in the arteries, the usual response is decreased heart rate and vasodilation. When pressure in the arterial system stimulates these receptors, information is transmitted to the vasomotor center of the brainstem, and this inhibits the sympathetic nervous system so that the parasympathetic nervous system causes the heart rate to temporarily decrease and vasodilation to occur. Decreased pressure in the arteries causes the opposite effect, increased heart rate and vasoconstriction.

117. D: A common age-associated change in the cardiovascular system is decreased number of pacemaker cells in the SA node to the point that patients older than 75 years may have only one-tenth the normal number of pacemaker cells. While this number of cells may be adequate, the decrease of pacemaker cells increases the risk of sinus dysrhythmias. Other changes include decreased cardiac reserve, decreased cardiac output, decreased stroke volume, and decreased contractility of the heart because of increased collagen and decreased elastin in the heart muscle.

118. A: On the DASH diet, a patient may have ≤5 servings of sweets and added sugars per week. One serving is equal to 1 tablespoon of sugar, jelly, or jam, one-half cup of sorbet or gelatin, or 1 cup of lemonade. Patients should have 4 to 5 servings per week of nuts, seeds, and legumes, as well as 7 to 8 servings/day of whole grains, 4 to 5 servings/day of vegetables and fruits, 2 to 3 servings/day of low-fat or fat-free dairy foods, 2 or fewer servings/day of lean meats, poultry, and fish, and 2 to 3 servings/day of fats and oils.

119. B: Mended Hearts is a national support organization for patients with cardiovascular disease and their families/caregivers. Programs include the visiting program in which volunteers visit patients in the hospital and make contact per the Internet and telephone. Some chapters have regular meetings that provide emotional and educational support. Mended Hearts publishes *Heartbeat* magazine for members as well as a variety of other educational resources, including newsletters and online information, such as information about clinical trials.

120. C: Exclusion criteria for therapeutic hypothermia for a patient who experienced sudden cardiac arrest and resuscitation is major surgery within the previous 2 weeks because of increased risk of bleeding and infection associated with hypothermia. Other factors that may increase risk to the patient during hypothermia include preexisting bleeding diathesis (although not thrombolysis) and systemic infections. Additionally, therapeutic hypothermia is usually avoided in patients with a DNR order. Various cooling methods can be used to reduce the body temperature to 32°C to 34°C over a 3- to 4-hour period.

121. D: If the cardiac/vascular nurse is serving as a preceptor for a nursing student and feels that the student lacks essential skills, the cardiac/vascular nurse should first meet with the student to outline concerns. While the student may, in fact, lack essential skills, the student may also feel stressed or intimidated and afraid to demonstrate skills effectively. The cardiac/vascular nurse should avoid using an accusatory or critical approach but should focus on what the nurse has observed.

122. B: The primary treatment focus for patients with dilated cardiomyopathy is controlling heart failure by improving myocardial contractility and decreasing afterload. Patients may take a variety of medications, including diuretics, nitrates, ACE inhibitors, beta-blockers, antidysrhythmics, and anticoagulants. However, dilated cardiomyopathy does not readily respond to medications, and patients may experience repeated episodes of heart failure. Some patients may receive a ventricular-assist device, especially while awaiting transplant.

123. A: If a physician with whom the staff is very friendly is admitted to the cardiac unit with a myocardial infarction, and a number of nurses, who are not assigned to the patient, review his laboratory findings by reading over the shoulder of the physician's assigned nurse (shoulder surfing), this is primarily a HIPAA violation and is a major violation of privacy, as well as an unprofessional activity. Both the nurse accessing the patient's file and those looking over the nurse's shoulder are in violation of the law and may be disciplined or fired.

124. B: If a patient experienced a severe adverse reaction to a drug while left unattended because of suboptimal staffing, this problem will likely be referred to risk management, which will determine liability issues and further courses of action. Depending on policies in place in the organization, the patient/family may or may not be apprised of the staffing problem or may not understand the implications. Incident reports are generally not included in the patient's record but are filed separately.

125. C: Using the SBAR communication technique, the cardiac/vascular nurse will begin the report about Ms. Jones to the physician in this order:
- (S) Situation: "Ms. Jones has increasing shortness of breath, cough, and chest pain for the past hour."
- (B) Background: "Ms. Jones recently had cardiac catheterization and angioplasty, and Ms. Jones has a pulse of 130, BP 140/60, and respirations of 32 per minute."
- Assessment: "I believe that Ms. Jones may have a pulmonary embolism or cardiac event."
- (R) Recommendation: "I recommend immediate oxygen and physician examination."

126. A: As a patient advocate, any time a cardiac/vascular nurse observes a patient being mistreated, the best initial response is to immediately intervene, such as by stepping in and offering to assist the patient. The cardiac/vascular nurse should avoid reprimanding the other nurse in the patient's presence but may confront the nurse later and/or report the nurse's behavior to a supervisor. There is no circumstance in which being verbally abusive to a patient is acceptable.

127. C: If a patient is awaiting surgical intervention for a dissecting aortic aneurysm, prior to surgery, the patient's systolic blood pressure should be maintained at 110 to 120 to ensure adequate perfusion of the patient's organs while preventing undue pressure on the dissection. The patient should receive medications to reduce pain and anxiety as these symptoms may increase the blood pressure. Antihypertensive agents should be administered under close supervision with constant monitoring of ECG recordings and vital signs.

128. D: If the cardiac/vascular nurse proposes forming an interdisciplinary team to work on process improvement, the best members are likely to be those who have needed knowledge/skills. While the temptation is often to form a team of friends or like-minded staff members, if they lack the necessary expertise, the team may not be productive, and friends may be reluctant to offer a different perspective. When forming a team for any purpose, the cardiac/vascular nurse should look for the best-qualified members.

129. A: Because Medicare restricts coverage for home health care to patients who are essentially homebound, a patient who is able to walk for 1 mile around her neighborhood would not be classified as homebound. A patient may, with effort and/or assistance, walk for a short distance (such as down the block), and may visit physicians and attend rehabilitation programs and adult daycare programs and still qualify. Patients may also attend church or other religious programs with assistance.

130. C: If a close personal friend of the cardiac/vascular nurse is a patient on the cardiac unit, and the cardiac/vascular nurse trades assignments with another nurse in order to be assigned to the patient, this constitutes a professional boundary violation. It is very important for a nurse to treat all patients with the same degree of professional consideration and care, but it is very difficult to avoid showing preference when a personal relationship, such as family or friend, is involved.

131. D: If a patient with bradycardia of 30 bpm is to have a temporary transcutaneous pacemaker (TCP) until a transvenous catheter can be inserted and the cause of the bradycardia determined, in preparation for the TCP, the nurse should advise the patient to expect muscle contraction and discomfort with pacing. Most patients find these contractions uncomfortable and, if possible, should receive analgesia and/or sedation prior to application of the TCP to minimize discomfort.

132. A: Osler's nodes may be found with bacterial endocarditis, which is most commonly caused by *Staphylococcus aureus* or *Streptococcus viridans*. Osler's nodes are small painful red/purple lesions occurring on the fingertips or toes. Endocarditis is characterized by vegetations that adhere to the valves or endocardium. In about half of patients with vegetations, embolization will occur. Endocarditis is most commonly caused by aging, aortic stenosis, IV drug use, prosthetic valves, intravascular devices, or (about 20%) rheumatic fever.

133. B: If the mother of an 18-year-old patient with hypertrophic cardiomyopathy has been scheduled twice to attend CPR classes before her son is discharged but has failed to attend the classes, stating that the CPR class is "not necessary" and "a waste of time," according to Kübler-Ross's stages of grief, the mother is probably experiencing denial. Other stages in the grief process include anger, bargaining, depression, and acceptance. While some people go through all stages, some do not, and some become fixed at one stage.

134. D: If a patient makes a statement that is untrue or a distortion of reality, such as "The doctor promised that I didn't have to exercise today," the cardiac/vascular nurse should avoid directly agreeing or disagreeing but should comment on the distortion of fact in a way that presents the truth without being judgmental: "That's surprising because the doctor wrote an order for you to walk twice today." It is important to avoid arguing with the patient because patients retain the right to refuse treatment.

135. A: If the ECG shows a heart rate of 80 bpm with regular rhythm and normal P waves and QRS complex with a PR interval of 0.5 seconds, this finding is characteristic of first-degree atrioventricular block. It presents much like the normal sinus rhythm except that the PR interval is

extended (normal is 0.12 to 0.2), sometimes up to a full second or longer. The delay in conduction occurs in the AV node, but generally all impulses are conducted.

136. C: The primary difference between partnership councils and other forms of shared governance is that partnership councils (an evolution of shared governance that usually included only nursing personnel) include all disciplines and all levels and areas within an organization. One organization may have many partnership councils, such as at the unit level and department level with one member (usually the chairperson) a representative to a central council. The central council often serves as an advisory board to the administration and/or board of directors.

137. A: If a Middle Eastern female patient leaves all medical decisions about her treatment to her husband, this probably represents a cultural norm of patriarchal societies. Because the male traditionally makes decisions in Middle Eastern countries, when decisions about treatment are necessary, the discussion should be directed to the male, such as a spouse, son, or father, rather than directly to the female patient. It is important to remember that these practices are meant to protect and support the female even though they are counter to Western practice.

138. D: If a patient with coronary artery disease has a medication list that shows the patient is currently taking clopidogrel 75 mg daily, omeprazole 20 mg daily, metoprolol 50 mg twice daily, docusate sodium 1 capsule daily, and atorvastatin 80 mg daily, the drug that may pose the greatest risk of drug-drug interactions is omeprazole. Omeprazole may decrease the antiplatelet effect of clopidogrel by up to 50%, increasing the risk of a cardiovascular event. Omeprazole may also increase the effects of atorvastatin as well as the risk of adverse effects.

139. C: If a nursing diagnosis is "ineffective self-health management associated with lack of knowledge about condition and therapy," an appropriate patient goal is, "Patient can describe key elements of the disease process and therapeutic regimen." Self-health management must begin with knowledge and understanding about the patient's condition and therapeutic regimen, which should include the treatment plan, preventive measures (including lifestyle changes), medications, and any other treatments, such as diet and exercise.

140. A: The primary advantage of PCI with drug-eluting stents (DES) or bare-metal stents (BMS) is decreased restenosis and need for revascularization techniques with a DES more effective than BMS, although even BMS decreases restenosis by about 50% compared with balloon angioplasty. About 9 out of 10 PCI procedures now utilize stents. CABG is done much less frequently, and PCI with stents has almost completely replaced directional coronary atherectomy (DCA), which has higher rates of complications. Rotational atherectomy is still occasionally used for patients with severe calcifications that prevent balloon inflation.

141. B: A patient with an automatic implantable cardioverter-defibrillator should generally be advised to avoid MRIs because of the potential for harm to the patient or the device. However, some centers have successfully done MRIs on patients with ICDs when the MRI was deemed essential, such as with suspected brain tumors. While in some cases the threshold for pacing changed or the device required reprogramming, no deaths or severe injuries have been associated with MRIs in patients with ICDs. Patients should avoid prolonged exposure to metal detectors and anti-theft devices, but microwave ovens should cause no problem.

142. B: For a patient with an Unna boot, the most important factor in promoting adequate compression is ambulation because the pumping action of the calf muscles is necessary to increase compression. Nonambulatory patients should not have an Unna boot applied. Proper application is

also necessary because improper application may further impair circulation. Patients should be advised to elevate the leg with the Unna boot above the level of the heart for 10 to 15 minutes two or three times daily, and to assess the color and swelling of the leg and the toes and report tingling, numbness, or pain.

143. A: According to the ACCF/AHA/HRS Focused Update on the Management of Patients with Atrial Fibrillation, the goal for patients with atrial fibrillation is generally a ventricular rate at rest of 60 to 80 bpm and a ventricular rate of 90 to 115 bpm during moderate activity; however, targeted rates should be individualized depending on patient's age and condition. Patients treated for atrial fibrillation are usually maintained on warfarin as a preventive measure. Patients unable to tolerate warfarin may be treated with clopidogrel and ASA.

144. D: According to the AACVPR's *Guidelines for Cardiac Rehabilitation and Secondary Prevention Programs*, patients should be referred to a cardiac rehabilitation program if they experience an acute cardiovascular event, such as acute coronary syndrome or acute myocardial infarction. Once the patient is discharged, outpatient cardiac rehabilitation is usually done for a period of up to 36 weeks. Cardiac rehabilitation services can help ensure that patients adhere to treatment regimens and have access to needed resources.

145. C: If a patient has been admitted to the cardiac care unit with chest pain and atrial fibrillation, unlicensed assistive personnel can take daily weight. The cardiac/vascular nurse should assess the apical/radial pulse rate to evaluate the atrial fibrillation and should monitor the IV fluids. Additionally, the cardiac/vascular nurse should monitor the response to medications, such as analgesia. Assessment is outside the scope of practice of unlicensed assistive personnel.

146. A: If a patient is being treated for acute heart failure, the task that has priority is monitoring response to medications because acute heart failure is a life-threatening condition; physiological functioning is critical. The cardiac/vascular nurse must ensure that the patient's oxygenation is above 90% and that perfusion is adequate. The patient should be assessed for skin lesions once stabilized and the nurse should always check that the call light is within reach before leaving a patient unattended. Instruction in low-sodium diet has the lowest priority because this is information the patient will need for discharge.

147. B: Lidocaine is used primarily for treatment of ventricular tachycardia/fibrillation (VT/VF), both of which can be life-threatening dysrhythmias. Lidocaine can also be used for premature ventricular contraction (PVC) suppression, but PVC suppression is usually not recommended. Typically, for VT, lidocaine 1 mg/kg is administered IV as a bolus over 3 minutes and then followed by a 2 to 4 mg/min infusion. A repeat bolus of 0.5 mg/kg may be administered after 10 minutes. For VF or pulseless VT, lidocaine is administered as a 1.5 mg/kg bolus, repeated if necessary, and followed by infusion of 2 to 4 mg/min.

148. D: Opioid-induced hypotension does not respond to reversal agents, such as naloxone, so the medication should be held and a crystalloid bolus administered to reverse the hypotension. When pain medication resumes, smaller more frequent doses or a different medication should be used and fluid status optimized. Antihistamine (such as diphenhydramine) may be administered to help alleviate opioid-induced pruritus. If the itching is intractable and not responsive to the antihistamine, naloxone may be administered.

149. C: Non–Q-wave myocardial infarctions are characterized by contraction necrosis associated with reperfusion, which usually occurs spontaneously because infarct area tends to be small with

complete coronary occlusion occurring in only 20% to 30% of cases and mortality rates of about 2% to 3%. The non–Q-wave MI is usually non-transmural. Peak CK levels occur in 12 to 13 hours. Reinfarction is common, so 2-year survival rates are similar to Q-wave MIs, which have a higher initial mortality rate of about 10%.

150. A: If a patient is classified as having NYHA class I heart failure, the patient should expect no symptoms with activities because, while there are some changes in the heart, these changes remain asymptomatic. With class II, the patient may experience some shortness of breath and/or angina with activities of daily living. With class III, the patient will experience marked symptoms, such as dyspnea and angina while doing routine activities or walking a short distance and will only feel comfort at rest. With class IV, the patient will have severe symptoms even at rest.

Secret Key #1 - Time is Your Greatest Enemy

Pace Yourself

Wear a watch. At the beginning of the test, check the time (or start a chronometer on your watch to count the minutes), and check the time after every few questions to make sure you are "on schedule."

If you are forced to speed up, do it efficiently. Usually one or more answer choices can be eliminated without too much difficulty. Above all, don't panic. Don't speed up and just begin guessing at random choices. By pacing yourself, and continually monitoring your progress against your watch, you will always know exactly how far ahead or behind you are with your available time. If you find that you are one minute behind on the test, don't skip one question without spending any time on it, just to catch back up. Take 15 fewer seconds on the next four questions, and after four questions you'll have caught back up. Once you catch back up, you can continue working each problem at your normal pace.

Furthermore, don't dwell on the problems that you were rushed on. If a problem was taking up too much time and you made a hurried guess, it must be difficult. The difficult questions are the ones you are most likely to miss anyway, so it isn't a big loss. It is better to end with more time than you need than to run out of time.

Lastly, sometimes it is beneficial to slow down if you are constantly getting ahead of time. You are always more likely to catch a careless mistake by working more slowly than quickly, and among very high-scoring test takers (those who are likely to have lots of time left over), careless errors affect the score more than mastery of material.

Secret Key #2 - Guessing is not Guesswork

You probably know that guessing is a good idea. Unlike other standardized tests, there is no penalty for getting a wrong answer. Even if you have no idea about a question, you still have a 20-25% chance of getting it right.

Most test takers do not understand the impact that proper guessing can have on their score. Unless you score extremely high, guessing will significantly contribute to your final score.

Monkeys Take the Test

What most test takers don't realize is that to insure that 20-25% chance, you have to guess randomly. If you put 20 monkeys in a room to take this test, assuming they answered once per question and behaved themselves, on average they would get 20-25% of the questions correct. Put 20 test takers in the room, and the average will be much lower among guessed questions. Why?

1. The test writers intentionally write deceptive answer choices that "look" right. A test taker has no idea about a question, so he picks the "best looking" answer, which is often wrong. The monkey has no idea what looks good and what doesn't, so it will consistently be right about 20-25% of the time.
2. Test takers will eliminate answer choices from the guessing pool based on a hunch or intuition. Simple but correct answers often get excluded, leaving a 0% chance of being correct. The monkey has no clue, and often gets lucky with the best choice.

This is why the process of elimination endorsed by most test courses is flawed and detrimental to your performance. Test takers don't guess; they make an ignorant stab in the dark that is usually worse than random.

$5 Challenge

Let me introduce one of the most valuable ideas of this course—the $5 challenge:

You only mark your "best guess" if you are willing to bet $5 on it.
You only eliminate choices from guessing if you are willing to bet $5 on it.

Why $5? Five dollars is an amount of money that is small yet not insignificant, and can really add up fast (20 questions could cost you $100). Likewise, each answer choice on one question of the test will have a small impact on your overall score, but it can really add up to a lot of points in the end.

The process of elimination IS valuable. The following shows your chance of guessing it right:

If you eliminate wrong answer choices until only this many remain:	Chance of getting it correct:
1	100%
2	50%
3	33%

However, if you accidentally eliminate the right answer or go on a hunch for an incorrect answer, your chances drop dramatically—to 0%. By guessing among all the answer choices, you are GUARANTEED to have a shot at the right answer.

That's why the $5 test is so valuable. If you give up the advantage and safety of a pure guess, it had better be worth the risk.

What we still haven't covered is how to be sure that whatever guess you make is truly random. Here's the easiest way:

Always pick the first answer choice among those remaining.

Such a technique means that you have decided, **before you see a single test question**, exactly how you are going to guess, and since the order of choices tells you nothing about which one is correct, this guessing technique is perfectly random.

This section is not meant to scare you away from making educated guesses or eliminating choices; you just need to define when a choice is worth eliminating. The $5 test, along with a pre-defined random guessing strategy, is the best way to make sure you reap all of the benefits of guessing.

Secret Key #3 - Practice Smarter, Not Harder

Many test takers delay the test preparation process because they dread the awful amounts of practice time they think necessary to succeed on the test. We have refined an effective method that will take you only a fraction of the time.

There are a number of "obstacles" in the path to success. Among these are answering questions, finishing in time, and mastering test-taking strategies. All must be executed on the day of the test at peak performance, or your score will suffer. The test is a mental marathon that has a large impact on your future.

Just like a marathon runner, it is important to work your way up to the full challenge. So first you just worry about questions, and then time, and finally strategy:

Success Strategy

1. Find a good source for practice tests.
2. If you are willing to make a larger time investment, consider using more than one study guide. Often the different approaches of multiple authors will help you "get" difficult concepts.
3. Take a practice test with no time constraints, with all study helps, "open book." Take your time with questions and focus on applying strategies.
4. Take a practice test with time constraints, with all guides, "open book."
5. Take a final practice test without open material and with time limits.

If you have time to take more practice tests, just repeat step 5. By gradually exposing yourself to the full rigors of the test environment, you will condition your mind to the stress of test day and maximize your success.

Secret Key #4 - Prepare, Don't Procrastinate

Let me state an obvious fact: if you take the test three times, you will probably get three different scores. This is due to the way you feel on test day, the level of preparedness you have, and the version of the test you see. Despite the test writers' claims to the contrary, some versions of the test WILL be easier for you than others.

Since your future depends so much on your score, you should maximize your chances of success. In order to maximize the likelihood of success, you've got to prepare in advance. This means taking practice tests and spending time learning the information and test taking strategies you will need to succeed.

Never go take the actual test as a "practice" test, expecting that you can just take it again if you need to. Take all the practice tests you can on your own, but when you go to take the official test, be prepared, be focused, and do your best the first time!

Secret Key #5 - Test Yourself

Everyone knows that time is money. There is no need to spend too much of your time or too little of your time preparing for the test. You should only spend as much of your precious time preparing as is necessary for you to get the score you need.

Once you have taken a practice test under real conditions of time constraints, then you will know if you are ready for the test or not.

If you have scored extremely high the first time that you take the practice test, then there is not much point in spending countless hours studying. You are already there.

Benchmark your abilities by retaking practice tests and seeing how much you have improved. Once you consistently score high enough to guarantee success, then you are ready.

If you have scored well below where you need, then knuckle down and begin studying in earnest. Check your improvement regularly through the use of practice tests under real conditions. Above all, don't worry, panic, or give up. The key is perseverance!

Then, when you go to take the test, remain confident and remember how well you did on the practice tests. If you can score high enough on a practice test, then you can do the same on the real thing.

General Strategies

The most important thing you can do is to ignore your fears and jump into the test immediately. Do not be overwhelmed by any strange-sounding terms. You have to jump into the test like jumping into a pool—all at once is the easiest way.

Make Predictions

As you read and understand the question, try to guess what the answer will be. Remember that several of the answer choices are wrong, and once you begin reading them, your mind will immediately become cluttered with answer choices designed to throw you off. Your mind is typically the most focused immediately after you have read the question and digested its contents. If you can, try to predict what the correct answer will be. You may be surprised at what you can predict.

Quickly scan the choices and see if your prediction is in the listed answer choices. If it is, then you can be quite confident that you have the right answer. It still won't hurt to check the other answer choices, but most of the time, you've got it!

Answer the Question

It may seem obvious to only pick answer choices that answer the question, but the test writers can create some excellent answer choices that are wrong. Don't pick an answer just because it sounds right, or you believe it to be true. It MUST answer the question. Once you've made your selection, always go back and check it against the question and make sure that you didn't misread the question and that the answer choice does answer the question posed.

Benchmark

After you read the first answer choice, decide if you think it sounds correct or not. If it doesn't, move on to the next answer choice. If it does, mentally mark that answer choice. This doesn't mean that you've definitely selected it as your answer choice, it just means that it's the best you've seen thus far. Go ahead and read the next choice. If the next choice is worse than the one you've already selected, keep going to the next answer choice. If the next choice is better than the choice you've already selected, mentally mark the new answer choice as your best guess.

The first answer choice that you select becomes your standard. Every other answer choice must be benchmarked against that standard. That choice is correct until proven otherwise by another answer choice beating it out. Once you've decided that no other answer choice seems as good, do one final check to ensure that your answer choice answers the question posed.

Valid Information

Don't discount any of the information provided in the question. Every piece of information may be necessary to determine the correct answer. None of the information in the question is there to throw you off (while the answer choices will certainly have information to throw you off). If two seemingly unrelated topics are discussed, don't ignore either. You can be confident there is a relationship, or it wouldn't be included in the question, and you are probably going to have to determine what is that relationship to find the answer.

Avoid "Fact Traps"

Don't get distracted by a choice that is factually true. Your search is for the answer that answers the question. Stay focused and don't fall for an answer that is true but irrelevant. Always go back to the question and make sure you're choosing an answer that actually answers the question and is not just a true statement. An answer can be factually correct, but it MUST answer the question asked. Additionally, two answers can both be seemingly correct, so be sure to read all of the answer choices, and make sure that you get the one that BEST answers the question.

Milk the Question

Some of the questions may throw you completely off. They might deal with a subject you have not been exposed to, or one that you haven't reviewed in years. While your lack of knowledge about the subject will be a hindrance, the question itself can give you many clues that will help you find the correct answer. Read the question carefully and look for clues. Watch particularly for adjectives and nouns describing difficult terms or words that you don't recognize. Regardless of whether you completely understand a word or not, replacing it with a synonym, either provided or one you more familiar with, may help you to understand what the questions are asking. Rather than wracking your mind about specific detailed information concerning a difficult term or word, try to use mental substitutes that are easier to understand.

The Trap of Familiarity

Don't just choose a word because you recognize it. On difficult questions, you may not recognize a number of words in the answer choices. The test writers don't put "make-believe" words on the test, so don't think that just because you only recognize all the words in one answer choice that that answer choice must be correct. If you only recognize words in one answer choice, then focus on that one. Is it correct? Try your best to determine if it is correct. If it is, that's great. If not, eliminate it. Each word and answer choice you eliminate increases your chances of getting the question correct, even if you then have to guess among the unfamiliar choices.

Eliminate Answers

Eliminate choices as soon as you realize they are wrong. But be careful! Make sure you consider all of the possible answer choices. Just because one appears right, doesn't mean that the next one won't be even better! The test writers will usually put more than one good answer choice for every question, so read all of them. Don't worry if you are stuck between two that seem right. By getting down to just two remaining possible choices, your odds are now 50/50. Rather than wasting too much time, play the odds. You are guessing, but guessing wisely because you've been able to knock out some of the answer choices that you know are wrong. If you are eliminating choices and realize that the last answer choice you are left with is also obviously wrong, don't panic. Start over and consider each choice again. There may easily be something that you missed the first time and will realize on the second pass.

Tough Questions

If you are stumped on a problem or it appears too hard or too difficult, don't waste time. Move on! Remember though, if you can quickly check for obviously incorrect answer choices, your chances of guessing correctly are greatly improved. Before you completely give up, at least try to knock out a couple of possible answers. Eliminate what you can and then guess at the remaining answer choices before moving on.

Brainstorm

If you get stuck on a difficult question, spend a few seconds quickly brainstorming. Run through the complete list of possible answer choices. Look at each choice and ask yourself, "Could this answer the question satisfactorily?" Go through each answer choice and consider it independently of the others. By systematically going through all possibilities, you may find something that you would otherwise overlook. Remember though that when you get stuck, it's important to try to keep moving.

Read Carefully
Understand the problem. Read the question and answer choices carefully. Don't miss the question because you misread the terms. You have plenty of time to read each question thoroughly and make sure you understand what is being asked. Yet a happy medium must be attained, so don't waste too much time. You must read carefully, but efficiently.

Face Value
When in doubt, use common sense. Always accept the situation in the problem at face value. Don't read too much into it. These problems will not require you to make huge leaps of logic. The test writers aren't trying to throw you off with a cheap trick. If you have to go beyond creativity and make a leap of logic in order to have an answer choice answer the question, then you should look at the other answer choices. Don't overcomplicate the problem by creating theoretical relationships or explanations that will warp time or space. These are normal problems rooted in reality. It's just that the applicable relationship or explanation may not be readily apparent and you have to figure things out. Use your common sense to interpret anything that isn't clear.

Prefixes
If you're having trouble with a word in the question or answer choices, try dissecting it. Take advantage of every clue that the word might include. Prefixes and suffixes can be a huge help. Usually they allow you to determine a basic meaning. Pre- means before, post- means after, pro - is positive, de- is negative. From these prefixes and suffixes, you can get an idea of the general meaning of the word and try to put it into context. Beware though of any traps. Just because con- is the opposite of pro-, doesn't necessarily mean congress is the opposite of progress!

Hedge Phrases
Watch out for critical hedge phrases, led off with words such as "likely," "may," "can," "sometimes," "often," "almost," "mostly," "usually," "generally," "rarely," and "sometimes." Question writers insert these hedge phrases to cover every possibility. Often an answer choice will be wrong simply because it leaves no room for exception. Unless the situation calls for them, avoid answer choices that have definitive words like "exactly," and "always."

Switchback Words
Stay alert for "switchbacks." These are the words and phrases frequently used to alert you to shifts in thought. The most common switchback word is "but." Others include "although," "however," "nevertheless," "on the other hand," "even though," "while," "in spite of," "despite," and "regardless of."

New Information
Correct answer choices will rarely have completely new information included. Answer choices typically are straightforward reflections of the material asked about and will directly relate to the question. If a new piece of information is included in an answer choice that doesn't even seem to relate to the topic being asked about, then that answer choice is likely incorrect. All of the information needed to answer the question is usually provided for you in the question. You should not have to make guesses that are unsupported or choose answer choices that require unknown information that cannot be reasoned from what is given.

Time Management

On technical questions, don't get lost on the technical terms. Don't spend too much time on any one question. If you don't know what a term means, then odds are you aren't going to get much further since you don't have a dictionary. You should be able to immediately recognize whether or not you know a term. If you don't, work with the other clues that you have—the other answer choices and terms provided—but don't waste too much time trying to figure out a difficult term that you don't know.

Contextual Clues

Look for contextual clues. An answer can be right but not the correct answer. The contextual clues will help you find the answer that is most right and is correct. Understand the context in which a phrase or statement is made. This will help you make important distinctions.

Don't Panic

Panicking will not answer any questions for you; therefore, it isn't helpful. When you first see the question, if your mind goes blank, take a deep breath. Force yourself to mechanically go through the steps of solving the problem using the strategies you've learned.

Pace Yourself

Don't get clock fever. It's easy to be overwhelmed when you're looking at a page full of questions, your mind is full of random thoughts and feeling confused, and the clock is ticking down faster than you would like. Calm down and maintain the pace that you have set for yourself. As long as you are on track by monitoring your pace, you are guaranteed to have enough time for yourself. When you get to the last few minutes of the test, it may seem like you won't have enough time left, but if you only have as many questions as you should have left at that point, then you're right on track!

Answer Selection

The best way to pick an answer choice is to eliminate all of those that are wrong, until only one is left and confirm that is the correct answer. Sometimes though, an answer choice may immediately look right. Be careful! Take a second to make sure that the other choices are not equally obvious. Don't make a hasty mistake. There are only two times that you should stop before checking other answers. First is when you are positive that the answer choice you have selected is correct. Second is when time is almost out and you have to make a quick guess!

Check Your Work

Since you will probably not know every term listed and the answer to every question, it is important that you get credit for the ones that you do know. Don't miss any questions through careless mistakes. If at all possible, try to take a second to look back over your answer selection and make sure you've selected the correct answer choice and haven't made a costly careless mistake (such as marking an answer choice that you didn't mean to mark). The time it takes for this quick double check should more than pay for itself in caught mistakes.

Beware of Directly Quoted Answers

Sometimes an answer choice will repeat word for word a portion of the question or reference section. However, beware of such exact duplication. It may be a trap! More than likely, the correct choice will paraphrase or summarize a point, rather than being exactly the same wording.

Slang
Scientific sounding answers are better than slang ones. An answer choice that begins "To compare the outcomes..." is much more likely to be correct than one that begins "Because some people insisted..."

Extreme Statements
Avoid wild answers that throw out highly controversial ideas that are proclaimed as established fact. An answer choice that states the "process should used in certain situations, if..." is much more likely to be correct than one that states the "process should be discontinued completely." The first is a calm rational statement and doesn't even make a definitive, uncompromising stance, using a hedge word "if" to provide wiggle room, whereas the second choice is a radical idea and far more extreme.

Answer Choice Families
When you have two or more answer choices that are direct opposites or parallels, one of them is usually the correct answer. For instance, if one answer choice states "x increases" and another answer choice states "x decreases" or "y increases," then those two or three answer choices are very similar in construction and fall into the same family of answer choices. A family of answer choices consists of two or three answer choices, very similar in construction, but often with directly opposite meanings. Usually the correct answer choice will be in that family of answer choices. The "odd man out" or answer choice that doesn't seem to fit the parallel construction of the other answer choices is more likely to be incorrect.

Special Report: How to Overcome Test Anxiety

The very nature of tests caters to some level of anxiety, nervousness, or tension, just as we feel for any important event that occurs in our lives. A little bit of anxiety or nervousness can be a good thing. It helps us with motivation, and makes achievement just that much sweeter. However, too much anxiety can be a problem, especially if it hinders our ability to function and perform.

"Test anxiety," is the term that refers to the emotional reactions that some test-takers experience when faced with a test or exam. Having a fear of testing and exams is based upon a rational fear, since the test-taker's performance can shape the course of an academic career. Nevertheless, experiencing excessive fear of examinations will only interfere with the test-taker's ability to perform and chance to be successful.

There are a large variety of causes that can contribute to the development and sensation of test anxiety. These include, but are not limited to, lack of preparation and worrying about issues surrounding the test.

Lack of Preparation

Lack of preparation can be identified by the following behaviors or situations:

- Not scheduling enough time to study, and therefore cramming the night before the test or exam
- Managing time poorly, to create the sensation that there is not enough time to do everything
- Failing to organize the text information in advance, so that the study material consists of the entire text and not simply the pertinent information
- Poor overall studying habits

Worrying, on the other hand, can be related to both the test taker, or many other factors around him/her that will be affected by the results of the test. These include worrying about:

- Previous performances on similar exams, or exams in general
- How friends and other students are achieving
- The negative consequences that will result from a poor grade or failure

There are three primary elements to test anxiety. Physical components, which involve the same typical bodily reactions as those to acute anxiety (to be discussed below). Emotional factors have to do with fear or panic. Mental or cognitive issues concerning attention spans and memory abilities.

Physical Signals

There are many different symptoms of test anxiety, and these are not limited to mental and emotional strain. Frequently there are a range of physical signals that will let a test taker know that he/she is suffering from test anxiety. These bodily changes can include the following:

- Perspiring
- Sweaty palms
- Wet, trembling hands
- Nausea
- Dry mouth
- A knot in the stomach
- Headache
- Faintness
- Muscle tension
- Aching shoulders, back and neck
- Rapid heart beat
- Feeling too hot/cold

To recognize the sensation of test anxiety, a test-taker should monitor him/herself for the following sensations:

- The physical distress symptoms as listed above
- Emotional sensitivity, expressing emotional feelings such as the need to cry or laugh too much, or a sensation of anger or helplessness
- A decreased ability to think, causing the test-taker to blank out or have racing thoughts that are hard to organize or control.

Though most students will feel some level of anxiety when faced with a test or exam, the majority can cope with that anxiety and maintain it at a manageable level. However, those who cannot are faced with a very real and very serious condition, which can and should be controlled for the immeasurable benefit of this sufferer.

Naturally, these sensations lead to negative results for the testing experience. The most common effects of test anxiety have to do with nervousness and mental blocking.

Nervousness

Nervousness can appear in several different levels:

- The test-taker's difficulty, or even inability to read and understand the questions on the test
- The difficulty or inability to organize thoughts to a coherent form
- The difficulty or inability to recall key words and concepts relating to the testing questions (especially essays)
- The receipt of poor grades on a test, though the test material was well known by the test taker

Conversely, a person may also experience mental blocking, which involves:

- Blanking out on test questions
- Only remembering the correct answers to the questions when the test has already finished.

Fortunately for test anxiety sufferers, beating these feelings, to a large degree, has to do with proper preparation. When a test taker has a feeling of preparedness, then anxiety will be dramatically lessened.

The first step to resolving anxiety issues is to distinguish which of the two types of anxiety are being suffered. If the anxiety is a direct result of a lack of preparation, this should be considered a normal reaction, and the anxiety level (as opposed to the test results) shouldn't be anything to worry about. However, if, when adequately prepared, the test-taker still panics, blanks out, or seems to overreact, this is not a fully rational reaction. While this can be considered normal too, there are many ways to combat and overcome these effects.

Remember that anxiety cannot be entirely eliminated; however, there are ways to minimize it, to make the anxiety easier to manage. Preparation is one of the best ways to minimize test anxiety. Therefore the following techniques are wise in order to best fight off any anxiety that may want to build.

To begin with, try to avoid cramming before a test, whenever it is possible. By trying to memorize an entire term's worth of information in one day, you'll be shocking your system, and not giving yourself a very good chance to absorb the information. This is an easy path to anxiety, so for those who suffer from test anxiety, cramming should not even be considered an option.

Instead of cramming, work throughout the semester to combine all of the material which is presented throughout the semester, and work on it gradually as the course goes by, making sure to master the main concepts first, leaving minor details for a week or so before the test.

To study for the upcoming exam, be sure to pose questions that may be on the examination, to gauge the ability to answer them by integrating the ideas from your texts, notes and lectures, as well as any supplementary readings.

If it is truly impossible to cover all of the information that was covered in that particular term, concentrate on the most important portions, that can be covered very well. Learn these concepts as best as possible, so that when the test comes, a goal can be made to use these concepts as presentations of your knowledge.

In addition to study habits, changes in attitude are critical to beating a struggle with test anxiety. In fact, an improvement of the perspective over the entire test-taking experience can actually help a test taker to enjoy studying and therefore improve the overall experience. Be certain not to overemphasize the significance of the grade - know that the result of the test is neither a reflection of self worth, nor is it a measure of intelligence; one grade will not predict a person's future success.

To improve an overall testing outlook, the following steps should be tried:

- Keeping in mind that the most reasonable expectation for taking a test is to expect to try to demonstrate as much of what you know as you possibly can.
- Reminding ourselves that a test is only one test; this is not the only one, and there will be others.
- The thought of thinking of oneself in an irrational, all-or-nothing term should be avoided at all costs.
- A reward should be designated for after the test, so there's something to look forward to. Whether it be going to a movie, going out to eat, or simply visiting friends, schedule it in advance, and do it no matter what result is expected on the exam.

Test-takers should also keep in mind that the basics are some of the most important things, even beyond anti-anxiety techniques and studying. Never neglect the basic social, emotional and biological needs, in order to try to absorb information. In order to best achieve, these three factors must be held as just as important as the studying itself.

Study Steps

Remember the following important steps for studying:

- Maintain healthy nutrition and exercise habits. Continue both your recreational activities and social pass times. These both contribute to your physical and emotional well being.
- Be certain to get a good amount of sleep, especially the night before the test, because when you're overtired you are not able to perform to the best of your best ability.
- Keep the studying pace to a moderate level by taking breaks when they are needed, and varying the work whenever possible, to keep the mind fresh instead of getting bored.
- When enough studying has been done that all the material that can be learned has been learned, and the test taker is prepared for the test, stop studying and do something relaxing such as listening to music, watching a movie, or taking a warm bubble bath.

There are also many other techniques to minimize the uneasiness or apprehension that is experienced along with test anxiety before, during, or even after the examination. In fact, there are a great deal of things that can be done to stop anxiety from interfering with lifestyle and performance. Again, remember that anxiety will not be eliminated entirely, and it shouldn't be. Otherwise that "up" feeling for exams would not exist, and most of us depend on that sensation to perform better than usual. However, this anxiety has to be at a level that is manageable.

Of course, as we have just discussed, being prepared for the exam is half the battle right away. Attending all classes, finding out what knowledge will be expected on the exam, and knowing the exam schedules are easy steps to lowering anxiety. Keeping up with work will remove the need to cram, and efficient study habits will eliminate wasted time. Studying should be done in an ideal location for concentration, so that it is simple to become interested in the material and give it complete attention. A method such as SQ3R (Survey, Question, Read, Recite, Review) is a wonderful key to follow to make sure that the study habits are as effective as possible, especially in the case of learning from a textbook. Flashcards are great techniques for memorization. Learning to take good notes will mean that notes will be full of useful information, so that less sifting will need to be done to seek out what is pertinent for studying. Reviewing notes after class and then again on occasion will keep the information fresh in the mind. From notes that have been taken summary sheets and outlines can be made for simpler reviewing.

A study group can also be a very motivational and helpful place to study, as there will be a sharing of ideas, all of the minds can work together, to make sure that everyone understands, and the studying will be made more interesting because it will be a social occasion.

Basically, though, as long as the test-taker remains organized and self confident, with efficient study habits, less time will need to be spent studying, and higher grades will be achieved.

To become self confident, there are many useful steps. The first of these is "self talk." It has been shown through extensive research, that self-talk for students who suffer from test anxiety, should be well monitored, in order to make sure that it contributes to self confidence as opposed to sinking the student. Frequently the self talk of test-anxious students is negative or self-defeating, thinking that everyone else is smarter and faster, that they always mess up, and that if they don't do well, they'll fail the entire course. It is important to decreasing anxiety that awareness is made of self talk. Try writing any negative self thoughts and then disputing them with a positive statement instead. Begin self-encouragement as though it was a friend speaking. Repeat positive statements to help reprogram the mind to believing in successes instead of failures.

Helpful Techniques

Other extremely helpful techniques include:

- Self-visualization of doing well and reaching goals
- While aiming for an "A" level of understanding, don't try to "overprotect" by setting your expectations lower. This will only convince the mind to stop studying in order to meet the lower expectations.
- Don't make comparisons with the results or habits of other students. These are individual factors, and different things work for different people, causing different results.
- Strive to become an expert in learning what works well, and what can be done in order to improve. Consider collecting this data in a journal.
- Create rewards for after studying instead of doing things before studying that will only turn into avoidance behaviors.
- Make a practice of relaxing - by using methods such as progressive relaxation, self-hypnosis, guided imagery, etc - in order to make relaxation an automatic sensation.
- Work on creating a state of relaxed concentration so that concentrating will take on the focus of the mind, so that none will be wasted on worrying.
- Take good care of the physical self by eating well and getting enough sleep.
- Plan in time for exercise and stick to this plan.

Beyond these techniques, there are other methods to be used before, during and after the test that will help the test-taker perform well in addition to overcoming anxiety.

Before the exam comes the academic preparation. This involves establishing a study schedule and beginning at least one week before the actual date of the test. By doing this, the anxiety of not having enough time to study for the test will be automatically eliminated. Moreover, this will make the studying a much more effective experience, ensuring that the learning will be an easier process. This relieves much undue pressure on the test-taker.

Summary sheets, note cards, and flash cards with the main concepts and examples of these main concepts should be prepared in advance of the actual studying time. A topic should never be eliminated from this process. By omitting a topic because it isn't expected to be on the test is only setting up the test-taker for anxiety should it actually appear on the exam. Utilize the course syllabus for laying out the topics that should be studied. Carefully go over the notes that were made in class, paying special attention to any of the issues that the professor took special care to emphasize while lecturing in class. In the textbooks, use the chapter review, or if possible, the chapter tests, to begin your review.

It may even be possible to ask the instructor what information will be covered on the exam, or what the format of the exam will be (for example, multiple choice, essay, free form, true-false). Additionally, see if it is possible to find out how many questions will be on the test. If a review sheet or sample test has been offered by the professor, make good use of it, above anything else, for the preparation for the test. Another great resource for getting to know the examination is reviewing tests from previous semesters. Use these tests to review, and aim to achieve a 100% score on each of the possible topics. With a few exceptions, the goal that you set for yourself is the highest one that you will reach.

Take all of the questions that were assigned as homework, and rework them to any other possible course material. The more problems reworked, the more skill and confidence will form as a result. When forming the solution to a problem, write out each of the steps. Don't simply do head work. By doing as many steps on paper as possible, much clarification and therefore confidence will be formed. Do this with as many homework problems as possible, before checking the answers. By checking the answer after each problem, a reinforcement will exist, that will not be on the exam. Study situations should be as exam-like as possible, to prime the test-taker's system for the experience. By waiting to check the answers at the end, a psychological advantage will be formed, to decrease the stress factor.

Another fantastic reason for not cramming is the avoidance of confusion in concepts, especially when it comes to mathematics. 8-10 hours of study will become one hundred percent more effective if it is spread out over a week or at least several days, instead of doing it all in one sitting. Recognize that the human brain requires time in order to assimilate new material, so frequent breaks and a span of study time over several days will be much more beneficial.

Additionally, don't study right up until the point of the exam. Studying should stop a minimum of one hour before the exam begins. This allows the brain to rest and put things in their proper order. This will also provide the time to become as relaxed as possible when going into the examination room. The test-taker will also have time to eat well and eat sensibly. Know that the brain needs food as much as the rest of the body. With enough food and enough sleep, as well as a relaxed attitude, the body and the mind are primed for success.

Avoid any anxious classmates who are talking about the exam. These students only spread anxiety, and are not worth sharing the anxious sentimentalities.

Before the test also involves creating a positive attitude, so mental preparation should also be a point of concentration. There are many keys to creating a positive attitude. Should fears become rushing in, make a visualization of taking the exam, doing well, and seeing an A written on the paper. Write out a list of affirmations that will bring a feeling of confidence, such as "I am doing well in my English class," "I studied well and know my material," "I enjoy this class." Even if the affirmations aren't believed at first, it sends a positive message to the subconscious which will result in an alteration of the overall belief system, which is the system that creates reality.

If a sensation of panic begins, work with the fear and imagine the very worst! Work through the entire scenario of not passing the test, failing the entire course, and dropping out of school, followed by not getting a job, and pushing a shopping cart through the dark alley where you'll live. This will place things into perspective! Then, practice deep breathing and create a visualization of the opposite situation - achieving an "A" on the exam, passing the entire course, receiving the degree at a graduation ceremony.

On the day of the test, there are many things to be done to ensure the best results, as well as the most calm outlook. The following stages are suggested in order to maximize test-taking potential:

- Begin the examination day with a moderate breakfast, and avoid any coffee or beverages with caffeine if the test taker is prone to jitters. Even people who are used to managing caffeine can feel jittery or light-headed when it is taken on a test day.
- Attempt to do something that is relaxing before the examination begins. As last minute cramming clouds the mastering of overall concepts, it is better to use this time to create a calming outlook.
- Be certain to arrive at the test location well in advance, in order to provide time to select a location that is away from doors, windows and other distractions, as well as giving enough time to relax before the test begins.
- Keep away from anxiety generating classmates who will upset the sensation of stability and relaxation that is being attempted before the exam.
- Should the waiting period before the exam begins cause anxiety, create a self-distraction by reading a light magazine or something else that is relaxing and simple.

During the exam itself, read the entire exam from beginning to end, and find out how much time should be allotted to each individual problem. Once writing the exam, should more time be taken for a problem, it should be abandoned, in order to begin another problem. If there is time at the end, the unfinished problem can always be returned to and completed.

Read the instructions very carefully - twice - so that unpleasant surprises won't follow during or after the exam has ended.

When writing the exam, pretend that the situation is actually simply the completion of homework within a library, or at home. This will assist in forming a relaxed atmosphere, and will allow the brain extra focus for the complex thinking function.

Begin the exam with all of the questions with which the most confidence is felt. This will build the confidence level regarding the entire exam and will begin a quality momentum. This will also create encouragement for trying the problems where uncertainty resides.

Going with the "gut instinct" is always the way to go when solving a problem. Second guessing should be avoided at all costs. Have confidence in the ability to do well.

For essay questions, create an outline in advance that will keep the mind organized and make certain that all of the points are remembered. For multiple choice, read every answer, even if the correct one has been spotted - a better one may exist.

Continue at a pace that is reasonable and not rushed, in order to be able to work carefully. Provide enough time to go over the answers at the end, to check for small errors that can be corrected.

Should a feeling of panic begin, breathe deeply, and think of the feeling of the body releasing sand through its pores. Visualize a calm, peaceful place, and include all of the sights, sounds and sensations of this image. Continue the deep breathing, and take a few minutes to continue this with closed eyes. When all is well again, return to the test.

If a "blanking" occurs for a certain question, skip it and move on to the next question. There will be time to return to the other question later. Get everything done that can be done, first, to guarantee all the grades that can be compiled, and to build all of the confidence possible. Then return to the weaker questions to build the marks from there.

Remember, one's own reality can be created, so as long as the belief is there, success will follow. And remember: anxiety can happen later, right now, there's an exam to be written!

After the examination is complete, whether there is a feeling for a good grade or a bad grade, don't dwell on the exam, and be certain to follow through on the reward that was promised and enjoy it! Don't dwell on any mistakes that have been made, as there is nothing that can be done at this point anyway.

Additionally, don't begin to study for the next test right away. Do something relaxing for a while, and let the mind relax and prepare itself to begin absorbing information again.

From the results of the exam - both the grade and the entire experience, be certain to learn from what has gone on. Perfect studying habits and work some more on confidence in order to make the next examination experience even better than the last one.

Learn to avoid places where openings occurred for laziness, procrastination and day dreaming.

Use the time between this exam and the next one to better learn to relax, even learning to relax on cue, so that any anxiety can be controlled during the next exam. Learn how to relax the body. Slouch in your chair if that helps. Tighten and then relax all of the different muscle groups, one group at a time, beginning with the feet and then working all the way up to the neck and face. This will ultimately relax the muscles more than they were to begin with. Learn how to breathe deeply and comfortably, and focus on this breathing going in and out as a relaxing thought. With every exhale, repeat the word "relax."

As common as test anxiety is, it is very possible to overcome it. Make yourself one of the test-takers who overcome this frustrating hindrance.

Additional Bonus Material

Due to our efforts to try to keep this book to a manageable length, we've created a link that will give you access to all of your additional bonus material.

Please visit http://www.mometrix.com/bonus948/cardiacvas to access the information.